Raising and Caring for Animals

A HANDBOOK OF ANIMAL HUSBANDRY AND VETERINARY CARE

Raising and Caring for Animals

A HANDBOOK OF ANIMAL HUSBANDRY AND VETERINARY CARE

Guy Lockwood D.V.M.

Published by
CHARLES SCRIBNER'S SONS
New York

Revised Edition

Copyright © 1977 Guy Lockwood, D.V.M.

Library of Congress Cataloging in Publication Data

Lockwood, Guy C.
   Raising and caring for animals.

   Bibliography: p. 314
   1. Livestock.   2. Veterinary medicine.
I. Title.   II. Title: Self-sufficient living.
SF65.2.L6   1979   636.08   79-14025
ISBN 0-684-16299-7

First American edition published 1977. Printed in the United States of America.

1 3 5 7 9 11 13 15 17 19 M/P 20 18 16 14 12 10 8 6 4 2

ACKNOWLEDGEMENTS

I wish to thank all the people who helped me with this book. I especially thank Rene Baxter, whose idea it was for me to write it. Thank you to Dr. Bill Tyznik, Professor of Animal Science and Nutrition, Ohio State University, for editing the nutrition chapter, and to Lyle Cunningham, Architect, A.I.A., for editing the housing and ventilation chapter. I also want to thank all the kind people who contributed photographs for use in this book. And thanks to Vicki Lockwood for putting up with all the hours I spent away from my family while writing it.

Dedicated to Tom and Margaret
and Matt and Todd, the best
people in my life.

TABLE OF CONTENTS

Introduction

*Husbandry: providing a healthy total
environment for your animals*

This book is written for people who want to become completely self-sufficient and self-reliant on their own piece of land. Call it a homestead, a farm, a ranch or a retreat, it is all the same, your own place. There are many fine references and textbooks on homesteading and retreating as well as all phases of farming and livestock production. I will mention some of the ones I am familiar with in the last chapter. But most of the references you can find still leave you dependent on the local feed mill and the commercial hatchery. This book is intended to correct that dependency.

As a self-sufficient farmer, homesteader or retreater you really need a great deal of technical knowledge. First, you should assemble a very complete library of reference texts and literature. Then decide on the numbers, types and breeds of livestock to support the people on your place. Decide on the amount of land you need to support the crops and pasture for the people and livestock. Always allow for a surplus of land and animals to prevent an occasional shortage. Try to understand the principles of disease and parasite recognition, prevention and control. You must know how to sterilize equipment and disinfect areas and buildings. Become familiar with animal husbandry and feeding, and learn to calculate rations for periods of growth, pregnancy, lactation and fattening. You need to know how to control rodents, insects and predatory wildlife. You must design your fencing and housing, the farmstead layout, even before you bring your livestock onto the place. If you buy an operating farm, chances are that the buildings and fencing setups will not be suitable for self-sufficient farming for a family or small group so you will need to renovate it. You must plan on the types of equipment, machinery and tools that you will need and know what supplies you will need, such as salt and mineral supplements that cannot be produced on your farm. Those people who want complete self-sufficiency will want to store these items ahead. The most isolated ranches I know of are on the Aleutian Islands which extend out from the mainland of Alaska. Those ranchers are truly self-sufficient. They don't run down to the local feed store for a couple of blocks of salt because the nearest feed store is hundreds of miles away. You need to know how to treat injuries, cuts and wounds in your livestock and what medicines and drugs you should or shouldn't use. You need to know what animals to pasture together and what ones to separate. In short, you need to rediscover all the wealth of knowledge that the people of the land used to have plus those good parts of modern technology that agricultural science and veterinary medicine have to offer.

Good animal husbandry is mainly just good common sense. It's providing the right environment for your livestock. Your animals' needs are really very much like your own. They need space, food, water, shelter and sanitation. Don't crowd them. Let each one have some elbow room. They need abundant water 24 hours a day, even in winter. In general, a variety of fresh, growing food along with stored hay and grain will suffice but you should calculate the rations to be sure they are adequate, especially during pregnancy and lactation. Many areas of the world have mineral imbalances in the soil and you must become familiar with the requirements for your area.

My advice is to use your creativity. Take good care of your livestock but try to do it the easy way. You'll have hours of chores on a self-sufficient farm so set up everything ahead of time for minimum maintenance. Use your common sense and make the necessary investment in land, buildings and equipment. In this book I will try to show you ways to calculate your needs and to find the information you need for successful animal husbandry for self-sufficient living.

Raising and Caring for Animals

A HANDBOOK OF ANIMAL HUSBANDRY AND VETERINARY CARE

1
Livestock Housing and Ventilation

Housing and ventilation are more important to the health of your livestock than a visit to the average farm would lead you to believe. Most farmers are good livestock feeders through the help of feed company nutritionists but they are notoriously careless about their livestock housing. Visit a few farms and see what I mean. The animals' quarters in cold weather are invariably cold and damp. Cattle and hogs are up to their knees in barnyard mud. It is only because livestock are so hardy that they get by. Providing the best of housing facilities will help to insure your success and self-sufficiency. There is no reason why you should lose livestock to pneumonia and scours during severe weather. After all, you usually manage to take care of your own comfort. All you need do is have the same sensitivity for your livestock and apply some simple principles. Most types of livestock can survive the most severe weather and prosper even in such cold places as interior Alaska if they are cared for properly.

The principles of livestock housing and ventilation are simply to prevent horizontal drafts, including wind; provide for natural vertical ventilation of moist air; provide shelter from precipitation; provide insulation from the cold and provide for sanitation and pest control. Some animals require the addition of artificial heat but most species of livestock can keep themselves warm with proper shelter. Hogs are one species that need artificial heat in sub-freezing weather. Poultry, rabbits, ruminants (cattle, goats, sheep, etc.) and horses do well even in sub-zero weather with proper shelter because they produce plenty of heat and have heavy coats. But they all suffer losses with inadequate shelter and they all need more feed and constant fresh water in cold weather. Your animals get no water from a bucket of ice!

You may be saying that you don't have a fortune to invest in knotty-pine paneled stables. Don't be discouraged. You can usually build a suitable shelter for the same price that you would have spent on that cold, damp, unhealthy one. In some cases, my recommended housing is cheaper. If you already have your livestock barns you can usually renovate them fairly easily.

Insulation:

First you seal it up, then you open it up, as follows: Build or renovate your livestock housing so the walls are airtight. A lamb that gets crowded up against a crack in the wall admitting cold wind and rain will soon chill and die. The best, of course would be to have exterior and interior siding and provide an insulated wall with a vapor barrier. But the important thing is that the walls keep out the wind. This includes replacing damaged windows, shutters and doors. In the northern zones, it becomes important to insulate barn walls. Concrete or concrete block walls are so dense that the heat travels through them as fast as the animals produce it. Between about 35° and 40° latitude, it is sufficient to use

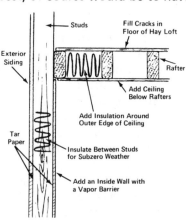

Outer barn wall and ceiling insulation

tar paper under the siding, on both sides of the studs. Above about 40°, you need to add insulation between the studs. Otherwise, the circulation of air between the studs carries the heat to the outside. Even if you live in southern latitudes, if the elevation is high enough that you have sub-zero weather, you definitely should have insulated barn walls and roof.

Fix the roof! The animals' coats will keep them warm unless they get wet. In cold weather, a wet animal is likely to get sick.

Ventilation:

The most often ignored moisture problem comes from the animals themselves. In both hot and cold weather, a group of animals exhale enough moisture to saturate the air around them in an enclosed building. In cold weather, this saturated air destroys the insulation properties of the animals' hair coats, which leads to chilling and lowered resistance. In hot weather, the added humidity from respiration adds to the heat and discomfort of the animals. Again, this can lead to illnesses on a flock or herd level. Proper ventilation is provided by the vertical movement of air by taking advantage of the fact that warm, moist air rises in cooler or drier air. The simplest application of this principle is to have one or two small windows at the top of the barn or hen house but these sometimes won't give adequate ventilation by themselves. The upper windows should be of a type called "Sheringham" windows, that are

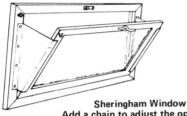

Sheringham Window
Add a chain to adjust the opening

hinged at the bottom and open inward. They have triangular boards beside them so when they are open, incoming air must flow upward towards the ceiling. For almost any size building, these windows should be only 60 square inches in area, such as 5" high x 12" wide. You need one opening for each 3500 pounds of livestock in the building. For our purposes, this will mean 1 or 2 Sheringham windows for any building since we are not going to have large barns or large numbers of animals. Put them on the side of the barn and opposite the prevailing wind. We will discuss the floor space for your number of animals under each species.

In conjunction with the high windows, you need a ventilation "flue" for each building. This is an ingenious affair similar to a fireplace and chimney and it draws air on the same principle. It may cost you the time and materials to install but it lasts as long as the barn and it requires no power or fan to operate. It must be built of light material such as wood because concrete or metal are too dense and cold and wouldn't "draw". The building must be fairly high so you get the drawing action. For best action, the entire flue should be at least 20' high. If the flue goes through a hayloft, you must insulate around the flue or the cold loft will stop the rising action. Regardless of the small size of the building, the inside cross section area of the flue should be a minimum of 400 square inches, that is, say 20″ on each side. This size will be sufficient for up to 8,000 pounds of livestock. It should have an opening at the bottom, inside the barn, like a fireplace. The top of the flue must extend 18″ above

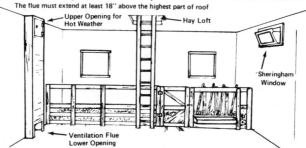

Interior of barn showing ventilation window and ventilation flue with adjustable upper opening

the highest part of the barn, like a chimney. It needs a rain-shield over it, another 18″ above the top of the flue. The flue needs a second opening inside the barn, near the ceiling, with a hinged door on it. Don't put more than one flue in a barn or they will compete and stop the circulation. In cold weather, close the ceiling door on the flue. The warm humid air near the floor will go up the flue through the bottom opening and fresh air will enter through the Sheringham window. The animals' body heat will warm up the barn but the ventilation will prevent a harmful build-up of humidity. In very cold weather, you must pay close attention to the ventilation to provide for your animals' comfort. You should adjust the ventilation by adjusting the opening of the Sheringham windows to keep the inside of the barns feeling fairly warm and dry. You should check it morning, afternoon and evening, increasing the ventilation in the morning because the animals' activity will increase; increasing it further for a sunny, warm afternoon to refresh the interior and decreasing it at evening because the animals' metabolism will be lowest at night. In hot weather, open the ceiling door on the flue so the hot air will exit near the ceiling. Of course, in hot weather you can open all the doors and windows. Just remember that when a cold rainstorm blows in you must close those windows, even if it's 3 A.M. If your flue is operating properly it will change the air at least 6 times per hour even though you will not feel a draft.

The ventilation flue will work for even small sheds or shelters, down to the size of a garage. Just extend the flue chimney above the shed so the total height of the flue from the ground is a minimum of

Cross-Sectional Area of Ventilation Flue According to
Height of Barn and Amount of Animals Housed.

Number of 1000-pound Animal Units in the Barn	Total Flue Area in Square Inches			
	Height, in Feet, from Barn Floor to Highest Part of Barn Roof			
	20 ft	30 ft	40 ft	50 ft
1 thru 8	400 sq. in.	400 sq. in.	400 sq. in.	400 sq. in.
9	408	400	400	400
10	455	400	400	400
11	500	400	400	400
12	544	422	400	400
13	592	457	400	400
14	636	493	415	400
15	682	527	445	400
20	910	704	594	525
30	1330	1055	890	788
40	1730	1370	1165	1045
50	2105	1660	1420	1275
60	2460	1940	1655	1490
70	2782	2205	1865	1692
80	3100	2455	2090	1880
90	3390	2670	2280	2055
100	3660	2870	2460	2225

20 feet. Most farms have a larger barn that has a hayloft on one side or above, so height is no problem except perhaps for the henhouse. If you do have a barn with a hayloft, be sure to close off the animal shelter area from the loft. Otherwise the heat they create escapes to the high part of the barn and they suffer with cold weather. Their area should be reduced in size with walls and ceilings so that they can keep warm. If your loft is above the animals, check the ceiling for cracks and drafts. Install a ceiling, hung under the beams, if there is none. In most barns, even if the animals have a ceiling under the beams, the wind blows through the cracks, and between the ceiling and the loft floor, and saps the animals' heat. Insulate around the outside of the ceiling to stop heat loss. Seal the floor of the loft if the boards have cracks between them. Hay above the animals will provide good insulation in cold weather. A large barn can be partitioned off to provide warm quarters in the winter for all your different species of animals, even the rabbits. In the summer, most of them can be returned to pasture.

Ventilation for a small henhouse is another matter. Some people have so few chickens that they build a small shed, maybe on stilts or skids. Then it isn't practical to attach a ventilation flue but there are lots of possible solutions. In moderate climates, you can put the hen house on stilts or skids and use a wire mesh floor. Most of the droppings and all of the ammonia go out through the mesh floor since ammonia is heavier than air. If you use a solid floor I recommend the built-up litter method, which won't produce as much ammonia, but you still need ventilation. Ammonia will build up from the droppings especially under the roosts. Use high windows like the Sheringham windows. If your hen house already has another type of windows, keep these closed in the winter and add the Sheringham windows anyway. Fix them so that you can adjust how far they stay open, such as with a chain and hook. Remember that you want the chickens to be able to keep themselves warm. Now install a small screened opening in one wall near the floor to allow ammonia gases to escape. Put it on the wall opposite the prevailing wind. Put the upper ventilation windows opposite the prevailing wind. Put a heavy wire mesh over the lower ventilation hole to keep out small predators and put a solid board a few inches in front of the hole inside the house so a direct draft won't blow in.

In hot climates a small, low hen house will be too hot in the summer. Here you must build a high-roofed shelter with lots of windows to open so the birds have cool shade. The shade of a big tree helps, too.

For ventilation and comfort you only need about 600 cubic feet of airspace per 1000 pounds of livestock in the barn. That would be an area 10 feet high, 6 feet wide and 10 feet long for a mature beef steer. In southern hot climates you should provide more than this because your biggest requirement is for cool shade. In cold northern climates, keep the size of the housing down to this figure so that the animals can keep the place warm with their own body heat. If your shelters are properly designed, with the proper insulation and ventilation, you won't be plagued with the typical winter scours and pneumonia and your animals will be snug and warm during the coldest blizzards.

I know of a farm in my home state that is a showplace, owned by a famous millionaire. In the winter, he always lost a lot of calves to pneumonia until his housing and ventilation were analyzed. The calf barn was well-sealed and had no ventilation. When the proper ventilation was installed, his calf illnesses stopped. Of course, he installed automatic electric fans, calculated to change the air the proper number of times per hour. Fancy, but no better than your self-powered ventilation flues. After you read the chapters on each species, you can calculate the number of animals you plan to keep and then you can plan their barns and shelters.

Sanitation:

Design your barns for easy cleaning. Sanitation is one of your hardest jobs on a farm. A lot of farmers just ignore sanitation most of the time. They seem to think that domesticated animals are somehow equipped to live in their own filth but it seems obvious to me that they are not. Wild animals don't foul themselves with their own manure and neither will livestock if given a choice. But since you are confining them, you must provide for their sanitation. Otherwise, you will have problems with foot rot, infected wounds, and other illnesses. It is common for veterinarians to see problems in livestock caused by poor sanitation. Urine contains urea which breaks down to ammonia in dirty litter. The ammonia is heavier than air and builds up near the floor. Chickens can become blinded as the moisture on their eyes absorbs the ammonia. Horses are very sensitive to it. The moisture in their skin absorbs it and it produces a skin rash. Most cases of infected wounds occur because the wound gets contaminated with manure. Mastitis in dairy animals is often caused by the animals' udders dragging in the filth as they step through knee-deep mud and manure in dirty barnyards.

For our purposes there are only two ways to provide proper sanitation. Either use hard floors such as concrete and clean and hose them every few days, or else use the built-up litter system. Commercial farmers use various types of automatic cleaning systems with cesspools or digesters but these are not practical for a small farm.

If it is managed properly, the built-up litter system is cleaner, warmer in winter, and much less work except when it comes time to clean out the barn, which is usually twice a year, spring and fall. If you do not have a tractor and front-loader to scoop up the accumulated, packed litter, you may want to clean more often so it is not so deep and heavy. The idea of deep litter is that you keep putting dry bedding over a buildup of used litter. The bacteria in the litter allow it to "work" just like compost. It absorbs the urine, has less odor problems than fresh manure and urine on a concrete floor, and the animals stay much warmer and cleaner. Start your built-up litter by spreading a deep layer of straw, corncobs or shavings, 6 or 8" deep on the floor. Then add a little straw several times a week to cover manure or wet spots. Don't let the animals spill their water on the bedding or get one spot completely soaked with urine. Add enough new litter to keep it clean and dry. If it gets soaked, the composting action stops and you start getting ammonia fumes. A big advantage to the built-up litter system is that your barns will be much cheaper because you don't need concrete floors. In fact, a porous floor will work much better. A base flooring of heavy rocks covered with coarse gravel, then fine gravel will be excellent and allow excess moisture to leach out. Just don't scoop out the gravel when you clean out the barn. This gravel bed should be about 12" thick.

Pest Control:

The last factor about shelter design or renovation is pest control. Rats and flies are terrible problems on most farms. Rats are amazing creatures. They will dig the mortar out from between the stones of a foundation to gain access. They can actually chew through aluminum and thin sheet metal. Fix both swinging and sliding doors so they are tight at the bottom when closed. Clean up junk piles and garbage and trash heaps so the rodents have less food and shelter. Clean up old piles of hay or corncobs in the barns. Put your grains in metal garbage cans or hoppers lined with sheet metal. Set up some rodent traps. There are lots of designs of traps which catch or drown the rodents. The important thing is to keep at it constantly. You don't notice rats and mice because they are shy and nocturnal. If you are seeing them in the daytime, your place is really loaded with them. To see how much of a problem you have, quietly go inside the barn at night and shine a flashlight in the corners and under things. You'll see their beady eyes shining back.

Rats and mice love henhouses because they provide such a banquet of their favorite foods. Many farmers put their henhouse up on concrete blocks but rats and mice climb these happily. I recommend that if you want to elevate the henhouse, use posts or stilts at least 2 feet high. Tack galvanized sheet metal around each post from the ground to the henhouse. It is too slippery for the rodents to climb. Also, a henhouse raised on stilts allows the chickens to get underneath it in the daytime for cool shade. If the henhouse is on the ground, put sheet metal around the bottom half of the door and doorjamb, put heavy wire mesh over the windows, and repair all ratholes by nailing sheet metal over them. Rats will climb all over a henhouse at night looking for an opening and they will chew through solid wood walls in a short time. Rodent control is a continual operation so just keep at it.

An excellent rat-proof grain bin can be built as in the sketch and it can be made in any suitable size. The inside is lined with galvanized sheet metal. This will make it rat-proof and will let the grain flow out more easily. All you have to do is put your bucket or cart under the outlet and raise the guillotine door. The grain will flow out by gravity. Many farmers have these bins on tall legs so that the space under them can be used for storage and is not wasted. You need a separate bin for each type of grain you will be storing. Some farmers have them arranged with chutes from each bin to a single outlet which goes into a feed grinder or into a scale. Be sure to cover the lid with sheet metal and don't let spilled grain accumulate on the floor under the bins.

Be sure to screen the windows of your henhouse to keep out wild birds as well as flies and mosquitoes, all of which carry diseases to your flock. In hot weather you may have a problem deciding whether to open up the henhouse for cool shade and ventilation or to darken the interior for fly control.

The best situation is to have a large tree nearby for cool shade and keep the henhouse fairly closed. Otherwise you'll have wild birds

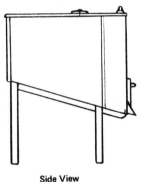 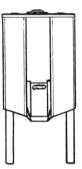 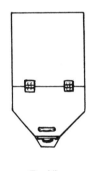

Side View   Front View   Top View

Grain bin. Line with galvanized sheet metal to keep out rats

and flies entering and depositing disease organisms in the feed and water in the henhouses. Or install a screen on the door and install a small 1' x 1' door for the chickens.

If you have dairy goats, fly control is one of your most important objectives. I recommend that you have a separate milking parlor which opens only into a dark area of your barn so that flies don't enter. Use a spring-closing screen door and screened windows in the milking parlor. Use slaked lime on the floor to kill microorganisms. These efforts are well worthwhile. If there are flies in the milking parlor, they walk on manure and then on the milk utensils and the intestinal bacteria from their feet will shorten the storage life of the milk and interfere with yogurt and cheese-making processes. Just remember that the flies' favorite hangout is a nice, fresh, juicy pile of manure.

Flies can be partially controlled by closing out the light. Flies don't like to fly into dark places so darken the interior by covering the windows and partially closing the doors. If this interferes with circulation, the alternative is to have well-fitting screen doors and windows. Large barn doors, which are used to admit tractors and implements, should have a smaller people-size door installed. The large door can then be closed and the small door screened.

2
Farmstead and Fencing Layout

If you are starting out on an established farm you are stuck with the layout of the major buildings, driveways, wells, sewage disposal, etc., but you will probably want to change the layout of some of the fields. People starting with raw land certainly have a lot of work ahead but they can lay out everything for best efficiency. Most farms are laid out with the house next to the road and the barns beyond the house. I guess this is from habit or maybe so they don't have to clear as much snow for the family car to get out to the road. Those farmers living on the upwind side of the road get all the odors from the barns in their back window. Pleasant dreams!

If you have not yet selected your land, I would recommend that you purchase as much acreage as possible for two reasons. First, extra land around your house will assure your isolation from noise, odors, or unpleasant neighbors. Second, you may want to use the extra land someday for commercial farming or for re-sale. Put your farm in the middle of the largest piece of land you can afford, even if you won't use the extra now. You can plant hardwood trees on part of it for future generations and you can have a clear area around your farm for observation and isolation.

There are several principles of fence and farmstead layout that

I would suggest for you to consider. These include the direction of the prevailing winds; the elevations and slopes of the terrain; the placement of the barns and sheds for your "traffic pattern" when you do chores; placement of fences, gates and lanes for moving animals and implements, and placement and size of fields for rotation between crops and pastures.

Winds and Elevation:

If your land has an elevated knoll, I would recommend that spot for your home unless you live in a very windy area. If you do, you may want to put the house on the lee side of a knoll or behind

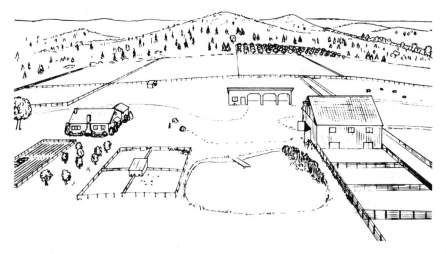

some large trees for a windbreak. I recommend having your house on the highest elevation so you can have full view of your land. Where I grew up, in Ohio, most of the old farmhouses had a cupola, a little room with windows on all sides on top of the house, so the farmer could inspect his grounds from the house.

Place your barns downwind from your house. Be sure to check with local people about the winds. In some areas, the prevailing winds change with the season. You want your barns far enough from the house to avoid odors and flies but close enough to make chores easy. In general, I'd recommend you have 50 yards between your house and the nearest animal shelter. No backyard homesteads, please! In my area of the country there are lots of people trying to become self-sufficient on their own little half-acre and one-acre suburban lots. They have horses, calves, goats, poultry and so on right in their backyard. In the summertime the flies are sometimes so bad that people can't sit out on their patios. The odors are bad, too.

Traffic Patterns:

I would recommend arranging your barns and sheds around a court or circular driveway to save steps. Put the henhouse and the milking parlor nearest the house because you will be visiting them most often.

Think through all the types of farming you will be doing and all the chores involved and try to arrange your daily schedules. Arrange your sheds and animal shelters so that you can have an efficient schedule and traffic pattern.

Water and Sewage:

As a general rule, the septic tank leach bed should be separated from your well by a distance equal to at least 10 times the depth of the well or the depth to the rock strata. The well should be a further distance from any other source of contamination such as the barnyard or a swampy marsh. I know of an instance where one person's septic tank was leaching to his neighbor's well. A person carrying typhoid visited the first family and everyone in the second household came down with typhoid. The source was traced by public health officials.

Be sure your house and well are not down-hill from your barnyards or a heavy rain will carry filthy water flooding down from the barnyard.

Lanes for Moving Livestock:

I would recommend that you have lanes going out between

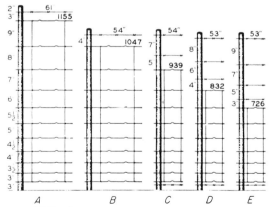

Types of Commercial Fencing

Cattle, horses & goats - A or B. The barbed wire strand at top keeps them from mashing fence down.

Hogs - C,D or E, without upper barbed wire. Bottom barbed strand prevents digging under.

Sheep - D or E, without barbed wire or use barbed wire with extended strand of wire at top to keep out dogs and coyotes.

your fields. Most farmers just have gates in all the fences and when they want to drive some animals from the barn to the back field, they drive them through all the fields in between. I'm talking about a roadway or lane down between the fields with fences on both sides and with access gates into each field along the lane. The lane will make it much easier to drive stock to a rear field and you won't contaminate the fields in between with parasite eggs from their manure. This will take at least 25% more fence but I think it's worth it. Be sure to make the lanes and gates wide enough to admit any tractors or implements you might use. Even though you may not have a big enough place to have a wheat combine or cornpicker, you might someday have a neighboring farmer bring his harvesting implements over.

Field Size for Crop and Pasture Rotation:

Make your fields small enough for pasture rotation for your different species of livestock. Consult the chapters on different species to determine how many animals you will have for your family and make the fields large enough to support them on pasture but small enough so that you have adequate numbers of separately fenced fields for rotation of pastures and rotation of the crops. The reason you want fences between your different crops is that you will be rotating grain crops with legume forages, like alfalfa, to rebuild the soil and each field must be able to contain pastured animals while it is planted to pasture grasses or legumes. Grains, especially corn, take a lot out of the soil so each field should be rotated through two years of legumes and animal pasturing within no more than every 5 years. Write out a rotation schedule and keep track of it so that you can keep track of the fields and the crops that were planted in the past years, such as the following 5 year plan:

Field #	1974	1975	1976	1977	1978	1979
1	pasture	oats	wheat	corn	pasture	(Repeat
2	pasture	pasture	oats	wheat	corn	of '74)
3	corn	pasture	pasture	oats	wheat	
4	wheat	corn	pasture	pasture	oats	
5	oats	wheat	corn	pasture	pasture	

On this rotation schedule, each field gets two years of pasture to build it up every time it has corn on it. If you have room for more fields, plant them to legumes and have your rotation schedule go as many years as you have fields. The legumes are the only plants that add nitrogen back into the soil. If you can't use all the legume crops, just let them grow or plow them under to add even more nutrients to the soil. The cost of their seed is the best fertilizer investment you can make.

Most people don't rotate their poultry on regular fields because the fields are usually larger than chickens need. There are several ways to set up your poultry pastures, called ranges. One way is to put the poultry house in the middle of a field and fence the field off into 3 or 4 smaller ranges with the house in the center. Install some small doors in the house, opening one into each field. Then you can just let the chickens out the appropriate door to rotate pastures. Another way is to have 3 or 4 small fields with big gates in the fences. Have the henhouse on skids and pull it into a new field with a tractor when you want to rotate ranges. Just don't do it with the hens inside or they'll probably stop laying!

To protect sheep from dogs and coyotes

Most farmers keep the vegetable garden separate from the cropland and pastures. It is safer to put only composted manure and not fresh manure on your garden because composting kills all the bacteria and parasite eggs from the livestock, some of which are pathogenic to humans. I recommend that you put a secure fence around the vegetable garden to keep out foraging animals. If you have a lot of trouble with woodchucks or other burrowing creatures, you may need to dig a trench all the way around the garden 12" to 18" deep, install the fence in the trench and then back-fill it to discourage the hungry varmits. In some cases you even have to lay a section of horizontal fence in the bottom of a wider trench for those varmits that burrow deeply. It's also a good idea to keep the dogs and cats out of the garden because of the parasite eggs that they might pass in their stool.

One last recommendation I would make for the self-sufficient farm is to plan one field that can be used as an airplane landing field. You may someday decide that air transportation is a worthwhile saving of time, especially if your location is quite isolated. You may take up flying yourself or you may find people with goods and services to offer who are also pilots. For those of you who are retreating because you foresee political or economic turmoil, remember that there will always be other farsighted, inde-

Grounding of woven wire fence with wood posts. Place pipe every 150 feet to arrest lightning.

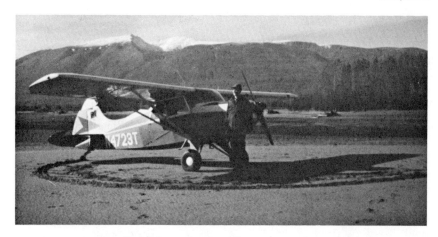

A bushplane like this can land on almost any unimproved strip.

pendent people who will survive and prosper. You may become acquainted with them and you may wish to trade goods or services with them. After all, this is the basis of private enterprise. An airplane shortens great distances easily. In the far north of Canada and Alaska, bush pilots still link isolated villages with the goods and services from outside.

If you worry about destroying your isolation by having a landing strip, you may put obstacles on it such as barrels or other obstructions which you can remove when wanted. In the far North, landing strips are unsafe during spring "breakup" or thaw due to mud and during fall freeze due to heaving of the permafrost. During these times, homesteaders put a few barrels at the ends and in the middle of their landing strips so visiting pilots won't land.

Plan your landing strip so it is at least a quarter mile long, in the direction of the prevailing wind. There are several makes of high-performance bush planes that can land in only a couple of hundred yards but if the area is available, clear it. The longer the landing strip the safer it will be. Plant the strip to pasture and you can graze animals on it in dry weather. Don't put animals on it in wet seasons or they will make it too rough and bumpy. Mow the strip to keep the weeds under a foot high.

Acreage for Crops and Livestock:

You can calculate the acreage you will need for crops and pasture by consulting the chapters on the different species of animals and deciding what species and how many animals you wish to have on your place. Those chapters give you an idea about how much grain, hay and pasture land will be required to support each animal per year and I will show you some examples of calculations in this chapter. Your yields of grains and hay will vary a great deal from one locality to another but here are some average yields along with the volume and weight figures.

Yields & Volumes:

Crop	Bushels/Acre Estimate	Pounds/Bushel	Pounds/ft ^{3}
Corn on Cob	100	70	28
Shelled Corn	80	56	44.8
Wheat	20 - 50	60	48
Oats	40 - 80	32	25.6

Alfalfa and clover hays -- Average 3 tons per acre in most areas. Some mild climates get 6 or more cuttings at a ton per cutting per acre.

As an example of calculating acreage needed, let's take a family of four people. Suppose that they want dairy goats for milk, yogurt, cheese, etc. In the chapter on goats, we note that one goat, while lactating, will need about 500 lbs. of grain, 500 lbs. of hay, and pasture in warm weather. We also note that the grain could consist of half corn and half oats. Therefore 250 lbs. of oats at 32 lbs. per bushel and 40 bushels per acre calculates out to 7.8 bushels or 0.19 acre per year. (250 lb. ÷ 32 lb./bu. = 7.8 bu. ÷ 40 bu./A. = 0.19 A.) The 250 lb. of corn at 56 lb. per bushel and 80 bushels per acre means 4.5 bushels and 0.05 acres of corn. Most families keep two or three does in case one fails to produce. If they have three does and a buck goat, then they need about 3/4 acre of oats, 1/5 acre of corn and about 1 acre of hay if they are getting one ton of hay per acre.

For pasture, you can usually feed 5 to 8 goats per acre even in a dry year, 10 to 16 in a wet year or wet climate. In southern climates you may have year-around pasture, eliminating the need for the hay. Also, in warm climates you can get 4 to 6 or more cuttings of legume hay per year, of at least a ton per cutting. Therefore, the four goats may need an acre for grain and anywhere from 1/3rd to 2 acres for hay and pasture, depending on the growing season and climate.

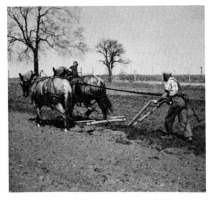

Two-Horse Hitch for Garden Plow
Courtesy Charles H. Ross, Jr., Galena, Kan.

Most back-to-the-landers like to keep chickens. You can estimate that an average laying hen will eat 90 lbs. of mixed grains per
year. If you have a flock of 40 chickens for four people, you will
have plenty of chickens and eggs for your family and usually a surplus for the hogs. You can make up your own chicken ration but as
an example, let's use 50% corn, 40% wheat, and 10% oats. The 40
birds will need 3600 pounds of feed per year (40 x 90). The corn will
calculate to 1800 lb., wheat 1440 lb., and oats 360 lb. Dividing by
the pounds per bushel and the bushels per acre gives 0.40 acre for
corn, 0.96 acre for wheat and 0.2 acre for oats or about 1½ acres for
the chickens:

Corn: 50% x 3600 = 1800 ÷56 lb/bu = 32 bu ÷80 bu/A = 0.40 Acre
Wheat: 40% x 3600 = 1440 ÷60 lb/bu = 24 bu ÷25 bu/A = 0.96 Acre
Oats: 10% x 3600 =   360 ÷32 lb/bu = 11 bu ÷50 bu/A = 0.2 Acre

If you have rabbits, you can estimate that a 10 or 11 pound
buck or dry doe will eat 100 to 120 lb. grain and maybe 40 lb. hay
per year. A pregnant or lactating doe will eat closer to 200 lb. grain
and maybe 50 to 80 lb. hay per year. The bunnies are raised strictly
as meat except for breeding replacements. They nurse for about 8
weeks and during that time will probably eat 5 pounds of grain and
a couple of pounds of hay each. If you have 3 does and a buck, you
will probably get 8 bunnies per doe every 3 months, or 96 bunnies
per year. The bunnies average 4 pounds at 8 weeks of age so you are
producing 384 pounds of live rabbit per year, probably all the average family can consume. So we can estimate their feed needs as
follows:

3 does x 200 lb. grain   = 600 lb., and 50 lb. hay = 150 lb.
I buck x 120 lb. grain   = 120 lb., and 40 lb. hay = 40 lb.
96 bunnies x 5 lb. grain = 480 lb., and 2 lb. hay = 192 lb.
       Total grain   = 1200 lb., and total hay = 382 lb.

If you used a concentrate of 1/3 oats, 1/3 wheat and 1/3 corn, you
would calculate it as follows:

oats   1/3 x 1200 lb = 400 lb. ÷32 lb/bu = 12.5 bu ÷40 bu/A = 0.3 Acre
wheat 1/3 x 1200 lb = 400 lb. ÷60 lb/bu = 6.7 bu ÷25 bu/A = 0.26 Acre
corn   1/3 x 1200 lb = 400 lb. ÷56 lb/bu = 7.1 bu ÷80 bu/A = 0.08 Acre
hay   ---   ---   382 lb   ---   ---   ÷ 2000lb/A = 0.18 Acre

In other words, 1/3 acre oats, 1/4 acre wheat and 1/10 acre corn,
with 2/10 acre for hay which is probably just leftovers.

Hogs are the hardest to estimate their needs because of the variations in what you may have to feed them and the pasture available.
If you have a 700 pound sow, you should give her about 2 pounds of
grain concentrate per 100 pounds of body weight per day while she
is pregnant and lactating. This would mean 14 pounds of grain per
day for 114 days of gestation plus 56 days of lactation. However let's

assume you are feeding her swill and you put in vegetables and trim-mings from the garden and food scraps from the kitchen, so we can reduce the grain to 10 pounds per day for 170 days or 1700 lbs. Sup-

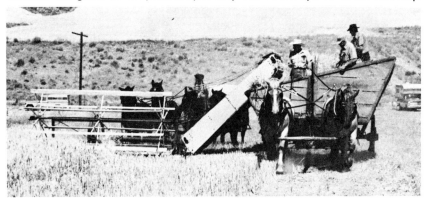

Two Belgians pulling a header box, with four Percherons pushing the header. Photo by Durland, courtesy David Horner, Forest Grove, Oregon

pose it is 80% corn and 20% oats:

corn   80% x 1700 lb = 1360 lb ÷ 56 lb/bu = 24.3 bu ÷ 80 bu/Acre = 0.30 Acre

oats   20% x 1700 lb = 340 lb ÷ 32 lb/bu = 10.63 bu ÷ 40 bu/Acre = 0.26 Acre

Or about 1/3 acre of corn and 1/4 acre of oats. When the sow is not pregnant or lactating you should still give her swill with some grain plus vegetables, table scraps, surplus milk or eggs, etc. so you need more grain but as you can see the figures are small. If you are quite isolated, you will need to keep a boar and some of the pigs for breed-ing replacements.

If we total our figures for all the animals we get:

	Corn	Oats	Wheat	Hay	Pasture
goats	0.05 A	0.17 A	--	1.0 A	0.5 A
chickens	0.40 A	0.20 A	0.96 A	--	0.5 A
rabbits	0.08 A	0.30 A	0.26 A	0.18	---
hogs	0.30A	0.26 A	--	--	1.0 A
Totals:	0.83 acres	0.93 acres	1.22 A	1.18 A	2.0 A
	= 6.16 total acres required				

These figures are intentionally inflated and fail to allow for the fact that most farmers supplment their larder with fish and game. In most areas 5 acres under cultivation are plenty for crops, livestock and vegetables for a family of four. Also, your growing season, cli-mate and rainfall will dictate your hay, grain and pasture yields. You can use your own figures for yields per acre in these formulas to cal-culate your needs. If you don't know the yields for your locality, talk to the county agricultural extension agent. The figures for the amount of feed each animal will eat per year will also vary widely according to your climate and housing. You will have to keep track of the amount of feed you are using by weighing it or calculating the weight from the volume of your grain bins. Keep good records for at least the first few years of operation so you can plan your crops according to your needs. The figures I use for pounds of grain per bushel are standard. The point of this exercise is to calculate how many animals you want and then to estimate the acreage of crops that you will need to support them.

You can calculate the bushels of grain in a bin by measuring it in feet, calculating the volume in cubic feet then multiplying by 0.80. The formula for a rectangular grain bin is "Bushels = volume in cubic feet (height x length x width) x 0.80." Here are some figures

One Section equals One Square Mile, which contains 640 Acres. Each side of a section equals One Mile.
One Mile = 1760 yards = 5280 feet = 320 rods = 1609.3 meters = 1.6 kilometers

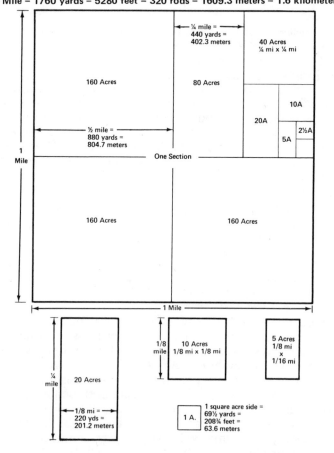

for calculating amounts of roughage in your barn and storage space needed.

Type	Loose		Bailed		Chopped	
	ft³/ton	lb/ft³	ft³/ton	lb/ft³	ft³/ton	lb/ft³
alfalfa	450-500	4--4.4	200-300	6--10	285-360	5.5--7
non-legume						
hay	450-600	3.3--4.4	250-330	6--8	300-400	5--6.7
straw	670-1000	2--3	400-500	4--5	250-350	5.7--8

Here are some figures for measuring your fields for acreage:
1 township = 36 sections = 23,040 acres
1 square mile = 1 section = 640 acres
1 acre = 160 square rods = 4840 sq. yards = 0.4046 hectare
1 Hectare = 10,000 sq. meters = 2.471 acres
1 Are = 100 sq. meters
1 Centare = 1 sq. meter

The most important principle to remember in your field layout and crop planning is that you should always plan for a surplus of everything you grow or raise. That way, if you have bad weather or crop failures, you can survive on stored food or surpluses from other crops or livestock. This is not wasteful; it is simply good insurance for self-sufficient living. Your surplus animal and dairy products can be well-utilized by your hogs and surplus crops can be saved for emergency and then put back on the fields as fertilizer. If you live in an agricultural community you can sell your surpluses or use them for barter.

3
General Nutrition and Calculation of Rations

The food you feed your livestock is the most important single aspect of animal husbandry. Your ability to feed your animals properly will probably mean the difference between your success or failure at self-sufficiency. Let's start the discussion of nutrition with some definitions. The general term for animal foods is feedstuffs. The ration is the specific diet you are feeding one group of animals at any one time and it includes everything they are eating. The ration consists of three parts, the forage or roughage, which is the hay or pasture; the concentrate, which is the grains; and the supplements, which may be vitamin, mineral, trace mineral or protein supplements.

The rules of thumb in livestock feeding have always been to feed a variety of fresh, growing foods along with hay and grain and to feed each individual animal by "eye." The good husbandryman watches his animals so closely that he can tell whether each one is gaining or losing weight. He increases the ration for those that are lagging and decreases it for those that are overweight. Besides providing variety, fresh foods and feeding by eye, there are some other principles that are very important, including those about water, protein, energy, minerals, vitamins, cracking hard grains and avoiding poisonous plants.

Water:

A continuous water supply is mandatory. You should provide clean water at a comfortable temperature twenty-four hours a day. Your animals will do best if their water is around 50° to 60° F. (10° to 15.6° C.) Animals need extra water in severely cold weather to keep themselves warm. The extra water is needed to metabolise additional food for warmth. Of course, they also need extra water during hot weather. Your two biggest problems are to keep the water from being fouled by urine or manure and to keep it from freezing in the winter. A watering trough for sheep or goats can be protected from contamination by placing it behind vertical slats or rods that the animals must reach through. Put the slats far enough apart to admit their heads. Goats are so particular that they need to have a fresh container of water several times a day or else a supply of running water. If you wish to have running water, allow the water supply to trickle into the trough and pipe the runoff away so it doesn't go into their pasture or bedding. For pigs you should build a platform or slab of heavy wood or concrete around their water or they will splash it out and make a mudhole. Their watering trough must be bolted down or else be heavy enough that they can't dump it. Horses and cattle can use high tanks, say three to four feet off the ground. Be sure to check all your watering troughs or buckets every day. Whenever one gets manure or urine in it, it should be emptied and rinsed

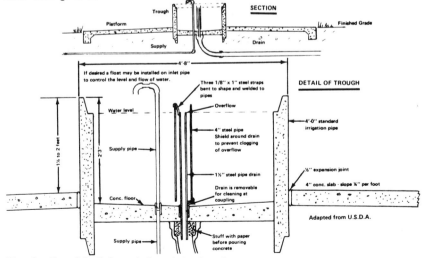

Watering Trough built from drain or irrigation pipe

out, then refilled. If you are using buckets or pans check them at least twice daily so the animals don't run out. A few hours of hot, humid weather without water can cause heat stroke.

To prevent freezing in cold weather, you must have running water, have heated tanks or refill the water containers regularly with warm water. Never use an electric immersion heater for livestock even if the manufacturer says it is safe. A malfunction or an animal chewing the insulation could cause electrocution of animals or people. Safe commercial or homemade heated water tanks have the heating element outside the water. If your place has no electricity and is in a cold climate, you may be able to avoid carrying warm water by providing continuous running water to keep the ice off the water troughs. Of course, your water pipes must be buried underground below the frost line and you must use freeze-proof or heated water hydrants.

Poisonous Plants:

You must be sure your animals are not eating any poisonous plants in their pasture or feed. There are hundreds of species of plants that can be poisonous. Usually they are dangerous only during a certain part of their growing cycle or during certain seasons. Poisonous plant varieties vary from one part of the country to the next. There are so many of them that their descriptions fill volumes. Collect literature on the poisonous plants of your locality from the county agricultural extension agent or from the nearest college that has agricultural services. This information is usually available even for very isolated areas. Be sure to get books and pamphlets with good pictures of the plants. Few people can recognize an offending plant from a mere description or a sketch. See if the county agent or college has a collection of preserved specimens so you can see them first-hand. Then go on a field trip in your own fields and look for specimens. If you find plants you think may be offensive but aren't sure, take them in and have them identified. All this leg work will be well worth it. If you find some poisonous plants in your area, dry and preserve them in a picture frame or shadow box. Keep them for future reference.

In most cases livestock won't eat the poisonous plant varieties even when plentiful. Probably most of them taste bad to the animals. But if you have a dry year and the poisonous plants are all that are available you can have a disastrous outbreak of poisoning. Most of the plant poisonings have no antidotes so prevention is the only key.

Cracking and Grinding Grains:

The physical presentation of your concentrate feeds is very important. Hard grains like corn and hard wheat are very poorly utilized unless they are cracked. If you feed whole kernel corn you will see many kernels come through intact in the manure. Even whole oats are not digested well because of their protective hulls. For chickens and rabbits it is almost mandatory that you crack the larger grains. Commercial rations always have the hard grains cracked or ground and the soft grains like oats crimped or rolled to open the hulls for better digestion.

I recommend that you set up some type of grain grinder. Farmers always used to have feed grinders but they seldom use them now because they get all their rations at the feedmill, premixed and computer-calculated for nutrition and cost. You can probably pick up a used feed grinder at a farm auction. While you're visiting auctions you may be able to pick up a hand powered corn sheller, too. If you have no electricity for an electric-powered grinder, devise some other source of power. You may even want to build a wind or water-powered stone mill. You'll often see millstones as decorations in farmers' yards and at auctions. A stonecutter, such as a person who makes cemetary headstones, could even make a custom millstone for you. The millstone is mounted on an axle and arranged so it rolls in circles over a large, flat stone. It can be powered by any means, even draft animals. There are a number of old, historic mills still operating and they are certainly worth a visit. There is a var-

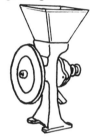

Small-capacity
grain grinder

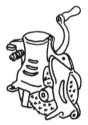

Cast iron, hand-powered
corn sheller

iety of small flour and grain mills and grinders available from farm supply outlets and from natural food and gardening sources. Some of these are hand cranked, some electric and some can be hooked up to other sources of power. Some of these are suitable only for household flour because of their small volume and fine grind. You can purchase a larger grinder from any farm implement source.

Grind your grain regularly so it is fresh. It loses its vitamin and nutrient values to oxidation more quickly after it is cracked. The hulls act to preserve it. In hot weather, grind grain every other day. In cool weather, grind enough grain to last a week at a time. For most of your livestock just run the grain through for coarse grinding. Crack most of the kernels of corn and wheat and just break the hulls open on oats and other soft grains. For chickens and rabbits you should grind the grain fairly fine but not to a powder and mix the ration well before feeding; The purpose of fine grinding is both for better digestion and so they don't pick out their favorite grain and leave the rest. Finely ground feed for chickens is called mash. You can also feed chickens some cracked or coarsely ground feed called scratch but they will eat this in preference to mash and they will waste a lot so don't overfeed it.

Fresh Feeds:

If your place is in an area with long, hard winters you should know that your stored hay and grain lose much of their vitamin and nutrient content from oxidation and deterioration over the winter. Late winter is the most unhealthy time for livestock because of this. One way to correct this problem is to make up some sprouting crocks or trays and sprout seeds. They can be sprouted in crocks or jars in the dark for plain sprouts or they can be placed on trays in front of a window for green growth. Another way to correct the problem is to add vitamin supplements to the feed in the winter.

Protein:

Protein is one of the most important nutrients for your livestock. An adult animal doing no work needs a small amount of protein but growing, fattening, pregnant and lactating animals need much greater amounts. You shouldn't underfeed protein or you'll have problems but you shouldn't overfeed it either. Extra protein is metabolized and changed to carbohydrates and fat and the resulting nitrogen waste puts added work on the animals' kidneys. It's a matter of waste versus efficiency. You can calculate your rations for the proper percentage of protein and other nutrients if you know the composition of the feedstuffs. The Nutrient Table gives average analyses for some of the common feedstuffs. You can use these figures or, better, figures from your own farm or area to calculate a ration for each species of your livestock in each stage of growth and production. You may wish to have samples of the feedstuffs you are growing analyzed for nutrient composition. You can get this done at most agricultural colleges or state universities. This might be worthwhile so you can get a firm basis for calculating your rations. Remember however that even your own crops will vary from field to field and year to year.

Consult the chapter on the species of livestock you are feeding and find the protein requirement for the animals' present needs. Then write down a trial ration of the grains and forage you have available and calculate the crude protein by consulting the Nutrient Table or your own analyses. If your trial ration is not suitable, change it and calculate it again. Suppose you were feeding pregnant and lactating doe rabbits and you want to provide 17% to 20% crude protein and a calcium to phosphorus ratio of about 1.2 to 1. See the Nutrient Tables at the end of this chapter and calculate a trial ration as follows:

Feedstuff	Pounds	X	% Crude Protein	=	lb. C.P.
Cracked Corn, yellow dent	10 lbs.	X	8.8%	=	0.88 lb.
Crimped Oats	10 lbs.	X	11.8%	=	1.18 lb.
Whole Wheat, Hard	10 lbs.	X	13.5%	=	1.35 lb.
Alfalfa Hay, Early	20 lbs.	X	15.5%	=	3.10 lbs.
Totals	50 lbs.				6.51 lbs.
					Crude Protein

Divide the total weight of the crude protein by the total pounds of the ration to get the final percentage in your trial ration: 6.51 lbs. crude protein ÷ by 50 lbs. X 100 = 13% crude protein.

As you can see by this trial calculation, you don't have enough protein in this ration for reproduction and lactation. By noting the protein content of these feedstuffs you can see that there is no way to juggle this formula to get it. Therefore you must add a protein

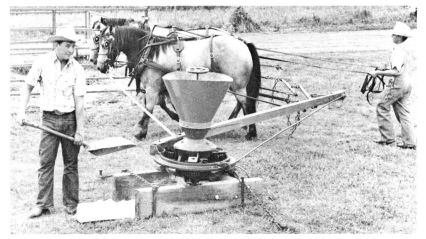

A "horsepower" being used to grind grain. Photo by Waltner, Freeman, South Dakota 57029.

supplement to this ration. If you are in a farming community just go to the feed mill and buy a bag of soybean oil meal, linseed meal or cottonseed meal and add some to the ration. Again calculate a trial ration adding soybean oil meal which is high in crude protein: Soybean Oil Meal (S.B.O.M.) 10 lbs. X 45% crude protein = 4.5 lbs. Adding these figures to the above chart adjusts the totals to 11.01 lbs. of crude protein in a total ration of 60 lbs. Then, 11.06 lbs. crude protein ÷ 60 lbs. X 100 = 18.35% crude protein. This will give you your needed protein but there are two problems. First you don't know what percentage of the ration they will eat in hay. They may eat more or less than you estimate. Hay is very important for providing protein if it is a high protein hay such as the legumes, clover or alfalfa. Look at the protein content of the various legumes in the Nutrient Table. The other problem is for those people who are so isolated that they don't have access to feed mill products. Their answer is to feed surplus home-grown protein supplements such as eggs and dairy products and roughages that are high in legumes. Whole fresh eggs are 13% crude protein and about 66% water. Hay and dried grains are about 10% water so if we analyze eggs on the basis of about 90% dry matter, like the hay and grains, we can calculate the eggs at about 29 or 30% protein and use them like protein supplements. Milk and milk products also supply good protein. The trouble with the use of eggs and milk products in your rations is that after you mix them with the concentrate they will soon spoil so you must clean out any leftovers later in the day. Another way to increase the protein is to use high amounts of oats and wheat, which are higher in protein than most grains. A natural feedstuff exceptionally high in protein is ladino clover pasture or early-cut hay.

Lactating goats, cows, sheep and other ruminants are very efficient at utilizing low quality protein. They can produce milk on a mixture of grains and low quality hay, sometimes on hay alone. They will give more milk, however, if you add extra protein supplement or high quality legumes to bring their ration up to 18% to 20% crude protein. Calculate a trial ration such as follows for a dairy goat:

Feedstuff	Pounds	X	% Crude Protein	=	Pounds Crude Protein
Corn	5 lb.	X	8.8%	=	0.44 lb.
Oats	10 lb.	X	11.8%	=	1.18 lb.
Wheat	5 lb.	X	13.5%	=	0.68 lb.
Alfalfa Hay	10 lb.	X	15.5%	=	1.55lb.
Ladino Clover	10 lb.	X	21.0%	=	2.10 lb.
Totals	40 lb.				5.95 lb. Crude Protein

Then, 5.95 lb. C.P. ÷40 lb. X 100 = 15% crude protein.

Although wheat is high in protein, you can not use an all-wheat concentrate because it is low in fiber and seems to cause bloat when fed in too high a proportion. It is especially dangerous to horses. I would recommend you not use over 20% of your grain concentrate as wheat and you will be safer if you don't feed any wheat to horses.

If you study the Nutrient Table closely, you'll see a disparity in the percentages of digestible protein in different feeds. In some feeds the digestible protein is only about half the crude protein and in other feeds the crude protein is almost all digestible. Compare the column marked, "crude protein" with the one marked, "digestible protein." It is really better to calculate your rations on the basis of digestible protein but most textbooks and publications on nutrition quote figures for crude protein when they tell you how much to use. Be sure you know which type of figure is being discussed when you are deciding on a specific ration for your livestock. If a source recom-

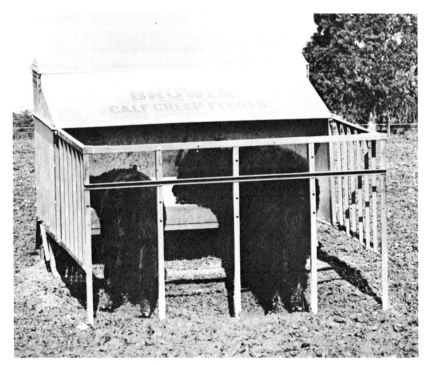

Angus calves at the creep feeder

mends 15% *digestible* protein for your lactating sow and you give her a ration with 15% *crude* protein, you will really shortchange her. Mistakes like this lead to mastitis and agalactia (lack of milk) especially in sows. To calculate digestible protein use the same formula as for crude protein but use the figures from the tables marked digestible protein. The only requirement is that you know the range of crude or digestible protein the animals need for their particular stage of their life cycle. The chapters on the different species of animals will outline their needs. The National Academy of Science, National Research Council, 2101 Constitution Avenue N.W., Washington, D.C. 20418, publishes tables of nutrient requirements for all the domestic species of livestock in all stages of their life cycles.

Energy:

The most important function of food is to provide energy. All organic nutrients, fats, carbohydrates and proteins, can be utilized by the body for energy. Most people are familiar with the measurement of energy in human foods in Calories. Animal feedstuffs can be measured for energy value in many ways, some of which are useful only to the research scientist. Most literature on the practical aspects of feeding livestock speak of total digestible nutrients, or T.D.N. This is expressed in pounds of the given food and it is written in tables as a percentage figure. For instance, No. 2 yellow dent corn is listed as approximately 81% T.D.N. which means that 100 pounds of the corn provide 81 pounds of total digestible nutrients. The various feedstuffs can thus be compared for their energy values. The National Research Council tables include energy requirements for livestock. These N.R.C. tables may be helpful especially if you are raising large numbers of animals. For a small operation you should become familiar with the energy content of the feedstuffs you are using and be aware of the general principles of energy utilization by each of your species of livestock. With this background you can feed by eye and keep each of your animals in top condition.

Note that the grains are generally higher in T.D.N. than forages. Corn and milo sorghum are about the highest, wheat is lower and oats are much lower in T.D.N. This means that animals get more energy, faster, from the grains, especially corn and milo. However, we must consider the differences in physiology, that is, the digestion and energy utilization, of different species of livestock. The major difference is between the ruminants (cattle, sheep, goats, etc.) and the monogastrics (horses, swine, rabbits, dogs, cats, humans, etc.).

The ruminants are aided in digestion by fermentation in the rumen or first compartment. Here, microorganisms ferment or break down the food, including plant cellulose, producing heat energy and readily available nutrients for the host animal. Because of this bonus process, mature ruminants can maintain themselves even in the coldest weather on poor quality roughages alone as long as the quantity is adequate. Any type of production such as growth, pregnancy, milk production or fattening requires extra energy, though, in the form of either higher quality roughages or grains. Insufficient energy intake in your ruminants will show up as retarded growth, low milk production, loss of weight or poor reproduction.

Monogastrics miss most of the benefits of fermentation so they need more grain in their rations both for maintenance of body heat in cold weather and for production and work. Insufficient energy intake in monogastrics shows up as retarded growth, loss of weight, poor reproduction, loss of the young from insufficient milk production, susceptibility to disease or reduced stamina.

Horses are very sensitive to rapid changes in the energy content of their rations. A sudden increase in a horse's energy intake will often give it severe colic and/or founder. Founder or laminitis causes severe damage to the hoofs. Such an increase in energy can easily occur by overfeeding grains. Since corn and milo are compact, high in T.D.N. and easily digested, feeding accidents can happen very easily with these grains. A new

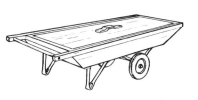

Home-made feed mixing and feeding cart. Line cart and lid with galvanized sheet metal to exclude rodents.

helper may misunderstand your directions or someone may accidentally feed the grain twice to the same horse. People often overfeed their work horses on their day off as a treat. Horses that are worked heavily should be given half-rations on a day that they do no work. Horses are notorious for overeating if they get loose in the cornfield or the grain bin. Never increase a horse's grain suddenly. Change it slowly, working up or down over days or weeks.

Minerals:

When you make up a ration you should calculate the calcium to phosphorus ratio as well as the protein content. Calculate the calcium and phosphorus from the Nutrient Table and the formula just as with protein and compare them. Here is an example using the last ration we calculated for the dairy goat:

Feedstuff	Amount	X	% Calcium	=	Pounds Calcium
Corn	5 lb.	X	0.03%	=	0.0015 lb.
Oats	10 lb.	X	0.10%	=	0.0100 lb.
Wheat	5 lb.	X	0.05%	=	0.0025 lb.
Alfalfa Hay	10 lb.	X	1.48%	=	0.1480 lb.
Ladino Clover	10 lb.	X	1.25%	=	0.1250 lb.
Totals	40 lb.				0.2870 lb.

Again, for phosphorus:

Feedstuff	Amount	X	% Phosphorus	=	Pounds Phosphorus
Corn	5 lb.	X	0.27%	=	0.0135 lb.
Oats	10 lb.	X	0.35%	=	0.0350 lb.
Wheat	5 lb.	X	0.40%	=	0.0200 lb.
Alfalfa Hay	10 lb.	X	0.23%	=	0.0230 lb.
Ladino Clover	10 lb.	X	0.35%	=	0.0350 lb.
Totals	40 lb.				0.1265 lb.

The Ca : P ratio for this ration, then, is 0.2870 : 0.1265 which equals 2.2 : 1. The ideal Ca to P ratio is 1.2 : 1. The acceptable ratio varies easily from 2 : 1 to 1 : 1, as long as an acceptable level of vitamin D is present. The above ration is a little low in both calcium and phosphorus, however, because the total calcium, 0.2870 lb. ÷ 40 lb. total ration X 100 = 0.72% and the total phosphorus, 0.1265 lb. ÷ 40 lb. X 100 = 0.32%. As a rule of thumb you need about 1% of the ration in calcium and 1% in phosphorus. This will usually supply adequate Ca and P for growth, reproduction and lactation. Maintenance of adult animals doing no work or production requires less, one-half per cent or less of each mineral. Laying and reproducing hens, however, need much more calcium, 2.25% to 2.75% of the total ration. Since most rations are too low in both minerals you will usually need to add mineral supplement.

Note the different types of mineral supplements in the Nutrient Table and the relative amounts of calcium and phosphorus in each. Dicalcium phosphate has the highest relative phosphorus while feeding-grade limestone has almost no phosphorus at all. Many areas of the country are deficient in phosphorus in the soil so the plants grown there are deficient for animal feed and phosphorus must be added to the ration. Your local conditions will dictate the type of mineral supplement you should use so you must investigate the local requirements.

Vitamin, Mineral and Trace Mineral Imbalances:

Trace minerals include all the minerals other than calcium, phosphorus, magnesium and salt (sodium chloride). Vitamins and trace minerals are important to the health of your livestock. There are volumes of material written on the deficiencies and excesses of the various vitamins and minerals. Unfortunately the symptoms of these imbalances vary with different species of animals and even from case to case. The trace mineral imbalances are geographically located, depending on the trace mineral content of the soil.

I would recommend that you do two things to arm yourself with the necessary knowledge about vitamin and mineral imbalances in your livestock. First contact your county agricultural extension agent or the nearest agricultural college and get information about vitamin and mineral problems in your locality. Second, buy three or four textbooks on animal and human nutrition. The reasons I suggest more than one are that in each book you will find details that are lacking in the others and because many authors tend to repeat classic symptoms of a deficiency disease without mentioning in which species of animals the symptoms appear. The study of nutrition is arduous but very interesting.

There are several vitamin and mineral problems that I think are common or serious enough to need discussion. The requirements for calcium, phosphorus and vitamin D are intricately related. A gross deficiency of any of the three can cause symptoms like rickets in any of the domestic animals, with softness and buckling of the bones, lameness, slow growth, enlarged painful joints, and spontaneous bone fractures. This is common in calves and pigs raised indoors due to vitamin D deficiency. The body makes its own vitamin D when exposed to sunshine. In cattle, a severe phosphorus deficiency can cause a depraved appetite, called pica, where the animals eat wood, rocks, cloth or anything at all. A severe calcium deficiency can cause tetanic spasms of the muscles and even convulsions and death if the blood calcium level gets low enough. While each animal has need for a specific amount of calcium and phosphorus in grams per day, the ratio between them is more important than the amount. This is because if the ratio is incorrect, as with way too much phosphorus, the calcium won't be absorbed at all. If you feed a ration containing several times as much phosphorus as calcium, the extra phosphorus will tie up the calcium in the intestines in insoluble forms so it can't be absorbed. If you feed a horse a diet of mostly bran, which has 0.14% calcium and 1.2% phosphorus, you can produce a type of rickets with soft, deformed bones, called bran disease, because he is absorbing hardly any calcium. Grains are generally lower in calcium than phosphorus while forages, especially legumes, are higher in calcium. Your total ration must never contain more phosphorus than calcium.

Be sure that your mineral supplement is feeding grade, such as the ones mentioned in the Nutrient Table. Rock phosphates and dicalcium phosphate are well utilized by all livestock but are naturally so high in fluorine that they are poisonous. Be sure your rock phosphate is defluorinated feeding grade. Don't let anyone sell you soft rock phosphate or phosphatic limestone, both of which contain too much fluorine. Fluorine toxicity from feeding untreated rock phosphate causes symptoms in domestic livestock except chickens. They get soft teeth that wear down and sometimes are mottled chalky-white and brown. In cattle and sheep the teeth get so sensitive they can't eat or drink. A few areas of the U.S. have excess fluorine in the soil or water. One to two parts per million in the water is safe.

Bone meal is an excellent mineral supplement but be sure it has been sterilized. There have been some infamous outbreaks of anthrax and other diseases in livestock from contaminated bone meal.

Mineral supplement should be fed free choice in a box which is protected from rain or other moisture. The animals will usually take what they need and this is easier than mixing powdered mineral sup-

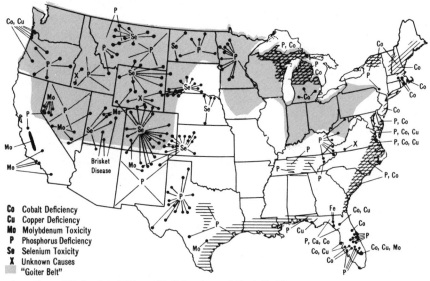

Co   Cobalt Deficiency
Cu   Copper Deficiency
Mo   Molybdenum Toxicity
P   Phosphorus Deficiency
Se   Selenium Toxicity
X   Unknown Causes
     "Goiter Belt"

Locations of Soil-related Mineral Deficiencies and Toxicity Diseases.

plement in the feed. As a rule you cannot hand-mix a ration well enough to properly distribute something like mineral or salt which is present as only one or two per cent. One animal would get too much and the next one too little.

Excess calcium can be as serious as a deficiency. There are areas where the soil has excessive calcium thus the feeds grown there contain excess calcium. High calcium in the feed depresses the assimilation of zinc, magnesium, iron, iodine, manganese and copper. Too much calcium in the soil or too much limestone (calcium) spread on the fields commonly causes a zinc deficiency disease in pigs called parakeratosis. This appears as crusts and folds of dry skin on the necks, sides, ears and faces of the pigs. Yet they have no odor and no itching. The signs of parakeratosis can include lameness, diarrhea and slow growth. Chickens are also affected with this type of zinc deficiency with slow growth, poor feathering and short, thick bones.

Livestock on a small farm will no doubt spend enough time outdoors to avoid a vitamin D deficiency. However in climates with long, cold winters it is a good idea to feed a vitamin D supplement in winter. Adding too much vitamin D, however, increases the absorption of calcium and can cause the excess-calcium problems discussed. Never add more supplement to the feed than is recommended on the container label. Vitamin D is produced in green forages when they are properly cured in the sun as ultraviolet light acts on the sterols in the plants.

Vitamin A deficiency is common and causes a great variety of signs. It causes night blindness in all species, an eye discharge in adult cattle, blindness in calves and dry, infected eyes in chickens. It causes a generally decreased resistance to infection in all species. It causes poor growth of bones and teeth by a different mechanism than does vitamin D deficiency. It can cause a myriad of other symptoms such as dead or deformed newborn, poor reproduction, muscle incoordination and nervous symptoms in cattle, sheep, swine and horses. Vitamin A is present as its precursor, carotene, in green forages, green, leafy hays, yellow corn, carrots, sweet potatoes, and green, leafy vegetables. Livestock utilize the carotene by converting it to vitamin A. Old, brown hay has lost its carotene content and thus its vitamin A value to oxidation.

A great area in a belt across the northern U.S. and Canada has a deficiency of iodine in the soil. Chronic iodine deficiency in livestock causes goiter, an enlargement of the thyroid glands. It occurs in most species and is especially noticeable in the newborn. Calves, lambs and kids are born weak or dead with big goiters in their necks. Pigs are born hairless with thick skin and puffy, swollen necks. Animals born with iodine deficiency symptoms do not respond to treatment and never do well even if they live. The only course is prevention by feeding iodine supplement which is easily fed as iodized salt. Feeding too much calcium or too much soybeans or peanuts contributes to iodine deficiency.

Iron is absolutely necessary for all livestock for red blood cell production. Iron deficiency anemia is seen most often in baby pigs and chicks raised in commercial indoor housing. The commercial farmers give each baby pig a dose of iron orally or by injection or they put a scoopful of sterilized dirt in the pen for each litter to root through. They need extra iron because milk is deficient and they aren't born with enough to carry them until they start eating solid food. If they are on pasture with their mothers they get enough from the soil to meet their needs.

There are some areas in California, Florida and Manitoba which have excess molybdenum in the soil which interferes with copper and sulfur utilization. Grazing animals in these areas get copper deficiency disease with diarrhea, loss of weight, stiff gait, anemia and changes in the skin and hair. Sheep wool becomes limp and glossy, losing its crimp. Cattle with black hair begin to turn brown and sheep wool loses its color. Lambs may be born with paralysis of the throat and be unable to nurse. Older lambs may develop swayback. Pigs may show slow growth, poor skin, lameness, weak bones and anemia. These areas need extra copper and sulfur supplements.

Sodium and chloride deficiencies produce lowered appetite, slow growth, poor production and poor reproduction in all livestock. Salt, sodium chloride, is a traditional condiment as well as a nutritional necessity. But it is also possible to have salt poisoning. This usually occurs when a heavy rain has disolved the salt from a salt box into a nearby puddle. Pigs, especially, will eagerly drink the salty water and become ill, sometimes fatally. Be sure to prevent this accident by protecting your salt boxes from rain.

There is only one B vitamin deficiency I will mention. There is a substance in raw egg whites called avidin which binds the B vitamin, biotin. High level feeding of raw whole eggs may produce a biotin deficiency in pigs and fowl but rabbits and ruminants synthesize enough biotin to prevent the problem. The deficiency in pigs produces loss of hair, dry, rough skin with a brown exudate on it, spastic muscles of the hind legs and cracking of the hoofs. Chickens have dermatitis, poor growth and poor hatchability of the eggs. Cooking the egg whites deactivates the avidin and prevents the biotin deficiency syndrome.

You can seldom diagnosis a specific B vitamin deficiency by the symptoms. In fact, most nutritional deficiency problems have very similar symptoms. The animals experiencing a deficiency usually begin to have a decreased appetite and then they decrease their growth and production. Lameness is common with deficiencies. Skin and haircoat symptoms frequently occur and diarrhea usually occurs late in the course of the deficiency syndrome.

Since it is usually difficult to diagnose the exact deficiency, the best thing is to prevent it. Most plants don't need the trace minerals. They just carry them from the soil to the animals. Therefore we seldom add trace minerals to the soil but directly to the livestock ration. Feed your livestock free choice mineral supplement for calcium and phosphorus and free choice iodized, trace-mineralized salt. Feed properly air dried grains and sun cured hay and try to provide some fresh growing greens at all times. Get to know your area and its specific mineral deficiencies or excesses.

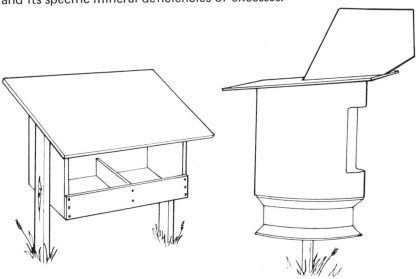

Two-compartment salt and mineral feeder. Use generous roof overhang to exclude moisture.

Weathervaning salt feeder. Made of steel drum on old wheel and axle. Swivels with the wind to keep out the rain.

NUTRIENT TABLE

Average Nutrient Compositions 1., 2.

Feedstuff	% Dry Matter	% Crude Protein	% Dig. Protein for			% T.D.N. for			% Ca	% P
			Cattle	Sheep	Swine	Cattle	Sheep	Swine		
A. Concentrates										
Barley grain, U.S. Gr. 1	89	12.1	9.1	9.5	9.4	73	76	72	.24	.36
Corn, ground ears, Corn and cob meal	87	8.1	4.0	4.4	5.8	78	68	70	.04	.27
Corn, shelled, flint	89	9.9	7.4	8.4	7.9	81	89	82	.02	.21
Corn, shelled, U.S. Gr. 2 yellow dent	89	8.8	6.7	6.9	7.1	81	87	82	.03	.27
Millet grain	90	12.0	7.4	5.9	8.8	69	55	66	.05	.28
Milo sorghum grain	89	11.0	6.3	8.6	7.8	71	84	78	.04	.29
Oats grain	89	11.8	8.8	9.2	9.9	68	67	65	.10	.35
Oats grain, white Canadian Western	86.5	11.4	8.6	8.9	9.6	67	68	60		
Rye grain	89	11.9	9.4	9.4	9.6	76	76	75	.06	.34
Safflower seed	93.1	16.3	13.0	12.9		83	82			
Wheat bran, dry mill	89	16.0	12.5	12.0	12.2	62	59	57	.14	1.17
Wheat grain, Pacific Coast	89.2	9.9	7.7	7.7	9.1	78	78	82	.12	.30
Wheat grain, Durham	89.5	13.4	10.5	10.5	12.4	78	78	82	.15	.40
Wheat grain, hard red spring	86.5	13.5	10.9	10.9	12.8	76	76	79	.05	.40
Wheat grain, hard red winter	89.1	13.0	10.2	10.2	11.9	78	78	81	.05	.40
Wheat grain, soft	90	10.8	8.5	8.5	9.9	79	79	83	.09	.30
Wheat grain, soft red winter	89.1	11.0	8.2	8.2	10.1	78	78	82	.09	.29

Feedstuff	% Dry Matter	% Crude Protein	% Dig. Protein for			% T.D.N. for			% Ca	% P
			Cattle	Sheep	Swine	Cattle	Sheep	Swine		
B. Forages										
Alfalfa, fresh pre-bloom pasture	21.1	4.3	3.4	3.4		13	13		.48	.06
Alfalfa hay cut early bloom	90.0	16.6	11.4	13.0		51	52		1.12	.21
Alfalfa hay cut mid-bloom	89.2	15.2	10.8	11.8		52	50		1.20	.20
Alfalfa hay cut mature	91.2	12.4	8.7	8.9		50	50		1.48	.23
Beets, sugar, fresh	16.7	2.7	2.0	2.0		11	11		.17	.04
Beets, dried sugar beet pulp	91.0	9.1	4.1	4.6	3.7	66	66	65	.68	.10
Bermuda grass, fresh pasture	36.7	4.2	2.9	2.9		23	24		.19	.08
Bermuda grass, hay	91.1	8.1	4.4	4.1		39	45		.42	.18
Bluegrass, Ky. early bloom pasture	35.7	5.3	3.7	3.8		25	22		.16	.14
Bromegrass, smooth, hay	92.8	5.4	1.8	2.5		54	50		.40	.20
Cabbage, fresh	11.7	2.6	2.2	2.2		10	10		.06	.03
Carrot roots, fresh	11.9	1.2	0.6	0.9	0.9	10	10	10	.05	.04
Clover, Alsike, fresh pasture	22.6	4.0	2.8	2.6		15	14		.29	.07
Clover, Alsike hay	87.9	12.9	8.2	8.6		53	49		1.15	.22
Clover, Ladino, fresh pasture	18.8	4.7	3.3	3.1		13	12		.25	.07
Clover, Ladino hay	91.2	21.0	13.2	13.0		56	52		1.25	.35
Clover, Red, early bloom pasture	19.6	4.1	3.0	2.8		14	12		.44	.07
Clover, Red hay	87.7	13.1	7.8	8.0		52	51		1.41	.19
Lespedeza, fresh early bloom pasture	25.0	4.1	3.0	3.1		17	15		.34	.05
Lespedeza hay cut pre-bloom	92.1	16.4	11.4	11.5		58	56		1.05	.24
Mangels, Mangel beets, roots	10.6	1.4	1.0	0.5		8	9		.02	.02
Potatoes, tubers, fresh	24.6	2.2	1.6	1.4	1.0	19	21	21		

Feedstuff	% Dry Matter	% Crude Protein	% Dig. Protein for			% T.D.N. for			% Ca	% P
			Cattle	Sheep	Swine	Cattle	Sheep	Swine		
Ryegrass hay	88.0	8.4	2.8			50			.45	.28
Soybean hay	89.2	14.5	9.0	10.0		46	48		1.15	.20
Sudangrass hay	88.9	11.3	4.9	5.8		52	46		.50	.28
Timothy hay, cut, early bloom	87.7	7.6	4.4	4.1		52	49		.53	.23
Trefoil, Birdsfoot, fresh pasture	20.0	5.6	4.6	4.6		15	15		.44	.05
Trefoil, Birdsfoot hay	91.2	14.2	9.8	9.8		56	55		1.60	.20
Turnips, fresh roots	9.3	1.3	0.9	0.8		8	8		.06	.02

C. Protein Supplements

Feedstuff	% Dry Matter	% Crude Protein	% Dig. Protein for			% T.D.N. for			% Ca	% P
			Cattle	Sheep	Swine	Cattle	Sheep	Swine		
Cottonseed meal - 36%	93.5	39.6	31.3	33.7	34.1	86	81	71	.19	1.02
Cottonseed Meal - 41%	94.0	41.0	33.2	33.2	34.9	73	69	67	.16	1.20
Chicken eggs with shells	34.1	12.8							1.50	1.10
Fish, Salmon	35.0	22.0								
Fish, Carp	22.0	18.5								
Fish, White Fish meal	92.0	63.2		58.8	58.1		68	66	7.87	3.61
Linseed Oil meal, mechanically extracted	91.0	35.3	31.0	29.7	31.8	74	73	77	.44	.89
Milk, Cows' fresh*	12.8	3.5	3.3	— species not stated —		16.3	— species not stated —		.12	.10
Milk, Goats' fresh*	13.2	3.6	3.4	"	"	17.1	"	"	.13	.11
Milk, Mares' fresh*	9.4	2.0	1.9	"	"	10.1	"	"	.08	.05
Milk, Ewes' fresh*	19.2	6.5	6.2	"	"	26.2	"	"	.21	.12
Milk, Sows' fresh*	20.1	7.3	6.9	"	"	26.7	"	"		
Meat and Bone scrap, dried	94.0	50.6	46.1	41.4	45.0	68	62	65	10.57	5.07
Peas, dry, ground	91.0	22.5	17.0	19.3	19.3	72	76	80	.17	.50
Peanuts with the hulls	92.0	19.1	15.1	15.1		99	99			.30
Peanut Oil meal, solvent extracted	92.0	47.4	42.7	43.1	44.5	71	76	77	.20	.65

Feedstuff	% Dry Matter	% Crude Protein	% Dig. Protein for			% T.D.N. for			% Ca	% P
			Cattle	Sheep	Swine	Cattle	Sheep	Swine		
Soybean Oil meal solvent extracted	89.0	45.8	39.0	41.3	41.7	72	71	75	.32	.67
Soybean Seeds	90.0	37.9	34.1	34.1	31.0	85	84	92	.25	.59
Soybean Oil meal, mechanically extracted	90.0	43.8	37.3	39.4	39.4	76	75	79	.27	.63

D. Mineral Supplements

Feedstuff	% Dry Matter	% Crude Protein	% Dig. Protein for			% T.D.N. for			% Ca	% P
			Cattle	Sheep	Swine	Cattle	Sheep	Swine		
Bone meal, steamed	95.0	12.1	8.2	8.2	9.4	15	15	15	28.98	13.59
Curacoa Rock Phosphate	99.0								33.0	14.5
Dicalcium Phosphate	96.0								22.2	17.9
Feeding grade limestone	100								33.84	.02
Defluorinated Rock Phosphate	99.0								29.57	13.55

E. Energy Supplements

Feedstuff	% Dry Matter	% Crude Protein	% Dig. Protein for			% T.D.N. for			% Ca	% P
			Cattle	Sheep	Swine	Cattle	Sheep	Swine		
Molasses, Cane	75.0	3.2	1.8	0.9		68	54	56	.89	.08
Molasses, Beet	77.0	6.7	3.8	2.3		68	58		.16	.03

1. Percentages are on an "as fed" basis rather than a dry analysis.
2. Source: "United States - Canadian Tables of Feed Composition, Second Revision", National Academy of Sciences, 2101 Constitution Avenue, Washington, D.C. 20418,
* Taken from Frank B. Morrison: *Feeds and Feeding, Abridged*, 9th Edition, by special permission of the Morrison Publishing Company, Box 130, Orangeville, Ontario, Canada

4
Disinfection and Sterilization

Have you ever wondered why physicians, veterinarians and other medical people make such a fetish of sterilizing and disinfecting everything? Is it really that important? The story behind the answer goes back thousands of years, starting with the ancient Egyptians and the Hebrews when all scientific knowledge was held and passed on by the Priests. Their findings and beliefs about the spread of disease are known from the Hebrew Bible and Egyptian heiroglyphics. They instructed their people via religious taboos and rules. Not all of their ideas were correct but many were. The Hebrews forbade eating pork and seafood without scales, that is, shellfish and bottom fish. Their rules were wise because undercooked pork can transmit trichinosis and tapeworm. Shellfish can transmit human hepatitis. Kosher slaughter originated for the purpose of meat inspection so that only wholesome beef from healthy cattle is used for human food. But unfortunately, they did not surmise the cause of disease as microbial life forms. Only since the discoveries of microbes, that is, viruses, bacteria, rickettsia, protozoa, and fungal life forms, have we left the age of imagining disease and parasitism as bad luck or divine punishment. Even today, many people instinctively consider disease as divine intervention or that God is testing them.

Legend has it that some medieval surgeons discovered boiling their instruments reduced their problems of post-operative infections. People have known for centuries to cauterize infected wounds and amputations but they didn't know why except that it obviously stopped the bleeding. If we consider disease and parasitism as the transmission of the causative organisms from one creature to another, then we can concentrate on prevention rather than magic. Many disease organisms and parasite eggs can live quite a long time in the soil, in animal bedding, in dried manure on walls and fences and in caked animal discharges, including milk. These are the organisms we want to reach with disinfection and sterilization so that the organisms don't live to infect another animal or person.

"Disinfection" is a vague term that means the destruction of pathogenic organisms while sterilization means the killing of all forms of organisms. In actual practice, disinfection usually refers to the use of chemicals to kill bacteria on surfaces such as floors, walls, fence rails, buckets, watering troughs, and other surfaces after a sick animal has been in contact with them. Unfortunately most disinfectants do not kill all viruses or spores of organisms like anthrax and tetanus. "Sterilization" is usually used to refer to the treatment of surgery instruments or milking pails and strainers just before they are used so that there are absolutely no living organisms on them at the time they are used. "Concurrent disinfection" refers to the continuous and immediate disinfection of the wastes and discharges from a sick animal during the course of his illness. This is an excellent concept to keep in mind whenever you are nursing a sick animal. Remember that the discharges and wastes from a sick animal are loaded with the disease-causing organisms and that he will recover more easily if these extra organisms are removed from his environment. These are the same organisms, however, that you do *not* want to carry to your healthy livestock. When you are nursing a sick animal, you should use a chemical disinfectant on your boots and your hands and change your clothes before visiting the healthy livestock. I will recommend specific disinfectants for each purpose but first I would like to explain sterilization.

True Sterilization

The easiest way to sterilize small tools and utensils is in a pressure cooker. Most pressure cookers are designed to hold a temperature of a little over 250°F (121°C) and steam pressure of 15 pounds per square inch. Don't forget to add the water in the bottom of the cooker and don't let it boil dry. Pressure cooking for 20 minutes or more provides wet steam sterilization and will kill all exposed spores, bacteria, viruses, fungi, etc. However, the utensils being sterilized must be scrupulously clean. If they have dried organic matter such as milk, blood, pus or manure on them, some organisms may survive within the organic matter. You can only sterilize a clean surface.

Items too large for your pressure cooker could be sterilized with dry heat in your oven but this requires much higher temperatures than wet steam under pressure. You need 680°F (360°C) for 3 hours, which will damage most items and discolor even some metals so this method is not very practical. You would be better off buying a large pressure cooker or even an old autoclave from a hospital. An autoclave is nothing but an oversized pressure cooker. If you wish to sterilize something and keep it sterile until it is used, simply wrap it in two clean cotton towels and tie it with a string before you pressure-cook it. Afterwards, put it in a dust-free cabinet and it will remain sterile in the wrapper indefinitely.

Formaldehyde probably comes as close as anything except phenol and several sterilizing gases to a true chemical sterilizer. The gases require special equipment and precautions. Phenol is too toxic to bother with but formaldehyde is relatively safe and easy to use. Formaldehyde can be purchased from drug supply houses as a 36% or 40% solution. Mix one part formaldehyde solution with nine parts water to make a 4% solution. Keep it in a closed container and you can drop cleaned instruments or utensils into it for 20 or 30 minutes for almost complete sterilization. You must rinse the items afterward, though, because formaldehyde is very irritating to delicate tissues. Don't get it in a cut or you will think you have been set on fire. I will admit, though, that getting formaldehyde in an infected cut was the best cure I have ever found! But even formaldehyde is not a true sterilizer. Phenol is the bacteriologists' standard of comparison for strength of chemical germicides. You must soak the spores of tetanus, *Clostridium tetani,* in 5% phenol for 12 to 18 hours in order to kill them! Therefore you can't consider anything weaker than 5% phenol for 18 hours as adequate for chemical sterilization and most people wouldn't want to put up with the odor and danger of phenol since it is so toxic. If you spill full-strength phenol on your skin or clothing it will cause severe burns and toxicity. Many doctors use a solution of 4% formaldehyde mixed with ½% phenol together with some rust preventative for their scissors and fine instruments. Twenty minutes in this solution will kill all vegetative bacteria including tuberculosis. The rust inhibitor consists of adding 2 grams of sodium nitrite per quart of solution. This solution deteriorates and should be changed every week or two.

Another method of complete sterilization is the use of direct flame, such as with a blow torch. I recommend this for wooden nest boxes and hutches. Scrub them with hot soap and water, let them dry and then lightly scorch them with a blowtorch. This will burn up all the organisms on the surface and get rid of any hair or feathers that might carry organisms or parasites.

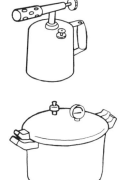

I would like to dispel the myths of boiling and using alcohol to "sterilize" things. Many farmers give their livestock vaccinations and antibiotic injections. They usually use the same old needle time after time and just wipe it off with alcohol. Tests have shown that some pathogenic organisms can live for days in pure alcohol. Other tests have shown that alcohol can inactivate some vaccines. You should never use a hypodermic needle on your livestock unless it is new in a sterile wrapper or you have sterilized it in your pressure cooker and kept it in a sterile wrapper. Boiling is adequate only for cleaning things. It may kill most vegetative bacteria but it does not kill spores such as those of botulism, tetanus, anthrax, etc. and it does not kill some viruses. For this reason I don't consider boiling as a method of sterilization. Remember, too, that at higher altitudes water boils at lower temperatures. Pressure cooking or autoclaving, however, combines a set temperature with steam pressure to kill organisms.

Sterilization And Disinfection For The Dairy:

Dry heat and steam under pressure are the only simple methods of true sterilization, that is, of killing *all* possible organisms on a surface. In practice, however, many people speak of sterilizing utensils and instruments, especially dairy utensils, with chemicals. Chlorine and iodine are good chemicals to use with dairy equipment and utensils because they are non-toxic. Chlorine is the best. Simply buy commercial laundry bleach, which is 5% sodium hypochlorite. One ounce in two gallons of water is sufficient. Let the chlorine solution remain in contact with the surface to be disinfected for at least

5 minutes. This will kill active, vegetative bacteria but probably not all spores and viruses so it is really a disinfectant, not a sterilizer. Chlorine is good for dairies because any residual chlorine left on the utensils is transformed to chlorides as soon as milk contacts it. There is no residual disinfectant left in your milk to interfere with yogurt or cheesemaking.

There are several brands of tamed iodine disinfectants available at rural and dairy supply stores. Chlorhexidine (Nolvasan) is another commonly used disinfectant. Quaternary ammonium types of disinfectants are also popular and commonly available. Quaternary ammoniums are sudsing and non-irritating to the skin. They cannot be mixed with soaps, however, or they will be inactivated. All these are good for wiping the animals' teats and udders before milking. Iodines, quaternary ammoniums and chlorhexidine are adequate for disinfecting utensils if left to soak long enough but then you must rinse them well so there is no disinfectant residue. For disinfecting your hands I would recommend that you wash them well several times with soap, rinse them well, then use a quaternary ammonium or an iodine disinfectant. Dry them with a clean towel or paper towels. For your boots, scrub them with a stiff bristle brush and any of the disinfectants mentioned.

Disinfection for Large Areas:

The most important thing to remember about disinfecting anything is that you must first scrub it thoroughly to remove all organic matter. Porous surfaces such as wood walls and fences are especially difficult because the organisms will survive in dried mucus, manure, pus, blood or milk in cracks and pores. Use a detergent and boiling hot water with a stiff brush to remove all dirt. Detergents and soaps remove dirt by breaking up fats and dissolving organic matter. The soap or detergent will remove much of the contamination but they do not have any disinfectant properties of their own. Rinse the surfaces and then apply your disinfectants. The cheapest effective disinfectant for large porous surfaces such as fences, stalls or the interiors of barns is hot lye solution, which is caustic soda, sodium hydroxide. Get 90% lye in cans and add 13 to 16 ounces of lye to 5 gallons of water. It will produce its own heat when mixed. Be especially careful when handling the dry lye powder. The dust is extremely dangerous to your eyes or if inhaled. Once it is mixed, it is not too caustic although it will burn your skin after a period of contact if not rinsed off. Any acid, such as vinegar, will neutralize it.

Recommended Spray Mixtures [*]

Disinfectant	Percent solution	Mixtures	Diseases
Cresylic [1]	4	4 oz. to 1 ga. water	Brucellosis Fowl plague Hog cholera Newcastle disease Shipping fever Swine erysipelas Tuberculosis Vesicular exanthema Vesicular stomatitis
Sodium carbonate (soda ash)	4	1 lb. to 3 gal. water	Foot-and-mouth disease
Sodium hydroxide (lye) Caustic soda	2	13½ oz. can to 5 gal. water	Hog cholera Foot-and-mouth disease Scrapie
Sodium orthophenylphenate (USDA approved)	1	1 lb. to 12 gal. water	Brucellosis Fowl plague Hog cholera
	2	2 lbs. to 12 gal. water	Newcastle disease Tuberculosis Vesicular exanthema Vesicular stomatitis
Sodium hydroxide (lye)	5	5 (13½ oz.) cans to 10 gal. water	Anthrax Blackleg

[1]See permitted list under ANH Division Memorandum No. 586.1.

[*] Animal and Plant Health Inspection Service, United States Department of Agriculture Hyattsville, Md. 20782

If you splash it in your eyes, rinse them with water, then with boric acid solution and call your physician! Lye is harmless to wood, rubber, and cotton but will damage varnished and painted surfaces. If not rinsed off, it will damage wool, silk and leather. The solution can be stored in most containers except aluminum but it should be air-tight or the lye will break down to sodium carbonate. You should add white wash, water-slaked lime, 2½ pounds per 5 gallons of your lye solution so you can see where you have applied the disinfectant. This also prevents breakdown of the lye solution. Most dairymen use this solution in their dairy barns at least once per year. Besides being economical, lye is very effective. It even kills anthrax spores and bacteria probably cannot build up a resistance to it.

Another effective method of disinfecting porous surfaces is with steam but this requires the construction or purchase of a steam jenny. Steam under pressure is especially good because it penetrates all the cracks and crevices and washes off the organic matter. The steam must remain in contact with each surface area for a period of time, though, so it probably doesn't usually contact the organisms long enough to do as good a job as lye. But nothing beats a steam jenny for cleaning, especially sheep pens which get coated with greasy lanolin from the wool. Just don't use a steam jenny in a barn in the winter or you will get your clothes dampened and catch pneumonia when you go outdoors.

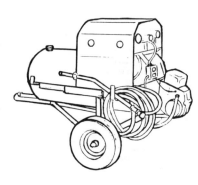

Another good area disinfectant is strong chlorine, which is available by using chloride of lime, U.S.P., available from drug supply companies. Mixing one pound in 3 gallons of water provides 30% available chlorine. This can be used in the same solution with detergents. Be careful when using strong chlorine solutions in a closed area because breathing the resulting chlorine gas can make you ill.

Steam jenny - Modern steam cleaner mounted on a trailer

There are several commercial area disinfectants that you can get for porous surfaces but they are more expensive and not much more effective than lye. One is sodium orthophenylphenate. Mix one pound in 12 gallons of water. This solution must be over 60°F. (15.5°C.) when applied to be effective. It cannot be used on a surface that previously had lye or other alkalies on it because they will deactivate it. There are several brands of cresylic disinfectants such as Lysol or you can get Saponated Cresol Solution, N.F. from a drug supply house and mix a 2% solution. You could also get Cresol, U.S.P. and mix 4 ounces in each gallon of hot water for a 3% solution. Cresols must be applied hot to be effective. The major differences between these disinfectants are as follows. Lye has better sporicidal activity for such organisms as anthrax when used at a 5% concentration but it does not kill T.B. bacilli. Cresols are very effective for T.B. but they should not be used in dairies because their strong odor may flavor the milk. Cresols are poisonous and must be handled with care. Saponated cresols are better but none of the cresols mix well with hard water because they precipitate with the minerals. Sodium orthophenylphenate kills T.B. and so is commonly used in dairies. All these can be applied to large areas such as floors with a sprayer.

Soil such as a field or barnyard cannot be disinfected or sterilized because the organisms sift or wash into it to a depth of several inches. Even burning will not reach more than a fraction of an inch into the ground. This is why pasture rotation is so important. Time and exposure will take care of most of the disease-causing organisms on a field, especially if the livestock are spread out and rotated enough that a heavy concentration of organisms or parasite eggs can't develop.

Disposal of Diseased Carcasses:

Burning or cremation is the best method of safely getting rid of carcasses of animals that have died of disease. Although burial is commonly practiced, it is not safe unless the carcass is buried under six feet of soil after being covered with quicklime, unslaked lime. You must not bury an animal in a low lying area because ground water or flood water can bring viruses and spores of organisms to the surface. In the winter when the ground is frozen, cremation may be the only method available. For large animals like sheep, goats, mature hogs, cattle or horses, cremation is the most practical way to dispose of the carcasses and get rid of all dangerous organisms that they may contain. On frozen ground or rock, bring in three or four logs, as large as needed to support the carcass. Put straw and kindling wood on top of the logs and put the carcass on top of that. Pile more kindling or straw around it and pour on old motor oil or kerosene to help ignite it all. Check the fire occasionally to keep it burning until the carcass is reduced to ash. If you can dig a hole at the site, make a central pit with ventilation ditches in four directions away from it, then place the logs and kindling over the central pit. The ditches will allow air to circulate under the fire and make it hotter. When it has completed burning, the ashes in the pit can be covered with dirt. Small animals like lambs or rabbits that have died of illness can be cremated on the hot coals of a hard-wood fire.

If you must bury an animal, dig the hole right beside the carcass. It must be over six feet deep. Roll the carcass into the hole then scrape the dirt in where the carcass was laying. Cover the carcass well with unslaked lime and then fill the hole. If you have a carcass that you can't dispose of immediately, cover it with unslaked lime or kerosene to keep other animals, insects and birds away from it. Remember that all this applies only to animals that die of disease. You cannot use these animals for human or animal food.

5
General
Disease and
Parasite Control

It would be lovely if we could live in perfect harmony with all of nature and invite the wild birds and wild animals to share our pastures and eat from our hands as in the fairy tales and the movies. Unfortunately the ecology of this world does not follow our dreams and wishes but has its own rules. The laws of ecology include the factor of disease. Disease is not an evil, a stroke of bad luck, or a mistake of nature. Disease is an expression of the ecology of the various animals, organisms and parasites and their balance or imbalance with the environment. Contagious diseases are those that pass from one individual to another. Zoonotic diseases are those that can pass from animals to man. There are three classes of disease you need to be constantly aware of on your farm. Those that can pass from wild animals to your livestock, those that pass from one of your animals to the others, and those that can pass to you and your family from the animals, either the livestock or wild. In the chapters on the different species of livestock we will discuss specific diseases that are dangerous to you and your livestock. In this chapter, we will discuss general principles of disease and parasite control.

In order to be successful, you must prevent losses due to disease. Those of you on a self-contained, self-sufficient farm are in a very enviable position compared to commercial farmers because you can avoid most of their sources of disease. Commercial farmers regularly buy and sell livestock and continuously introduce new sources of disease onto their farms. The rendering plant truck pulls into the barnyard to pick up a cow that died and in the process drips out fluids from an animal that died on someone else's farm. The commercial hog raiser buys a new boar and introduces an infectious disease that is passed by breeding. There are other examples but you can avoid all these problems by following the six basic principles: start with healthy breeding stock, quarantine new arrivals, keep your farm a closed system, isolate sick individuals, control wild or roaming varmits and pests that can carry disease and spread your livestock out with plenty of elbow room and pasture rotation.

Start With Healthy Breeding Stock:

Probably the hardest job of all is the selection of disease-free breeding stock. No farm animal is completely free of bacterial and fungal organisms. In fact, animals need certain organisms for digestion and they achieve a balance with the organisms in their environment. But you want animals that are free of all the damaging, disease-causing organisms and parasites. The problem is that you can't tell by just looking at an animal whether it is carrying certain diseases. The first step is to eliminate from your consideration any animal that looks thin or depressed. Never buy an animal from an auction or public sale barn where it will have been exposed to numerous animals from many sources. Never take a runt or a young animal with "just a little diarrhea" because you feel sorry for it. It's not your job to run an orphanage or animal welfare league. You must provide for your own welfare by getting only healthy, vigorous animals that will breed and produce healthy, vigorous offspring. Buy your breeding stock from a private farmer or livestock raiser. Try to find someone with a good reputation. If you drive out to his or her farm and you find a run-down, junky place with piles of trash and manure all over, don't even stop to talk. Just keep right on driving. A successful farmer will have a decent-looking place and will be more likely to have healthy animals. The unsuccessful farmer probably got that way because he couldn't produce healthy livestock. When you look at animals to buy, examine them closely. Watch them walk and run. If they are in a stall or small pen, ask the owner to let them out so you can see them move. If he complains, indicate that you aren't interested in an animal until you've seen how it moves. Stand back and look at an animal to get an overall picture. Does it look like the picture of a normal, healthy animal of that breed and species? If you don't know what it should look like, you must study your animal science books before you go shopping. Does it walk or run easily and smoothly? Examine its legs well for straightness and strength of bone. The joints should not be enlarged or "sloppy" in their action. The animal's back should appear strong, not sunken, and the backbone and ribs should be well-covered with flesh. The ribs and backbone shouldn't show in any species except dairy animals. The head should be carried well, not hung. The animal's face should look alert and its eyes should appear bright and shiny. It should not look sleepy or dull. There should be no discharges from the nose or eyes and no crusts of exudate around the nose or eyes. Calves will have a normal clear mucus from their nose and mouth but it should not be milky or yellow like pus. There should be no signs of diarrhea around the animal's rear end. An animal with diarrhea will have feces all over its tail or down the back of its rear legs. The animal should breathe easily and silently. If an animal makes noises when it breathes or if its ribs and sides move in and out as if it is having difficulty breathing, you don't want it or any other animals from that farm.

Tell the owner that you are looking for healthy, sound breeding stock and let him have his say. He might be able to give you some good advice but listen critically. He obviously likes the breed he is

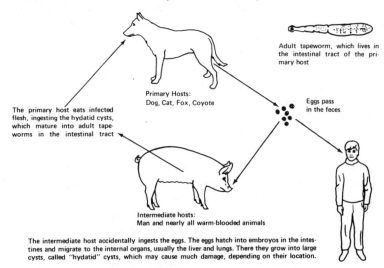

Adult tapeworm, which lives in the intestinal tract of the primary host

Primary Hosts:
Dog, Cat, Fox, Coyote

Eggs pass in the feces

The primary host eats infected flesh, ingesting the hydatid cysts, which mature into adult tapeworms in the intestinal tract

Intermediate hosts:
Man and nearly all warm-blooded animals

The intermediate host accidentally ingests the eggs. The eggs hatch into embroyos in the intestines and migrate to the internal organs, usually the liver and lungs. There they grow into large cysts, called "hydatid" cysts, which may cause much damage, depending on their location.

Echinococcus granulosus **Tapeworm Lifecycle**

selling and he naturally wants to sell his stock. During your discussion of livestock and breeds, ask the farmer the weak points of his breed. If he is conscientious and honest, he will tell you, along with all the good points. People who work livestock and the land generally seem to be honest, hard-working and intelligent. Don't be ashamed to admit it if you are inexperienced with livestock. He'll know that anyway, as soon as he sizes you up. Whatever you do, don't ask a lot of unnecessary questions or try to snow him with your knowledge of animals. There's nothing a farmer likes less than a city smart-alec. But he'll invariably be helpful and friendly if you are friendly. He won't sell his best stock because those are the foundation for his breeding program but if he likes you, he will help you pick out the best breeding specimens that he has for sale.

While I recommend buying young stock, this isn't absolutely necessary. You may be able to get good older animals that the farmer is replacing in his breeding program. Just be more critical and more careful that you aren't getting a sick animal or a problem breeder. With chickens and other fowl, however, never get anything but babies because of their several serious diseases, as we'll discuss later.

Quarantine New Arrivals:

Since there are so many diseases that your animals can be carrying when you buy them, you must quarantine them for a period of time before you put them on your fields or expose your other livestock to them. The principle of quarantining new arrivals is based on the fact that most diseases have an incubation period wherein the disease organisms grow in the animal's body before any external signs appear. The best procedure would be to quarantine them off your farm, with suitable shelter and plenty of feed and water, on ground that hasn't had any other animals on it for a year or more. If this isn't possible, then fix up an area on your farm such as a small shed and pen in a corner of a field well away from your regular barns or other livestock and use this as your isolated quarantine pen for new arrivals. Keep new stock in quarantine for three weeks and watch them closely during that time. Be sure they are properly fed and protected from inclement weather so you don't make them ill. While they are quarantined, take samples of their manure to a veterinarian and ask him to do a microscopic examination for internal parasites. Explain to him that you are setting up a new farm and that you want to have your breeding stock perfectly healthy and free of parasites. If the stool samples contain parasite eggs, treat the animals before you release them from quarantine. One treatment won't eliminate 100% of the parasites so keep these animals in separate fields from any others of the same species, re-treat them several times and rotate their pastures until they are free of all parasites.

During the quarantine, inspect them closely for any external parasites such as ticks and lice, as discussed under each species. Even if you are an organic gardener, this is one time to bend your rules and use insecticide. Get rid of any external parasites immediately before all your livestock are infested. If your animals are free of lice and mites they won't ever get them once you close your farm to new arrivals. Ticks and poultry parasites are an exception, unfortunately, for they can be brought in by wild birds or animals.

If you are buying dairy animals, have a veterinarian test each one for brucellosis and tuberculosis. Most authors state that goats don't get t.b. but the microbiology textbooks report rare infections of goats with both avian and bovine tuberculosis in other countries. Personally I'd rather be safe than having my case written up in a medical journal for having contracted t.b. from goat's milk. Milk pasteurization standards are based solely on the criteria of killing tubercle bacilli.

There are some diseases that can be carried in your livestock with no immediate symptoms and there are some that can be

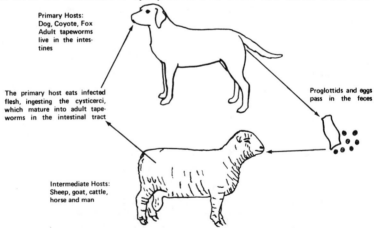

Primary Hosts:
Dog, Coyote, Fox
Adult tapeworms
live in the intestines

The primary host eats infected flesh, ingesting the cysticerci, which mature into adult tapeworms in the intestinal tract

Proglottids and eggs pass in the feces

Intermediate Hosts:
Sheep, goat, cattle, horse and man

The intermediate host ingests the eggs, and the hatching embryos migrate into the body, going to the spinal cord and brain to form cysts. This intermediate cyst stage, *Coenurus cerebralis*, is 5 cm. or more in diameter and its development in the brain and spinal cord causes nervous symptoms called "gid."

Multiceps multiceps **Tapeworm Lifecycle**

brought in by wildlife or roaming domestic animals so the quarantine won't solve all of your problems. But it is an absolute necessity for starting a new, clean livestock operation. Even after you are in operation, always use the quarantine period for any new arrivals of any livestock and use it for any animals that become ill.

Once you have selected your seed stock and have quarantined them, tested them for internal parasites and inspected them for external parasites, you are free to follow your own breeding program to support your family and improve your line of livestock. Surprise! Your disease control program has only started. You now are in the ideal situation to maintain a completely closed system as far as disease control. This is a continual thing, though, and requires constant attention.

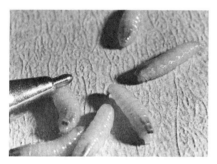

Screwworm larvae, entering through untreated wounds, can kill a full-grown steer within 10 days

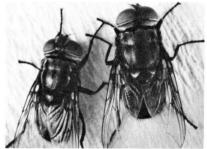

Male and female screwworm flies. Eggs laid on livestock wounds hatch into larvae which burrow and destroy living flesh

Keep a Closed System:

Many people are going back to the land because they think that our current economic system is near collapse or that national and international famine are about to occur. If these catastrophes do occur, epidemic diseases will spread their destruction through the animal and human populations. North America is one of the few places on earth that is relatively free of debilitating diseases. We are free of some of the species of insects that carry epidemics and the diseases themselves that make successful livestock operations impossible in places like Africa and Asia. It is the factor of disease which prevents the accumulation of wealth by commercial farmers in many other countries.

In general, most contagious diseases are spread by food or fomites. Fomites are simply all the things other than food that carry diseases, such as insects, manure on your boots, mucus on your hands, pus on your livestock tools, etc. In most countries in the world, you can still see deformed children who contracted tuberculosis of the spine from infected milk. Human brucellosis, called *undulant fever*, was a common debilitating disease even in the U.S. until recently. We have a continuous program to eliminate tuberculosis and brucellosis from our cattle and hogs. Many areas of the country are completely free. Hog cholera, a rapidly-spreading, highly fatal disease of hogs, has been almost eradicated from the U.S. Screwworm, a destructive maggot of a certain species of fly, used to cause millions of deaths yearly in range livestock. This flesh-eating fly maggot has been eradicated from most of the U.S. with only a few outbreaks. The list of contagious and epidemic diseases and dangerous foreign diseases is almost endless. These crushing foreign diseases and the insects that carry them are as close to you as the nearest international airport. They could be introduced easily and at any time from an airplane or ship arriving here. There have been many cases of disease introduction from one country to another. Foot and mouth disease was brought into the U.S. several times and was recently introduced to England, which was free of it. Hog cholera has been brought in via garbage from foreign ships. England is free of rabies, but rabid animals are imported every so often while they are incubating the disease. If our disease eradication efforts should break down or fail to be effective, diseases of people and livestock would become one of our biggest worries. Be aware that when famine strikes a country, epidemics soon follow.

The principles of protecting yourself and keeping your farm a closed system are the principles of isolation and non-exposure. Once your farm is self-sufficient, protect it from disease by strict self-discipline. Don't visit a commercial farm or a livestock auction yard, for you may bring home diseases on your clothing, hands, or boots. If you visit a friend's farm, scrub and disinfect your boots and hands and change clothes before you return to your own livestock area. Never feed any type of garbage or waste from off your farm, even if you intend to cook it first. Even if it's free, the price is too high. Garbage feeding was the main source of transmission of hog cholera. The disease virus was transmitted in pieces of raw pork in improperly cooked garbage until garbage feeding became illegal.

Don't invite visitors to have contact with your animals. If friends come to call, keep them out of the barnyards and animal areas. They might be carrying organisms of a new epidemic on their boots from their farm to yours. Don't let their misfortune become your own.

Control Dangerous Visitors:

Visitors also include animals. Roaming neighborhood dogs and cats as well as wild creatures can bring you the gift of disease. I will explain some of the specific diseases in the chapters on the different species, but one that should be emphasized is rabies. Rabies is endemic to North America, that is, it is present here now, alive, and thriving. It is kept going in a carrier state in wild animals. We know for sure that bats and skunks can carry it for quite a while without showing symptoms. Apparently the affected bats can expel the rabies virus for quite a long time, while skunks only expel it for a few days before they die of rabies. There are cyclical outbreaks of rabies in foxes and other wild animals, and sometimes it spills over into the domestic population. I mention rabies because it is endemic and your livestock can get it. It is extremely dangerous because a horse or cow can get it and we don't always recognize the disease until we have exposed ourselves. Many a rural veterinarian has had his hand in a rabid cow's mouth looking for the piece of wood or wire that must be in there, making the cow salivate and bellow. Rabies is transferred by the bite of a rabid animal. The virus is shed from the victim's nervous system into the salivary glands and out with the saliva, but only during the last few days of the course of the illness. Never approach a wild animal such as a raccoon, fox, or skunk if it appears to be friendly. Wild animals usually lose their natural caution only if they are ill or disoriented. Tell your children never to approach or pick up baby or "friendly" wild skunks, raccoons, coyotes, oppossums, foxes or similar creatures. Tell them never to play with bats in the barn, since these creatures can be approached and caught in the daylight. If you see a fox, skunk, etc., attacking your livestock, shoot it immediately. Just don't shoot it in the head! You can then send it or just the head to the state health laboratory. They will appreciate the data and will let you know if it had rabies. When the rabies cycle is in its peak years, you will hear of numerous incidents of rabid wild animals approaching people or livestock. The rest of the time, you won't hear of many such cases. It is documented in almost every state every year, though.

I would recommend that you don't encourage wild visitors by feeding them or allowing them access to your garbage, because there are lots of disesases they can carry besides rabies. Leptospirosis is commonly carried by wild mammals, and it can affect both you and your livestock. Wild birds are probably the only way that you will get avian tuberculosis on your farm, and yet it is very common for poultry to get it. I will outline the control procedures in the Poultry Chapter, but let me mention here that you shouldn't provide the opportunity for pigeons or other wild birds to take over your barns and haymow and contaminate your livestock feed. You can keep most of the birds out of the barns and loft by keeping the barn repaired and keeping the doors closed. If you have an upper door where the hay is put into the loft, keep it closed. Repair the ventilators and holes in the siding. Keep ventilators and windows screened. Don't use poisons or you will kill birds such as sparrows and barn swallows which eat their weight in insects. Keep rodents out of your barns and your feed bins as mentioned in Chapter 1. They contaminate your grains with urine and feces and thus pass diseases. Hobbyists and experimenters might be interested to know that rodent urine

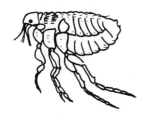 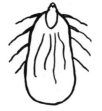

| Flea, side view, enlarged | Adult female tick, engorged with blood | Adult male tick |

fluoresces in the dark under ultraviolet light. You could construct a battery-operated ultraviolet lamp and use it to inspect your feed bins for evidence of rodent contamination.

Blood-sucking arthropods are probably the most dangerous vector of disease for the farmer. You can control most sources of contamination, but it is very hard to control mosquitos and ticks. Several years ago, an epidemic of a foreign disease, Venezuelan Equine Encephalomyelitis, which is carried by mosquitos, broke out in southern Mexico and spread clear into Texas within a few months' time. It was stopped by massive horse vaccination programs and area insecticide fogging. The historically famous tick-born disease, cattle tick fever or piroplasmosis, caused large losses and chronic unthriftiness in cattle in the U.S. until the causative organism and its transmittal by ticks was discovered in the late 1800's. The disease was eradicated by massive programs of dipping cattle to kill the ticks. I would recommend that you take precautions to keep down ticks and mosquitoes. Use screening on barn and henhouse windows to keep out mosquitoes and eliminate marshy areas on your farm by filling them in. If you have stagnant water areas that you can't drain or fill, you can kill the mosquito larvae by pouring a small amount of light oil on the water. The oil prevents their breathing at the surface and they die. The oil applications will have to be repeated as needed. Ticks are brought onto your land by roaming animals so you will have less tick problems if you have good perimeter fencing around your property. Ticks can cover quite a distance by walking, though, so they can enter your property from outside. They get on livestock by climbing up on bushes and weeds and sitting there with their front legs extended, waiting for an animal to brush against them. If you have a tick problem, it will help to mow your pastures and remove weeds and bushes. Keep it mowed to a few inches until the tick problem subsides. Some years are worse than others for ticks, depending on the weather. The adults are killed by frost in the fall.

Isolate Sick Animals:

If one of your animals becomes sick, isolate it well away from the others as soon as you see the signs of illness such as diarrhea, coughing, runny eyes or nose or depression and loss of appetite. Isolate them just like the quarantine for new animals. Remember that flies and other pests can carry disease from one pen to the next.

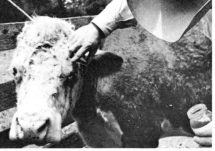

Prompt treatment of a screwworm infested wound is necessary

Fever is one of the cardinal signs of most illnesses. An animal's body temperature will vary according to the time of day and according to its physical activity. At the end of the day or after exercise, the temperature can easily be one-and-a-half degrees above normal. In fact, it is very common to cause heat stroke in pigs by chasing them around the barnyard on a hot summer afternoon. But if the animal's body temperature is two degrees or more above normal or even one degree in the morning at rest, consider it a fever. I recommend that you purchase several heavy-duty, ring-top livestock thermometers. These have a small ring on the end so you can tie a string to them. Attach a spring-loaded clamp to the other end of the string, like the kind you use to hold papers. Smear vaseline on the thermometer and gently introduce it into the rectum. Clip the clamp to the hair at the base of the animal's tail. This way, if the thermometer drops out, the clamp and string will prevent it from falling to the ground. They break easily! Leave it in three minutes, then take it out and read it. The average normal temperatures for different species of livestock are as follows although you will find an occasional animal whose normal temperature is different than the average:

Horse	100.5°F	= 38.1°C	Dog	101.5°F	= 38.6°C
Cow	101.5°	= 38.6°	Cat	101.5°	= 38.6°
Sheep	103.0°	= 39.4°	Rabbit	102.5°	= 39.2°
Goat	104.0°	= 40.0°	Pig	102.0°	= 38.9°

If an animal dies of illness, bury or burn the carcass. Never allow dogs or cats or other livestock to come in contact with the dead carcass or the fluids from it. If it dies in a barn, don't drag it across the livestock pasture or the fluids from the carcass will contaminate the ground. Put it on a wagon or a sledge and if possible, put plastic under it to prevent dripping fluids. If the carcass is small enough, just wrap it up and take it out for burning or burial. Be sure to bury the layer of soil it was laying on where it died and while you were digging the hole. Disinfect the wagon or other items that were contaminated while moving the carcass. The point of all these precautions with sick animals or dead carcasses is that when an animal first becomes ill, you don't know whether it is just an individual case or the beginning of a herd outbreak. If the illness is contagious, you certainly don't want to lose the whole flock or herd. If it is at all possible, have sick or dead animals examined by a veterinarian. If you must take it to him, wrap the carcass in ice to slow post-mortem changes which may prevent a diagnosis. It may not be economically feasible to pay the veterinarian just to save one animal since his fee may be more than the worth of that individual. But if the veterinarian can diagnose a contageous disease or a nutritional problem and thereby save the rest of your herd, then his fee is well worthwhile. Both commercial and self-sufficient farmers must consider veterinary and diagnostic services on the basis of economics. Of course, many people bring in a farm animal for care because they feel sorry for it. This is fine as long as you realize the economics of the situation and you don't make such a pet of the recuperating animal that you can't use it for its intended purpose when it is time.

Rotate Pastures and Prevent Crowding:

One of the best ways to prevent and control parasites and diseases is to have lots of pasture land, spread the animals out on it and rotate them onto clean land every month or so. Have, say, four different pastures so each one is rested quite a while before the animals are put back on it. Ultraviolet rays from the sun and physical exposure and drying will destroy most of the organisms and parasite eggs on the field. With plenty of elbow room, the animals will not be getting into each other's excretions and the natural cycles of most of the diseases and parasites will be broken.

Remember that disease organisms can be carried on your apparel or your hands or tools, by roaming domestic animals, by wild birds or animals or by flies, mosquitoes, ticks or other anthropods. There are even some diseases that can be transmitted through the air by aerosal when the sick animal coughs.

I recommend that you take every precaution and be constantly careful to avoid introducing parasites or diseases onto your farm. Your health and success are well worth the efforts.

6
Care of Wounds and Injuries

Restraint

Most of the wounds that you encounter in your livestock are minor cuts and scrapes from the animals kicking or butting each other or getting into fence wire or broken fence boards. One of the most important jobs on your farm is to keep your fences mended and sharp pieces of wood, wire, glass, or sheet metal picked up from the fields and barnyard. These cuts and scrapes are not usually serious by themselves but they often become irritated by flies or infested with maggots and infected with bacteria. You should inspect your livestock regularly for wounds and injuries and start treatment immediately when an injury is found. The most important treatment for minor wounds is careful and regular cleaning. Most of the wounds seem to occur on the faces and legs of livestock. The hardest part of treatment is restraining the animal while you treat it. For small animals like dogs, goats, or sheep, lay them down on their sides or sit sheep on their rumps. Goats can be put in a milking stanchion. Cattle must be placed in a narrow chute. See Chapter 14 for cattle chutes. Put their heads in a stanchion or use a nose clamp and tie the clamp and the halter to a *heavy* post. Horses are the hardest animals to restrain because they instinctively fight being tied. Never tie a horse to a small or thin post or to a steel fence post set in earth or in a few inches of concrete. Terrible injuries occur when a horse pulls such a post up and runs wildly, flailing the post about his chest and legs. Be sure to use a thick cotton rope and run the rope up through the halter on one side of the head, around behind the ears and down through the halter on the other side. Tie it under the chin with a

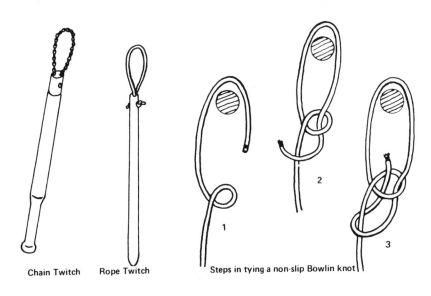

Chain Twitch   Rope Twitch   Steps in tying a non-slip Bowlin knot

non-slip knot such as a bowline knot. A cotton rope of one inch diameter is very strong and won't burn the skin if they fight it. You may need to restrain the horse by putting a twitch on its nose. This is a short shovel handle with a loop of rope or chain on one end of it. The loop is put over the horses' upper lip and twisted until it is tight. This keeps the horse occupied while you work on the wounds. If you have large animals like cattle or horses on your place you absolutely must build a heavy chute or tie-stall to restrain them while you work on them. This is constructed by sinking poles or heavy beams into the ground and having doors or removable rails on the sides so that you can get to the animal.

Minor Wounds

Once you have the animal restrained, take a clean cloth or piece of cotton and a bucket of warm soapy water and carefully clean the wound. Pick out any pieces of dirt, grass, straw or other foreign matter and soak the wound long enough to soften any scabs or dried blood or serum around the wound. Remove scabs and dried fluids because these are excellent places for infection to grow. After the wound is cleaned, rinse it well with warm, clear water. Then pat it dry and if it is in a location where it can be bandaged, bandage it with strips of cotton fabric or gauze and then adhesive tape. If you are bandaging a wound on a leg, be sure the bandage is loose enough that it doesn't constrict the blood flow. If the wound is near the foot, start the bandage at the hoof and wrap it a little above the wound. Your worst problem here is to keep the bandage from slipping off. Have the adhesive tape cover some of the hair as well as the bandage so it will stay in place. You must change the bandage every day and clean the wound with warm water as long as it is "weeping." Repeat this process until the wound is pink and dry, which means that the healing tissues have covered the wound. If the wound is on a part of the body that can't be bandaged, clean it the same way and, after drying it, cover it with a thick layer of antibiotic or antiseptic ointment, such as carbolated vaseline. In warm weather, it helps to use a fly repellent wipe or spray over the dressed wound. Your worst enemy with minor wounds is just plain dirt, especially with wounds near the feet. This is really the main reason we bandage wounds, as well as to keep off flies. If there are no flies, such as in the winter, and the wound is in a location where it won't pick up dirt, just keep it clean and dry until it heals.

Severe Wounds

If one of your animals gets a severe laceration, a fracture, or a deep, penetrating wound, I would recommend that you call a veterinarian. His ability to evaluate the severity of the injury and initiate the proper treatment are well worth his fee. If your place is in a community with veterinary service, you should get to know the veterinarian and let him know that your purpose is self-sufficiency so that he can advise you on the economic aspects of the various veterinary services. The rural veterinarian recognizes the value of livestock and he can tell you in most cases whether you are better off to treat the animal or to slaughter it for food.

If you are in such a remote area that no veterinary services are available, then there are some principles of the care of injuries that I can outline for you. With severe wounds and injuries, you must deal with several or all of the problems of hemorrhage, shock, debriding and cleaning the wound, suturing or holding it together, infection, and proper after-care of the injury.

Control of Hemorrhage

If you are lucky enough to be there, there are three main ways that you can stop severe hemorrhage. Restrain the animal and put pressure on the bleeding wound. Use a piece of cloth, hopefully something freshly laundered and clean. Sterile gauze pads are the ideal but they probably won't be where you can get them in an emergency. If the bleeding vessels are not too large, local pressure on the wound for ten or fifteen minutes will usually stop the bleeding. I do not recommend a tourniquet except for a short period while you prepare some other method because of the frequent damage that tourniquets do to the legs and feet of animals. If you have a deep wound and you are getting spurts of bright red blood from it, that means that an artery is open. Put a roll of cloth over the wound and apply pressure to it by hand or by putting a strap such as your belt or a rope around the part. If this fails to stop the flow, and the wound is on a leg, go ahead and put a tourniquet just above the wound. The best method to stop bleeding from arteries or veins is to clamp them with a self-retaining surgery clamp, called a hemostat, and then tie off the vessels above the clamp with sterile suture material. Perhaps your veterinarian can help you purchase a few emergency instruments such as hemostats and show you how to prepare a sterile emergency pack with hemostats, gauze pads, and silk or other suture material. Remember that you can sterilize the pack in your pressure cooker. Just don't leave the pack laying around on a dusty shelf. The problem with using hemostats is that you need to probe around in the wound to find the bleeding vessels and most people won't have the experience or the fortitude to do this. You may also lack the experience to judge the severity of the bleeding. A little blood goes a long way and most people think their animal is bleeding to death when it has just a superficial wound with minor bleeding. I would suggest that you can probably control most of your bleeding problems with continuous pressure on the wound until it stops or reduces to a slow "oozing", which will stop later by itself. Another time-honored method of controlling bleeding is cautery, which is simply burning the wound or the ends of the bleeding vessels with a red-hot piece of iron. Even amputations on humans used to be treated with this method to control hemorrhage. It also kills bacteria at the site but the pain may contribute to shock. If the cautery is applied too liberally, there will be a lot of dead tissue due to burning and this will contribute to later wound infection. You must also be careful not to touch any nearby nerves or large vessels with the hot iron or you will have more problems than you started with. Nevertheless, if you have a wound such as a severed ear or tail, and you wish to cauterize the bleeding arteries, the easiest method is to use a *clean* soldering iron with a fine-pointed tip. Just be sure there is no solder or acid left on the tip. Apply the hot tip directly onto the bleeding vessel for only a second or less. Repeat the momentary applications until the bleeding stops. In using this method, you need your sterile gauze pads to blot away the blood so you can see where the ends of the bleeding vessels are.

Clear airways

The other immediate problems with injuries besides hemorrhage are shock and breathing difficulties. If the injury is around the nose or throat, the animal may be having difficulty breathing. Try to open the animal's mouth and inspect his throat for foreign matter such as food or blood clots. Remove these with long tongs or forceps. Inspect the nasal openings for blockage. Horses cannot breathe through their mouth when their nose becomes swollen shut such as with rattlesnake bite of the nose. A short piece of garden hose forced into each nostril can save a horse's life in such a case. When inspecting the animal's mouth or throat, be sure you aren't bitten. Any of your livestock can really mash your fingers without even intending to. An injured animal will often respond to your probing in his mouth by closing his jaws. If an animal has an injury or swelling to its nose or mouth and you can see that he is in distress and that his gums and tongue are getting bluish-gray due to lack of oxygen, you may want to attempt the heroic procedure of a tracheostomy. This is done by making a slit at the very midline of the throat, into the trachea or windpipe, so that the animal can breathe through this hole. By the time you realize that this procedure is necessary, the animal has collapsed from lack of air, so restraint is no problem. But you must use a sharp blade and confine the cut to the middle of the throat so you don't sever the main arteries or veins on either side of the windpipe. Force the blade between the cartilage rings of the trachea and twist it to open the hole enough to allow air to pass. Find some type of clean tubular device to insert into the hole to keep it open until you can correct the reason for the original asphyxiation.

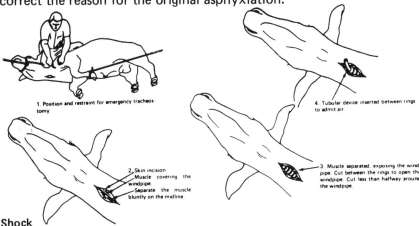

1. Position and restraint for emergency tracheostomy

2. Skin incision
Muscle covering the windpipe.
Separate the muscle bluntly on the midline.

3. Muscle separated, exposing the windpipe. Cut between the rings to open the windpipe. Cut less than halfway around the windpipe.

4. Tubular device inserted between rings to admit air.

Shock

Shock is one of the most complicated and least understood medical situations. Shock is usually associated with pain and the release of toxins due to an injury. It is often complicated by or caused by blood loss. An animal suffering from shock after an injury will be depressed and weak. It may collapse and be unable to stand up. It may thrash around on the ground or just lie still. Pull up the lip and the eyelid to inspect the color of the pink membranes. An animal in shock will have very pale or even white gums and membranes. Push hard against the gum with your thumb and then move your thumb away quickly. An animal in shock will have a white spot for more than 3 seconds where you pressed your thumb against the gums. If you're in doubt, try it on one of your normal animals to see the rapid return of color to the gums. The best you can do yourself is to keep the animal warm, dry and comfortable until it can recover or until you can get professional help. Blanket the animal or take it into a warm barn in winter. Get it out of the heat in summer. Give it soft, dry bedding. Try to get it to drink to provide the fluids it needs at this time. If it will drink, it may be helpful to add a level teaspoon of salt and a half teaspoon of sodium bicarbonate per liter (or per quart) of water. This will help the acid balance and the need for fluids. If the animal can't get up, roll it from one side to the other to change position every hour until it can sit up. If it is a ruminant you must keep it upright on its sternum so it doesn't bloat.

Fractures

If one of your livestock fractures a leg bone, you may want to have the fracture set by a veterinarian if the animal is a valuable breeding animal. If not, I would recommend that you slaughter it for food immediately. If you can transport it for care or get a veterinarian to your place it will help if you can temporarily

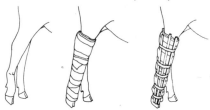

Temporary splint for a fracture requires plenty of padding. Extend the splint above and below the adacent joints. Loosen it to allow for swelling.

immobilze the fracture. Restrain the animal and wrap the entire leg with soft material such as rolls of cotton or terry cloth towels. Hold this padding in place with adhesive tape. Then tape thin, stiff sticks, such as grape-stakes on all sides of the padded leg, to keep it from bending at the fracture. Try to arrange the padding such that the outside of the padding is smooth and there are no pressure-points under the splints. Tape them on tight enough to stay in place but not so tight that you cut off the circulation in the leg. Remember that while you are waiting for professional help, the fracture site will swell and you may need to loosen the tape holding the splints. With the leg properly splinted, you can move or transport the animal without causing further damage to the leg. Fractures to some parts of the body, such as the nose or ribs, usually heal by themselves. Other fractures usually require veterinary care.

Debriding Severe Wounds

Deep wounds often contain dirt, debris, hair, and often have strings of devitalized tissue along the borders of the wound. To prevent this dead tissue from causing infection, take a sterile scissors and forceps or tweezers and cut off the pieces of dry, torn, or discolored skin and muscle and connective tissue. Trim it back until the edges of the wound bleed. This process, called debridement, is very important to the success of dealing with severe wounds.

Suturing Wounds

If a wound is too large to close with tape or bandages, you need to draw the deep tissues together and suture the edges of the wound. Do not close the skin over a pocket in a deep wound, because it will fill with fluid and become seriously infected. If you do not have proper veterinarian's needles and sutures, you can use sterilized nylon fishing line or sterilized silk. Nylon suture is preferable because silk acts as a wick for moisture and bacteria. See chapter 4 on methods of sterilization. Use a pair of forceps or needle-nose pliers to pull the needle through tough animal skin and tissue. Remove suture in ten to fourteen days or whenever the wound heals.

Aftercare of Serious Wounds

Fluids often seep from a wound and collect on the skin, drawing flies and collecting dirt. If possible, bandage the wound with absorbent cotton or gauze and clean the wound several times a day by holding a warm-water compress on it until the dry discharges soften and can be wiped off with a clean towel. Continue cleaning twice a day until the wound stops discharging. I recommend that a veterinarian attend severe wounds and infections, since problems can easily develop.

Burns

Livestock occasionally suffer burns from hot ashes, from touching electrical wires, from contact with lye, or from rubbing of rough ropes when you try to restrain them. Animal burns usually do not blister like those of humans. If the burn is superficial, you will see reddening of the skin with local pain. More severe burns will cause thickening and discoloration of the skin. Deep burns will cause a blackened, dead appearance to the skin. The superficial burns usually don't need treatment but a coating of vaseline will help the pain. Another treatment you may have available for burns is the juice of the succulent plant, *Aloe vera.* Cut off a "leaf" of the plant, split it open and apply the juice or the whole leaf to the burn. The aloe chemical is excellent for stopping the pain of burns. Deep burns of animal skin will slough off and leave a raw, open wound after a few days. These must be treated like any other wound to prevent infection. The wound should be gently washed with warm soapy water every day. After the wound is washed and dried, it can be covered with a dry bandage to keep out dirt and flies or if it is infected cover it with a water-soluble or hydrophilic antibiotic ointment and then bandage it. Do not use greasy or oily medications on severe burns.

If the burn covers more than 15% of the animal's body surface, you will need the help of a veterinarian because local treatment won't be adequate. The animal will need additional therapy. If the burn covers 50% or more of the animal's body surface, it won't survive and it should be put to sleep to avoid further suffering. If the animal chews or scratches at the wound during healing, you must devise some method of tying or restraining it so it doesn't mutilate the area or remove the dressings. Increase the protein in the animal's diet while it is recovering from a severe burn.

Friction burns such as rope burns can usually be treated with petroleum jelly or antibiotic ointment but they must be watched closely and kept clean because they can get infected and end up being very serious. Bandage them daily with clean dressings if they are on an area that can be bandaged.

Sunburn

Sunburn can occur in your livestock under certain conditions. It usually is seen only on white skin with white hair because there are no pigments to protect it from the sun. The pigments in colored hair and skin are protective and prevent sunburn. Sunburn is common on freshly-shorn sheep, on white hogs, on white horses, especially around the eyes, and on the udders of dairy cows and dairy goats. Hereford cattle commonly get cancer around the eyes and this is believed to be due to their lack of skin pigment there. I do not recommend white hogs or horses with white skin or white spots for any of the southern climates because of their sensitivity to the sun. White animals are particularly sensitive if they have not been exposed to the sun lately. If they have been kept in a barn for awhile, or in the case of freshly shorn sheep or freshly clipped goats or dogs, let them out for only short periods of time for a few days. Increase the duration of exposure over a week so that they can get used to it. If some of your animals get sunburned, the skin will be reddened and painful. They may act depressed and lose their appetites. The skin may blister or peel. Often their eyes become swollen and reddened and discharge excess tears. Severely burned pigs can develop fever and collapse. Remove the sunburned animals to the shade. Keep them in the barn or under shade until completely healed. It may help to dust the burned area with cornstarch or coat it with calamine or zinc oxide lotion. Severe sunburn will require veterinary care.

Heat Injury

All domestic animals can suffer from sunstroke or heatstroke. This can occur in a pasture with no water or shade or in a closed shed or barn on a hot day. High humidity contributes to it.

Heat cramps

Working dogs and horses can get heat cramps when working

hard on a hot day due to loss of salt. They will get severe muscle spasms and act lame or ill. Horses suffering heat cramps will stop sweating and may then suffer heat exhaustion.

For cramps on a hot day, take the animal to a shady spot and give it saline, that is, water with a teaspoon of salt per quart. If it will not drink, let it rest and give it some salt with its next feeding. Thereafter, make sure that salt is available free-choice near its feeding area and do not work it so hard on hot humid days.

Heatstroke

Heatstroke is common in dogs left in a closed automobile on a hot day due to extremely hot temperatures and lack of ventilation. The animal will often vomit and may collapse. It goes into shock and its body temperature may reach 110°F (43.3°C). The emergency treatment is to immerse it in cold' water to reduce its body temperature. Put it in a tub or watering trough. Put ice in the water and hold ice packs on its head. Use a rectal thermometer and continue cooling the animal until you get its body temperature down to normal. As soon as the temperature is reduced, rush it to the veterinarian's office for further treatment. If you are close to a veterinarian, take it there first. I can't tell you how often people take their dog shopping with them, leave it in the car and return to find it passed out from heatstroke.

Heat exhaustion

Heat exhaustion is seen especially in draft horses, cattle and hogs. It is a form of shock due to exposure to high heat coupled with physical activity. The animals become weak, tremble and collapse. They may breath rapidly and have a very rapid pulse. The onset of heat exhaustion is usually slow, over a period of time, and the animal's body temperature may not be elevated as it is in heatstroke. I recommend that you do not do any rounding up, vaccinating, castrating or de-horning in the middle of a hot day. Don't work your draft horses or run a riding horse in the middle of a hot, humid day. If it appears that an animal is suffering from heat exhaustion, move it to a cool, shady place or barn. Sponge it down with cool water. Don't shock it by blasting it with a hard spray of cold water. Let it rest and recover. Try to get it to drink some water with a teaspoon of salt and a half teaspoon of bicarbonate per quart. If the animal is valuable and seems severely weak, get veterinary attention if possible.

Lightning

Livestock occasionally are struck by lightning. It usually occurs when they are standing under a tree or are near a wire fence. Sometimes a rancher or farmer finds one or more dead cattle under a tree and doesn't realize what happened. There may be no external marks on the animal although it usually has some singed hair or skin and there are usually signs of lightning damage to a nearby tree or structure, although lightning can travel for miles down a metal fence if it isn't grounded. Lightning doesn't always kill the animals. Survivors may die later or they may completely recover. They may act depressed or excited and they may be dizzy and deaf but they usually recover from these signs. Their legs may be swollen and sore. If the animal cannot get up, roll it onto soft straw bedding, bring it food and water and change its position.

Frostbite

Your pets or livestock may suffer from frostbite if they are caught outdoors in a severe winter storm or if they are wet or undernourished. Pigs, especially baby pigs, can get frostbite especially of the ears and tails if they don't have proper shelter in cold climates. Chickens sometimes get their combs frosted. Cats lost outdoors in the winter often lose the tips of their ears and tails due to frostbite.

Superficial frostbite acts like a burn. The frosting causes the skin to lose its blood supply. This is followed by redness, heat, pain, and swelling of the area. The spot may be itchy and more sensitive to cold after it heals. Severe frostbite (freezing) affecting a whole ear, tail, or other part causes the part to swell painfully when it thaws. Later, the damaged area shrivels up and sloughs off. The line between the dead, sloughing part and the live tissue often becomes infected. Severe damage like this requires professional attention because the damaged part usually needs to be amputated. I would recommend that you be very careful to protect your animals during cold weather, especially during freezing rainstorms or blizzards.

Preventive Medicine

Since serious injuries are so hard to treat and so time-consuming, the best advice I can give you is to be vigilant and prevent the problems before they happen. Watch your livestock and if you find certain individuals that fight or attack the others, separate the troublemakers. Pasture them separately or get rid of them. Check your barns and fences for sharp wires, exposed nails, or sharp, broken boards. Don't leave sharp stubs or stumps of weeds or saplings in the fields. Don't bale hay with wire if you can help it.

7
Livestock Medications

These days any discussion dealing with drugs is automatically controversial. The subject of owners buying drugs to use on their pets and livestock is no exception for several reasons which we will discuss in this chapter.

Anyone who has been farming or raising livestock for any length of time knows that he can buy certain drugs from feed stores and similar farm outlets. Those people who are just starting will soon find out the same thing so there is no reason for me to ignore the subject of drug use by owners. Instead I would rather discuss medications in general, explain why many veterinarians are against your purchasing your own drugs and try to give you some guidelines on what medications you can use, when and why, and what medications you should not use and why.

The medications you can buy in the feedstores will vary from state to state but generally, farmers can get quite a variety. The main problem veterinarians have is that when they are called to look at an ill animal, the owner may not admit that he has already been treating it for several days. There are several reasons for this problem. First, the owner is no different from anyone else. He wants to save a few bucks whenever he can. So if he thinks he knows what is wrong with the animal, he may want to treat it himself to save the cost of professional care. One reason he may not admit treating the animal himself is that a doctor may have chewed him out for doing this in the past. Yet another reason is that he may not want to admit that he tried and failed. Whatever the reason, the owner's failure to tell the veterinarian about recent medication can cause very serious problems. One of the problems is drug interference or antagonism. Some of the medications the owner was using may remain in the animal's body and seriously interfere with the drug the veterinarian has chosen to use. Another problem is drug synergism. Something the veterinarian gives may add to or potentiate a drug the owner gave with serious, or even fatal, results. Another problem is that the owner's medication may mask signs which would be important to the doctor's diagnosis. When he examines an animal, the veterinarian considers everything he can find out and then he compares and weighs all the signs to arrive at the diagnosis. If an important sign, such as fever, is missing, it may throw off his diagnosis unless he knows what treatments or drugs were given before he arrived.

I will point out several classic examples from the veterinarian's point of view. It is very discouraging to be presented with an ill animal that has been made worse by the owner using the wrong treatments. For instance, aspirin is very toxic to cats and yet we frequently hear that someone has been using aspirin to reduce his cat's fever. Another common mistake is the misdiagnosis of constipation. An owner sees his animal straining as if to have a bowel movement. He thinks it is constipated, so he gives it a laxative. The fact of the matter was that the animal had diarrhea and was so sore and irritated that it kept straining. The owner made the case worse with the wrong treatment. A situation that makes every veterinarian cringe is to walk into the barn or the milking parlor and see a line-up of dirty syringes and tubes of mastitis medicine lying on a dirty ledge among cobwebs. He picks up a syringe and sees the needle covered with dried medicine and fly specks. The tube of mastitis medicine has the tip covered with dirt and dried exudate.

"Oh, yeah," the farmer says, "I was using that syringe on Old Bessie after she dried up. But it's o.k., Doc. I always wipe off the needle with alcohol."

Then imagine sticking the dirty tip of that tube of mastitis medicine into the opening of the cow's teat and expecting her mastitis to improve. If she recovers, it is in spite of her treatment, not because of it.

We frequently see the case of the seriously ill animal that the owner has been treating with antibiotics for four or five days. Often, the animal has gotten too ill to save while the owner was trying to treat it himself. This is because, of course, there is a great deal more to diagnosis and treatment than pumping the animal full of antibiotics.

In short, veterinarians become very upset and I suppose sometimes a little sarcastic because they see so many cases of mistreatment, misdiagnosis, and improper methods of treatment by owners.

In defense of the owners, however, let me say that it is your animal and you have the right to treat it as you wish, except for your moral obligation to any living creature to prevent suffering or cruelty. But you must temper your efforts with knowledge and care. If you are going to be so isolated that professional care is not available, then you must expect to spend a great deal of time studying and learning. You will need, more than anyone else, the help of a veterinarian to get your medicine chest set up and to learn what you should be able to do on your own. Establish a relationship with a large-animal doctor and confide in him. Then you can correspond with him about your problems. Or perhaps if you are that isolated, you will have a ham radio set-up and you can get a phone-patch when you need his advice. Realistically, you must expect to pay for his time and his advice just as if he spent that time actually working on your animal. Every day, strangers call the veterinarian and try to get free advice over the phone. But if you have established a relationship and a method of paying for his time and expertise, he will be glad to help you all he can.

In the case of those who are within range of professional care, again, it is your animal and you can do as you wish but I would recommend that you use these guidelines: whenever one of your livestock is seriously ill or injured, decide at the very beginning what is the value of the animal and whether it will be worth it to you to pay for professional care. Consider the possibility that an illness may be contagious and may spread to your other livestock. If you are in doubt, call the veterinarian, describe the situation, tell him what the animal is worth and ask him if it will be economical to treat it. He may not be able to say exactly what is the diagnosis or what it will cost to treat the case but he can give you an idea. The economics of livestock raising is part of the farm-animal veterinarian's job. He doesn't expect you to spend so much that you lose your profit, and he will so advise you. In fact, the cost of a house call is often more than the value of an individual animal so the veterinarian is more interested in spending some time with you, on your farm or ranch, going over your entire operation. He wants to advise you to improve your housing and management so that you can avoid those expensive "fire-engine" house calls. Following his advice may be expensive initially but it should save you money and maybe a great deal more in the long run. The most important point is don't let a serious problem go too long.

Now that we have discussed owner-treatment from both the owner's and the veterinarian's viewpoints, let's examine some of the drugs that are available and some considerations about them.

This chapter is not meant to be a complete or well-disciplined study of pharmacology. The scientific study of all the classes of drugs according to their actions and their chemical make-up is a monumental endeavor. Instead, I would simply like to point out some of the usages of the drugs and medications available to you, according to their modes of action.

There are so many different brand names of drugs that I will be using only the proper or common names of the active ingredients. Whenever you buy a medication, or any preparation, read the label to see what's in it. Never buy patent medicines that don't tell what's in them. If you do so, you are relying strictly on the manufacturer rather than on your own judgement.

Local and Topical Preparations to Use on the Skin and Mucous Membranes:

Emollients:

Emollients are fatty substances that are used to soften, soothe, and protect the skin. Antiseptics or other drugs are often mixed with the emollients. Lard and wool fat were probably the original emollients. Wool fat is anhydrous lanolin. For chapped skin, probably nothing beats good old-fashioned lanolin. White petrolatum is very commonly used. A familiar brand name is Vaseline. Yellow petrolatum is carbolated, that is, has phenol added as an antiseptic. Never use carbolated petrolatum on any species of the cat family, as they are extremely sensitive to the toxicity of phenol. Liquid petrolatum is mineral oil. The newest emollients are synthetics such as the polyoxyethylenes. These are liquid water-soluble hydrocarbons and are used to make the water-soluble creams. Then there are polyethylene glycols or carbowaxes that are ointments at room temperature and melt to liquid at higher temperatures such as body temperature.

These are used to make the "non-greasy" ointments. Glycerine or glycerol is a fat derivative that strongly absorbs water. If applied full strength, it will dehydrate the skin but it is often mixed with water (and scented) or mixed with medications. Vegetable oils are often used as emollients. Corn oil, cottonseed oil, linseed oil, and olive oil are often used. Cocoa butter, or theobroma, is a vegetable "butter" that melts at body temperature.

Demulcents

These are natural compounds of high molecular weight that are water soluble. They consist of the gums, mucilages and starches. Demulcents are used as coatings for irritated, abraded tissues. They are usually applied as a lotion, as a wet dressing for the skin, or as a drench, enema, electuary (a paste applied usually to the roof of the mouth) or nebula (a preparation that is sprayed with an atomizer)for the mucous membranes. The mucous membranes are the soft, moist tissues lining all the body openings.

Acacia U.S.P. is gum tragacanth. Glycyrrhiza U.S.P. is licorice root. These are plant gums that are usually put up as a powder and are made into a mucilage when added to water. Soap and barley water are common demulcents that are used in enemas. Corn starch is a good, old-fashioned healing powder for rashes. It may contain enzymes and vitamins that make it work so effectively.

Protectants and Adsorbants

These are insoluble or inert compounds used as powders, lotions, or protective coatings. An adsorbent is a compound that attracts and holds chemicals or toxins to its external surfaces. The old stand-by dusting powders were made with talc, a pulverized mineral. This is fine for absorbing odor or moisture but you must never use it on a sore or wound. We now know that when talc gets on raw tissues, the tissues react to it as a foreign body to wall-off each little particle. This can cause a great overgrowth of healing cells and scar tissue in a wound. It can cause an old wound to remain painful and itchy for a long time. In short, don't put talc on a wound. One of the most commonly used healing powders is Calamine U.S.P., which is zinc oxide powder, usually made up as a lotion. It is used for raw, itching lesions. Zinc stearate used to be popular because it clings to a wound and sheds water, but excessive amounts can be toxic. Boric acid used to be commonly used as a healing powder but is not used as much now because of toxicity. Betonite U.S.P., Fullers Earth, and

Kaolin N.F. are different forms of the natural clays of hydrated aluminum silicate. These become a gel with 7 to 10 parts water and a sol at 15 to 20 parts water. They are used as a liquid, mostly internally for diarrhea, and as a powder to absorb exudate or discharge from wounds.

Astringents

Astringents are strong chemicals that precipitate proteins usually just on the surface of a raw lesion or sore. The original astringents were derivatives of tannins from certain plants. There are also astringents of salts of silver, mercury, zinc and aluminum. The idea of the proper use of an astringent is to precipitate just the outer surface cell proteins of a wet or weeping wound. The precipitated proteins then form a protective film that stops drainage and resists infection. The only drawback is that astringents burn like fire when applied to an open sore. Astringents are also commonly used on the footpads of working dogs to toughen them. Sometimes dogs' footpads are soft and tender and need toughening to withstand snow, gravel, or other rough surfaces.

Antiseptics

Antiseptics are usually thought of as topical drugs that help kill bacteria and prevent or reduce infection. Since these are applied directly to a wound or burn, they cannot be overly strong. In order to avoid injuring the patient's living cells, the antiseptics are compounded in fairly weak strengths. They usually just inhibit the microorganisms so the body's natural defenses can take over.

Grain alcohol or ethyl alcohol has good antiseptic properties in high concentrations (70% or more) but it burns when put on a wound.

Chlorine bleach, which is usually 5% sodium hypochlorite, has good antiseptic properties but it should be diluted with water to no stronger than 10 to 1. Plain bleach is good for infectious hoof problems such as thrush.

Iodine tincture, iodine in alcohol, is a commonly-used antiseptic. It comes as 2% strength Iodine Tincture U.S.P., 7% Strong Iodine Tincture N.F., and Lugol's solution or Strong Iodine Solution U.S.P., which is 5% iodine with 10% potassium iodide. The 2% iodines are fine for most uses. Repeated use or application of bandages over even 2% iodine will cause blisters on the skin. Iodine is often helpful for fungal infections of the skin if it is used sparingly so it doesn't cause secondary problems. Never put a bandage over an area after applying iodine. Strong iodine mixed with glycerine is a commonly-used antiseptic, but be careful with it. It will burn raw or delicate tissues.

Carbolic acid or phenol is no longer used much but it is available in carbolated petrolatum (such as Carbolated Vaseline). In this form, it is a mild antiseptic. Phenol has a strong odor which can be absorbed by milk or other foods and it is very toxic to cats. Pine Tar U.S.P. is a phenol-containing antiseptic tar that is good for packing or painting over hoof wounds. It used to be used on livestock wounds to repel screwworms. It still can be used for this purpose if nothing better is available.

There are several dyes that have antiseptic properties and are widely sold in preparations for wounds. Scarlet Oil and Scarlet Red contain an azo dye that is active for the types of organisms from manure. Most of the other dyes, such as gentian violet, crystal violet and brilliant green are not effective for manure-origin bacteria and so are not much good for barnyard injuries. All of the dyes are inconvenient because they stain everything they touch. The staining properties tend to inhibit most people from cleaning the wound properly and regularly as they should because they want to avoid getting the dye on their hands and clothes.

Mercurial antiseptics such as mercurochrome are not very effective. Merthiolate, Thimersol N.F. and Nitromersol N.F. (Metaphen) are a little better.

Silver nitrate is a strong antiseptic but it stains the skin brown or black. It is commonly used in a caustic pencil or stick to cauterize wounds and to de-horn young ruminants. Don't let it get on your hands!

Hydrogen peroxide 3% solution is commonly used on wounds as an antiseptic. Actually, the oxidation of blood and exudates by the peroxide is very helpful for cleaning a wound but there is probably little antiseptic activity. Therefore, I would use peroxide to clean a wound the first time but I wouldn't bother with it after that.

Chlorhexidine (Nolvasan) is a synthetic antiseptic that is very good for a variety of bacteria and perhaps some viruses. It is good for wounds, for disinfecting teats before milking, and for disinfecting equipment.

Counterirritants

Counterirritants, linaments, and rubefacients are compounds that produce a mild irritation when applied to an external surface. The theory behind the use of counterirritants is that they increase the circulation to that area by dilating the skin vessels and superficial vessels, thereby speeding healing and the removal of toxins. When applied properly, liniments should be massaged in thoroughly. A good, long period of time spent massaging in the linament seems to produce significant results on mild sprains and sore tendons. Probably the massage is more beneficial than the liniment itself. Most liniments are mixtures of several aromatic or strong chemicals such as amonia, camphor, oil of turpentine, oil of wintergreen and others mixed always with alcohol. I would personally avoid the ones with a very high percentage of turpentine or kerosene.

There is a stronger class of counterirritants that are Blisters and Caustics. These were once widely used on livestock, especially horses. These produce severe damage to the skin by chemical burns. They may produce blisters or even raw burns that cause tissue to die and later slough off. Some of these are preparations of black mustard, cantharis (Spanish fly), strong tincture of iodine when covered with a tight bandage, mercuric iodide (red iodide of mercury) and capsicum (red or cayenne pepper). These preparations have nothing to recommend them and they are inhumane because they cause pain and often severe scars. About the only justification for them is that an owner occasionally cannot be made to rest his animal to give its lameness time to heal. A blistered leg is so obvious and ugly that the owner has no choice but to rest him while the blistered wounds, as well as the lameness, are healing.

The physical form of counterirritation, the "firing iron," on the other hand, still has its place for a few selected lamenesses where it helps to fuse or ossify a painful lesion. But it should be used only by a graduate veterinarian.

Digestive Tract Drugs

Most of the digestive tract drugs that are available for animals without a prescription act locally on the inside of the tract to soothe or protect it during bouts of vomiting or diarrhea or both.

Antacids

These are not usually needed for animals because most species of animals never suffer from hyperacidity as do humans. Perhaps the only time they may definitely need an antacid is when a ruminant (cow, sheep, goat, etc.) gets indigestion from overeating a large amount of grain or other rich food. A common antacid is aluminum hydroxide gel in aqueous suspension or tablets. This is helpful for indigestion, vomiting and diarrhea, as well as hyperacidity, because of its demulcent , coating, and mild astringent action. Calcium hydroxide solution (lime water) is also an antacid, but it is commonly helpful for diarrhea apparently because of its astringent action.

Antiemetics and Antidiarrhea Medications
Antiemetics (Antemetics) are drugs which stop vomiting.

1. Astringents
Common medicines for diarrhea usually contain plant extracts such as krameria, catechu, quercus (oak), rubus (blackberry), and sumac. These work primarily because they contain tannic acid or its glycosides, tannins. These are astringents which precipitate a thin film of protein over the surface of raw lesions in the intestinal tract. They thereby slow the loss of body fluids through the lesions, protect them, and allow them to heal. Tannic acid is also helpful in certain types of poisoning because it combines with heavy metals, alkaloids and glycosides, which are common plant and mineral poisons. The tannic acid forms insoluble complexes with these poisons and thereby inactivates them.

2. Protectants and Adsorbents
An adsorbent holds toxins or other chemicals to its surface. A protectant merely coats the part to protect raw or tender tissues. Bismuth preparations (such as Pepto Bismol) come as tablets and suspensions, mostly for human use for upset stomach and diarrhea, but these same ones can be used for animals. They produce a suspension in the digestive tract that coats and protects inflamed internal surfaces. For best results, use them often enough to coat the entire gastro-intestinal lining. Bentonite U.S.P, Fuller's Earth, and Kaolin N.F. are forms of hydrated colloidal aluminum silicate. They provide a protective coating for an irritated gastro-intestinal tract. They also have some activity as adsorbing toxic wastes or chemicals. Activated Charcoal U.S.P. is an excellent adsorbent for certain ingested poisons. Some research shows that it works better when given alone than when mixed with tannic acid powder as is often done in commercial poison antidotes. The theory behind the mixture was that between the two antidotes they should either adsorb or neutralize most common poisons, but they apparently don't work as well together as expected. In any case, Activated Charcoal U.S.P. is a good adsorbent for upsets and toxic indigestion. Pectin, from the in-

ner rinds of certain fruits, is commonly used as a protectant for the lining of the intestinal tract. It also seems to adsorb bacterial and break-down toxins. Most commercial preparations are combinations of protectants, adsorbants, and maybe some other drugs such as antibiotics or drugs to slow down the motility of the G.I. tract.

3. Antispasmodics, Anticholinergics, and others

With severe diarrhea or vomiting, the first things that are called for are a veterinary examination and a diagnosis. Vomiting is a common sign of many illnesses of both dogs and cats. It is a frequent sign in several serious illnesses such as distemper, as well as in mild upsets such as from over-eating or raiding the garbage can. Vomiting causes loss of chloride and acid from the stomach, thereby leading to acid-base and electrolyte imbalances. The imbalances can lead to weakness, prostration, and even death with continued frequent vomiting.

Most carnivorous species of animals such as dogs, cats, and birds of prey, can vomit or "regurgitate" quite easily. They have the proper mixture of types of muscle cells in the esophagus to regurgitate something they have ingested. This trait may have evolved with some of their rather indiscriminate eating habits. Swine can vomit, but less easily than dogs or cats. Ruminants regularly eructate or belch gas and regurgitate or return balls of food (their cud) from the rumen to the mouth. But they rarely vomit any volume of food when ill and they often bloat up and die rather than regurgitate when they overeat or get indigestion. Horses cannot vomit and will not actually do so unless they are dying. They may drip what appears to be vomited food when they have a blockage of the esophagus, called "choke". This can happen when they swallow a large ball of rough, dry food such as large pellets, apple cores, or similar matter and it sticks in their throat.

Severe, frequent diarrhea also causes dangerous imbalances. It allows great loss of body fluids, dehydrating the animal, and loss of sodium and other alkaline electrolytes, usually producing acidosis, the opposite acid-base imbalance as with vomiting. Together, frequent vomiting and diarrhea are rapidly disastrous. Mild vomiting and diarrhea can usually be controlled by any of the common preparations of protectants and adsorbents. But severe vomiting and/or diarrhea requires drugs that depress or slow down the hyper-motility of the digestive tract. On the other hand, a few types of diarrhea are due to paralysis of the digestive tract and require different treatment. This is another reason why veterinary diagnosis is worthwhile.

Some of the commercial preparations for diarrhea contain, along with the protectants, drugs that slow the motility of the digestive tract. These drugs are usually natural plant extracts such as hyoscyamine, scopolamine, stramonium, belladonna, and others. There are other belladonna derivatives and synthetics such as atropine and methylatropine salts. All these drugs are usually called antispasmodics or anticholinergics, and they help with serious vomiting and/or diarrhea.

Paragoric is no longer available over the counter (without a prescription). It is a narcotic and so is a controlled drug under the Federal government. It has always been and still is one of the best antidotes for severe, painful diarrhea but it may have the side effects of incoordination, drowsiness and, possibly, constipation. It could be habit-forming in animals, to the extent of developing a tolerance and a necessity for it to control the bowels. So, naturally, use it only temporarily to stop severe diarrhea or vomiting problems. There are other synthetic antispasmodics and anticholinergics but most of them are prescription items—that is, they are available only from your veterinarian, or with a prescription from him.

There are some drugs that act mainly as antiemetics, without many other effects. These are helpful especially for pets that get motion-sickness. Most antihistamines have some antiemetic effect. Two that are commonly used and are usually available are dimenhydrinate (Dramamine) and meclizine (Bonamine). Dimenhydrinate is recommended at the dosage rate of ½ to 1 milligram per pound for dogs, and meclizine at 1—2 mg per pound.

Most of the stronger antiemetics are tranquilizer-type drugs and are therefore federally controlled and unavailable except from your veterinarian.

Emetics

Emetics are drugs that make an animal vomit. Dogs and cats occasionally ingest a toxic substance and need to vomit to get rid of it. If the substance is irritating enough, it will cause nausea and vomiting naturally. But if not, such as when they eat certain kinds of poison, you need some way to make them vomit it. Some poisons, however, such as alkalies, acids, and gasoline-type vapor-producing chemicals should not be vomited because they will further damage the esophagus or be inhaled. If the animal is becoming weak, it should not be made to vomit because it is then more likely to inhale the fluids or it may become more toxic from the emetic drug.

Unfortunately, many of the commonly-recommended emetics are slow-acting and poisonous in themselves. Tartar emetic, ipecac, copper sulfate, and zinc sulfate are often recommended for emetics but they are very unreliable and, if the animal does not vomit them up, they are toxic. Ground mustard seed used to be commonly available and used as an emetic but it is seldom available today. Old dried-out mustard seed is not effective because it is the volatile oil of mustard seed that has the emetic activity. Fresh ground mustard seed, usually a tablespoonful or less in a cup of warm water, is given by drenching the animal. Be sure not to choke him. Regular table mustard doesn't work at all except if it irritates the throat sufficiently. For cats and dogs, the safest and most easily available emetic is regular table salt. Put about ¼ to ½ of a teaspoon of table salt in the palm of your hand and add one or two *drops* of water so it forms a ball. Carefully take this ball of salt and throw it into the back of the animal's throat. If necessary, have a helper hold the animal's mouth wide open. One or two of the balls of salt in the animal's throat will almost always induce vomiting within a few minutes. Before the salt treatment, however, it may be a good idea to feed the animal some milk or egg white to coat its stomach and esophagus as a protectant against the poison. Another emetic which often works well is hydrogen peroxide. Usually a teaspoonful in the back of a dog's mouth will make him vomit. The best emetic is probably apomorphine because it is quick and effective, but it is, unfortunately, a narcotic and not available to the public. Again, it is contraindicated for some types of poisoning.

In general, emetics are relatively dangerous because of the possibility that the animal might inhale the fluids or that the poison might further damage the esophagus when vomited. The most important is to determine what the animal ate. Then you can treat him correctly or get him to a veterinarian for treatment.

Emergency Poison Antidotes

Poisoning is a very serious matter and requires professional care. There are so many chemicals and plants that are toxic that it is impossible for me to list and discuss them all here. Many articles and textbooks have been written on poisonings and their treatments. Most major cities have poison control centers, usually located at large hospitals. There they have access to a number of textbooks and other literature so that they can advise you or your doctor. The most important thing is to find out what the poison was. If you have the package or container, take it to your veterinarian. If there is no veterinarian in your area, you may be able to get some help by phoning or radioing a poison control center in the nearest city, but you must know what the poison was. Should your animal come home sick and you suspect he has been poisoned, you must take him in or contact your veterinarian to try to determine the type of poison from his symptoms. In this case he may have been poisoned by some type of bait put out for coyotes or rats. I will discuss some emergency treatments for a few of the common chemicals and toxins that your animals might get into around the house or barn. Remember that these are merely first-aid measures. Then you must get the aid or advice of a veterinarian because the patient may need further treatment, antidotes, and supportive care for the poisoning and for shock, pain, and body fluid imbalances.

Acids: Do not make them vomit. Give milk of magnesia, aluminum hydroxide gel, bicarbonate of soda, or any antacid-protectant preparation at the rate of about one ounce per fifty pounds of body weight of the animal. Give it with lots of water.

Alkalis like ammonia, lye, or washing soda: do not induce vomiting. Give them vinegar in water. Cut it down to no more than a tablespoon of vinegar in 8 ounces of water, so that the animal can swallow it. Give at least 2 tablespoons of vinegar per hundred pounds of body weight, depending on the strength and amount of alkali. Then give them egg whites, as much as you can, depending on the size of the animal.

Volatile Chemicals like gasoline, kerosene, furniture polish pine oil, and turpentine: do not make them vomit. Give them as much milk as you can, then give them vegetable oil followed by protectants and a mild laxative, such as milk of magnesia.

Chlorine disinfectants or bleach: Give the animal as much milk as it can comfortably hold to neutralize the chlorine.

Carbolic Acid such as in Phenol disinfectants and Cresol disinfectants: Give milk, raw egg white, or activated charcoal, if available. Then induce vomiting. Repeat this process several times, then give more milk, egg whites, or activated charcoal, followed by a laxative or purgative, such as sodium sulfate.

Iodine and Iodine Disinfectants: Make a thin starch paste or solution with flour or cornstarch and force-feed it to the animal, as much as it can comfortably hold. Then induce vomiting if possible. Give water and repeat the vomiting until the fluid comes out clear. Then give the animal milk.

Spoiled food or food poisoning: Induce vomiting with an emetic if possible. Then purge the animal by giving sodium sulfate in water at the dosage recommended under "laxatives."

Arsenic poison: Give large amounts of milk and give activated charcoal or an internal protectant preparation. Then make the animal vomit. Give sodium thiosulfate orally, if available. Arsenic in poisonous amounts definitely will require professional care.

Strychnine poisoning: If spasms or convulsions have not begun, give milk, activated charcoal, or tannic acid preparations, induce vomiting, then give sodium sulfate as a laxative. If the animal is having the typical stiff, tetanic spasms or convulsions, veterinary care is a must. If he is having spasms, do *not* induce vomiting or give oral medications. With strychnine poisonings, any loud noises or other stimulations can bring on spasms or convulsions, so keep the animal quiet and avoid stimulation. Barbiturates, if available, will usually stop the spasms or convulsions but you will need further medical care for this potent poison.

Laxatives and Cathartics

In general, laxatives and cathartics are among the most misused drugs. Some people give their animal a laxative whenever it looks cross-ways. On the other hand, mild bulk laxative in the form of wheat bran is badly needed by most animals that are fed on prepared, packaged feeds. I will only recommend a couple of laxatives and their dosages. These should be used only if you think the animal is toxic or has eaten something poisonous. Most animals, however, will benefit from a regular addition of bran to their diet because it naturally softens and regulates the bowels and thereby prevents all types of disorders of the lower digestive tract. Bran is very helpful for animals, especially horses, that are raised in desert or sandy areas because bran seems to help them pass the sand that they accidentally ingest with their feed. Horses are prone to a build-up of sand in their large intestines and it can cause an illness commonly called "sand colic." Regular bran in the diet seems to help prevent this.

Mineral oil is a relatively safe laxative. It should be given to large animals with a stomach tube, but it can be drenched with a bottle if you are careful. If you give it by drenching, have the oil either warmer or colder than body temperature so that the animal can feel it going down its throat. Otherwise the oil may run down the windpipe with fatal results. Cattle and horses are usually given 1 to 4 quarts (1 to 4 liters). Sheep, goats, and swine get ½ to 1 pint

(¼ to ½ liter). Dogs get 1 to 6 tablespoonsful (15 to 90 ml) depending on the size of the dog. Cats can be given 1 to 2 Teaspoonsful (5 to 10 ml). This can be repeated daily until the stools are soft and oily. It should not be used regularly as it will interfere with nutrient absorption. It can be used to diagnose intestinal obstruction because it is easy to see when it comes through in the bowel movements. Never, therefore, give it as an enema, or you will ruin its diagnostic usefulness.

Milk of Magnesia is magnesium hydroxide, 8% suspension. This is commonly used as a laxative in small animals and young livestock, but it should not be used if there is a possibility of kidney malfunction or intestinal obstruction. The dosage for foals and calves is 1 to 2 ounces (30-60 ml); for lambs, kids, and pigs, 2 to 4 teaspoonsful (10-20 ml); for dogs, 1 to 3 teaspoonsful (5-15 ml); and for cats, ½ to 1 teaspoonful (2½ to 5 ml).

Glauber's Salt or sodium sulfate is one of the safest of the saline cathartics. The following amounts of sodium sulfate are mixed in a comfortable amount of water and given by drench or stomach tube: horses and cows get ½ to 2 pounds (250 to 900 grams); foals and calves, 1 to 2 ounces (28 to 56 grams); sheep and goats, 1 to 2 ounces; swine, 2 to 4 ounces (56 to 112 grams); dogs, 3 to 30 grams; and cats, 2 to 5 grams.

Epsom salts or magnesium sulfate is a strong cathartic or purgative. It will usually cause watery, sometimes projectile diarrhea within a few minutes of being given. Don't stand in the line of fire! This, like any other strong cathartic, should never be given if there is any possibility of an obstruction of the intestinal tract, or if the animal is weak or dehydrated. Magnesium sulfate will cause central nervous system depression and even death if there is an intestinal blockage so that a lot of it is absorbed. The epsom salts is dissolved in an equal volume of warm water and given by stomach tube or drench. This solution is given at the rate of ½ to 1 pint (¼ to ½ liter) for horses and cattle; 2 to 3 ounces (60-90 ml) for swine; 1 to 2 ounces (30–60 ml) for sheep and goats; 1 to 6 teaspoonfuls (5-30 ml) for dogs; ½ to 1 teaspoonful (2½-5 ml) for cats. These dosages are safer if they are diluted in as much water as the animal can comfortably take with it.

Wheat bran is high in fiber which passes through the digestive tract, holds moisture, provides bulk, and therefore stimulates normal peristalsis. Recent research indicates that all sorts of bowel diseases and cancers are due to low-residue diets and can be prevented with proper bulk such as from bran. The only problem you must be aware of is that bran is high in phosphorus. Therefore you must balance the diet with the proper amount of calcium. You can add bran to the rations as needed to control the animals' bowels so that they are soft and moist. Hard, dry bowel movements or straining to pass thick, pasty bowels indicate the need for bran or similar bulk fiber. As a general rule you can add bran to the ration up to about 30% by weight of the total ration. Increase it slowly over several days' time. When the bowels are normal you should cut down the bran to a smaller, maintenance level of 10% or less of the grain ration. Use the amount needed to maintain normal bowels.

Antibloat Medications

Bloat in ruminants is a very complicated and poorly-understood condition. A great deal of gas is produced by the normal process of fermentation in the stomachs of the ruminant. The fermentation is carried on by bacteria and protozoa which aid the animal in digestion of its food. Normally the animal gets rid of the gas by regular belching or "eructation." Bloat may occur with apparent paralysis of the muscles which perform this eructation. It may also occur with types of indigestion where all the food in the rumen gets worked up into a froth. Here, the gas can't escape or be belched up because it is distributed throughout the food as frothy bubbles. Since there are lots of theories and disagreements on the cause and physiology of bloat, there are no doubt many different causes, including perhaps toxicities, allergies, changes in diet, overeating, and others.

Read the discussion of treatment of bloat under "Goats," Chapter 9. The idea is to relieve the pressure of the excess gas in the rumen and then to administer antiferments or antifrothing agents.

Antifermentation agents are drugs that depress the bacteria in the rumen. Ethyl alcohol (the drinking kind) has been traditionally used, as well as very weak formaldehyde solution (given by stomach tube only). Most research discounts the effect of antiferments, however.

Antifrothing agents seem to be more helpful. These are agents which decrease froth by increasing fluid surface tension, thereby expelling the bubbles. The new highly-polymerized silicone agents are probably the most effective. They are available from feed stores and veterinarians. In the past, oil of turpentine and kerosene were used. Oil of turpentine is relatively effective at the rate of 30 to 60 millileters (2 to 4 tablespoonsful) for cattle and 5 to 15 milliliters (1 to 3 teaspoonsful) for sheep and goats but it can be toxic to the kidneys, even fatal. Safer and more commonly available antifrothing agents are such things as peanut oil, olive oil, soybean oil or even melted lard. Any of these agents is best given to the animal by stomach tube, especially since you will be passing a tube immediately to try to relieve the acute bloat, that is, the distension of the animal's stomach by the trapped gas. Strangely, these oils will prevent bloat in ruminants when sprayed onto the pasture or hay before the animals eat it. Perhaps it works here by depressing the amount of lush pasture or forage that the animals will eat.

Cough Medicine

Before considering the use of cough medicines, you must realize that coughing is not an illness. Coughing is a sign of a problem and the causative problem may be in the throat, respiratory tract or lungs. Suppressing an animal's cough frequently does more harm than good because, as often as not, he is coughing because he has something to get out of his lungs, bronchi or trachea. If the cough is "productive", that is, if it is useful to get rid of fluids, mucus or exudate, then suppressing the cough will be disastrous. The only times that coughing should be partially or completely suppressed are when it is non-productive and it is irritating the animal's throat, preventing the animal's rest, or damaging his heart or lungs by the coughing effort. It is certainly no excuse to suppress an animal's productive cough because the noise is interferring with *your* sleep. You really need to have a veterinarian examine a coughing animal. Often times even he will need diagnostic tests to determine the cause or seriousness of an animal's cough. I have known of such unusual cough cases as an animal that was presented to his veterinarian because of coughing and lack of appetite and the cause turned out to be a severe imbalance due to gastro-enteritis from having swallowed a rock that was stuck in the intestines!

The dry, nonproductive cough should of course be suppressed. Another type of coughing situation is when the animal has a severe infection of the respiratory tract and the mucus or exudate is too thick for him to move and cough up. This situation calls for something to break-up, liquify and mobilize the exudate. But this process must be done gently so you do not "drown" the animal. A cough can be caused by many different things but in general it is an infection or irritation of the respiratory tract. A productive or useful cough raises the excessive respiratory tract secretions to keep the tract open. A non-productive or useless cough is due to irritation of the tract with little or no secretions and it causes loss of rest, high blood pressure, a burden on the heart and discomfort to the animal. Severe forceful coughing can cause ruptures and hemorrhages. The useless or over-active cough can be treated with several types of medication:

1. Syrups: These are demulcents that soothe the throat. Honey, corn syrup, maple syrup and similar syrups coat the raw tissues of a sore throat and give some temporary relief from coughing which origin-ates from that area.

2. Expectorants: Syrups often contain substances called expecto-rants which increase the secretions of the respiratory tract. These may be helpful for a dry, unproductive cough if the secretion coats the irritated tissues and promotes healing or if they help dissolve and mobilize a thick, tenaceous exudate from a respiratory tract infec-tion. Expectorants include volatile oils of anise, eucalyptus, lemon, pine and others. These cause hyperemia (extra blood supply) to the respiratory tract as well as increased secretions which may help speed healing. Guaiacol, a wood tar derivative, and creosote increase respir-atory secretions if they are given in high enough doses although most proprietary cough syrups contain too low amounts to be helpful. The cough syrups with tars must not be used on cats because they may contain phenols, which are highly toxic to cats. The syrups may also contain salts such as potassium iodide or ammonium salts which increase respiratory tract secretions in the proper dosages.

Steam and nebulized water are two of the best expectorants because they dilute and mobilize the respiratory tract secretions. Nebulized water is a vapor made by a machine which produces ex-tremely fine droplets that can go deep into the small bronchioles. These droplets are smaller than made by a standard humidifier, which has little effect for a cough. Raising the humidity in extremely dry climates is often helpful; however I prefer the steam because the warmth along with the moisture may be beneficial to increase blood flow in the respiratory mucosa (lining). Steam decreases the viscosity of heavy secretions to help mobilize them. It is common practice to add volatile oils to the water being boiled, such as eucalyptus or com-mercial preparations for this purpose. These may be of some benefit.

3. Cough suppressants: Most commercially available cough medi-cines contain cough suppressants, usually dextromethorphan. This acts on the central nervous system at the site of control of the cough reflex. Prescription cough medicines often contain stronger cough suppressants such as codeine phosphate and Hycodan. These can be disastrous with a condition causing a copious secretion into the respiratory tract such as pneumonia because the animal will not be able to cough it up and get rid of it. He may, in fact, "drown" in his own fluids if coughing is stopped by strong medications. Thick, heavy exudates or secretions in other types of conditions can block portions of the respiratory tract and cause permanent damage to the lungs such as abscesses or emphysema.

In summary, you must not merely stop a cough. You must find and treat the cause of the cough and this usually requires professional help.

Antihistamines

Antihistamines are one of the most widely advertized types of drugs on the market. They are readily available in a wide variety in the famous and ever-present "cold medications" for humans. Antihistamines are among the most potent of non-prescription drugs.

Any injury to cells of the body causes the release of many natural but toxic chemicals, including histamines. These toxic products from damaged cells have various effects on different tissues in the body and in different species of animals. They can cause a severe drop in blood pressure, a constriction of the bronchioles causing asthma-type symptoms, spasms of the intestines, paralysis of the rumen, contractions of the uterus, hives of the skin, and many other severe signs. Histamines and their relatives are involved in allergies such as to drugs, plants and insects. Antihistamines are drugs that antagonize the toxic histamine-type chemicals by competing with them and replacing them at the cells where they act to do their damage.

Antihistamines are strong drugs and they often have significant side effects. They can cause such things as depression, salivation and drowsiness. Large doses or overdoses can cause central nervous system stimulation with confusion, incoordination, excitability, tremors and convulsions. They occasionally cause nausea, vomiting and diarrhea.

Antihistamines can be used in animals for allergic dermatitis which is especially common in dogs. They can be used for allergic coughs in dogs and cats and for heaves in horses. They are often used for laminitis in horses and cows. This is an inflammation of the growth tissues inside the hoof which causes damage to the feet. They are used in bovine "asthma" or pulmonary edema, an allergic reaction in cattle which can range from mild and transient to severe and even fatal. It is common in the northeastern U.S. and in southeastern Canada on moist pastures in the fall of the year. Antihistamines are often used in retained placenta and metritis after a difficult birth and for lots of other conditions associated with allergies and toxicities.

Since there are so many different antihistamines I won't list them and their dosages but as a general rule, large dogs usually get about the same dose as the human dose which is on the drug label. Small dogs and cats get proportionately less. Horses and cattle usually get 10 or more times as much, but these should be given by injection to be reliable in their effect. You may be able to get injectable antihistamines for animals in some states at rural or feed stores. Ask your veterinarian before starting an animal on antihistamines unless it is an emergency allergic reaction such as severe hives or pulmonary edema and you aren't able to contact him.

Antibiotic and Chemotherapeutic Drugs

Antibiotics are without a doubt the most misused and overused drugs on the market today. They are available in a wide variety of types and forms from feed stores, rural stores and mail-order companies. Their popularity has led to their being used almost anytime an animal coughs or stumbles. They were commonly fed in the feed in low levels on commercial feedlots but the "Fed's" have been outlawing many of the feed additives. Low-level antibiotics do increase feed efficiency but unfortunately they often leave a residue in the meat or milk. We now know that certain bacteria can transfer or spread their trait of resistance to a certain antibiotic. They can transfer it both to bacteria of their species and to bacteria of other species! Therefore we don't want antibiotic residues floating around because they may lead to more resistant strains of disease-causing bacteria.

Antibiotics are only one class of the drugs that are used to fight infection. Antibiotics are organic chemicals which are produced by molds or other microorganisms. Some of these chemicals merely suppress the growth or reproduction of certain microorganisms and are therefore called "bacteriostatic." Other antibiotics actually kill certain microorganisms and are called "bactericidal." Each antibiotic is commonly effective only against a certain group or type of organisms. Some of the common antibiotics are penicillin; streptomycin; the tetracycline group which includes chlortetracycline (Aureomycin), oxytetracycline (Terramycin) and tetracycline, U.S.P.; chloramphenicol; erthromycin; polymyxin; neomycin; bacitracin; tylocin and many others. New antibiotics are being discovered regu-

larly, both natural and synthetic forms. Some are very safe and non-
toxic to the patient even in high doses. Others are dangerous in doses
slightly above the therapeutic level, with some animals having toxic
reactions even at the proper dosage.

There are many other chemicals that have activity against
microorganisms besides the antibiotics. These are called chemotherapeutic agents. The major groups are the Sulfonamides and the Nitro-
furans but there are many others. Chemotherapeutic agents were successfully synthesized long before antibiotics in the search for drugs
to treat syphilis and other diseases.

Sulfas were first discovered in the early 1900's but weren't
put to use until the 1940's. Sulfas are mainly bacteriostatic in their
effect, allowing the animal's natural defenses to destroy the infective
organisms more easily.

The antibiotics and chemotherapeutic drugs are commonly ad-
ministered to animals in ointments or creams for topical application
to wounds of the skin, in ointments and solutions for infusion into
the eyes or mammary glands, in capsules, tablets or suspensions for
oral use, and in solutions or suspensions for injection. The drug and
its form dictate whether it can be injected into the muscle, under the
skin, or into the vein if it is an injectable drug.

One general rule that you should follow carefully is to avoid
using important antibiotics in any type of topical medication. In
other words, don't use ointments or creams containing penicillin,
tetracyclines, chloromycetin, or sulfas. Smearing these important
antibiotics all over the outside of your animals may lead to the
development of resistant strains of bacteria. These resistant bacteria
on your animals or your premises may then cause severe infections
which won't respond to the sulfas or antibiotics when you try to
treat them. Many of the feed-store and mail-order ointments and
mastitis medicines contain a mixture of 3 or 4 drugs including penicillin and sulfas. You should let your veterinarian make the decision
of what drugs to instill into the dairy animal's udder and let him
show you the proper way to do it. Use only topical ointments and
creams that contain drugs not usually used systemically (oral or injection) such as nitrofurazone (Furacin), bacitracin, neomycin, polymyxin, thiostrepton, or tyrothricin or else stick to the antiseptics
such as preparations containing iodine, phenol (carbolic acid), hexa-
chlorophene, chlorhexidine (Nolvasan), mercurials, or the many anti-
bacterial dyes like Scarlet Red.

When it comes to using injectable antibiotics or chemotherapeutics, I would highly recommend that you talk to your veterinarian before you institute therapy, even if you have to contact him by radio and phone-patch. Doing so may save you a lot of headaches later on.

It isn't necessary for me to state the dosages of all the antibiotics and sulfas here because when you buy them they come with a folded flyer or "throwaway" that gives the complete description of the drug, its indications, contraindications, side effects, dangers, and dosages for the species of animals for which it can safely be used. It also gives the withholding times for meat or milk from animals you use it on. Be *sure* that you follow the directions for not using meat or milk for the proper interval of time so that it does not contain the drug. If you don't you are toying with the possibility of someone developing an allergic, anaphylactic reaction. People can develop a sensitivity or allergy, especially to penicillin, even if they have no previous history of such reactions. When purchasing drugs from a store, never accept an antibiotic or sulfa that does not have these detailed directions with it.

The most commonly available injectable antibiotic for livestock is a combination of penicillin and streptomycin. It is marketed under a great many brand names. These two antibiotics work together synergistically and are very effective for most of the common infections. Their main advantage is that they can be given by intramuscular injection. You must be careful not to inject it into a blood vessel because it can cause a fatal reaction this way.

Members of the tetracycline group are available in a variety of forms. They come as powders for drinking water for swine and poultry, as tablets, capsules and boluses (large tablets) for oral use, and in injectable forms. Most of the injectable tetracyclines should be given intravenously, though. This is not feasable for the average owner. Most of the tetracyclines can be given by intramuscular injection to cattle and sheep if the injection is given in several small doses in different places but it is very painful when given intramusculary.

The sulfas come as powders for the drinking water, as tablets or boluses and as a solution for injection. Unfortunately the injection must be given intravenously or intraperitoneally. This is a job for the veterinarian unless he can teach you to do it yourself.

8
Meat Inspection On the Farm

Meat inspection, proper sanitation, and hygiene are extremely important to you and your family whether you are dressing wild game or your domestic livestock for meat. The object is to prevent the transmission of diseases through eating the meat or meat products or even to the person doing the slaughtering and butchering. Complete meat inspection includes inspection of the animal before slaughtering, called antemortem inspection; inspection of all the parts and organs after slaughter, called postmortem inspection; and all proper care during processing, which may be called processing inspection. In state and federally inspected slaughter houses, these inspections are supervised by a veterinarian and carried out by his trained assistants, called lay inspectors. My problem, and yours, is that there are so many facts, details and considerations about meat inspection that can't be explained in a book. You need to see healthy animals slaughtered to see what normal organs look and feel like. Then you need to see all the different pathological (disease) conditions in order to recognize them. Then you need to know what pathological conditions make the meat unfit for food and which ones only require that the diseased part be trimmed away. In effect, I'm saying that I can't give you enough information here to enable you to do a thorough job of meat inspection. But, I can give you some pointers and guidelines that will help you in this area. And abnormalities you find during slaughtering will help you manage your livestock herds and flocks and hopefully, let you know when to seek professional advice. At the very least, you should be able to learn from your own experience, over a period of time, what the meat and organs from a normal, healthy animal are like. Then, if you find an abnormality, you can take it to your veterinarian. If you live on an island or so far out in the bush that you can't get professional advice, then, as a rule of thumb, I would recommend that you simply discard any diseased looking meat or meat products.

Livestock slaughtering, carcass dressing and meat inspection are subjects which should be taught in person by an experienced, knowledgable instructor. For these skills you truly need first-hand experience. The best way to start would be to go to a small, custom meat packing plant and make some arrangements with them so you could work there or observe. State laws will probably require that you get a T.B. test and a food-handler's certificate before you can work in a packing plant. If there is no way for you to observe at a plant, try to find some farmers who will call you when it comes time to do some slaughtering on the farm. Most farmers these days, however, take their livestock to a custom packing plant or locker plant and have it slaughtered, butchered, frozen and stored there.

If there is no way for you to get reliable instruction and experience, then you must learn on your own, starting with small, manageable livestock like rabbits and chickens. If you are a hunter or have helped a hunter dress his game, just let me say that the way most hunters handle their game leaves a lot to be desired. At least I can say this for the ones I have seen. This, in fact is the real reason that so much wild game has a reputation for bad taste. Unfortunately, a lot of game meat ends up spoiled and unused (and in the garbage can). Of course, there is quite an art to preparing and cooking game to prevent strong odors and flavors.

There are really just three principles for the proper handling of any carcass. A live, healthy animal has plenty of dirt on his skin and hair and lots of organisms on the inside of his digestive tract. But between these two extremes, he is essentially sterile. If he was healthy and free of parasites, all of his meat and internal tissues are clean and wholesome until you do something to make them otherwise. So the three principles of handling a carcass are to avoid contamination from the outside of the animal, to avoid contamination from the inside of the digestive tract and to handle the carcass and butchered parts properly for storage, curing and cooking.

ANTEMORTEM INSPECTION

There are two complicating factors in the discussion of meat inspection. The first is that you may have an illness or injury in one of your animals and you want to know whether you can salvage it by slaughtering it and whether it will be suitable for human food. The second problem is that some serious illnesses show very few lesions in the dressed carcass so that you won't find any abnomalities at postmortem. This is why your antemortem inspection is important. If you are a hunter, you definitely want to take a thoughtful look at your game before you harvest it. Don't take an unhealthy looking individual or the laggard of the herd. Wild carnivores will take care of these. The one you take should be healthy because it will be for human food. In the case of domestic meat animals, an illness or injury may make it unfit for food, depending on the condition.

The first and most unequivocal condition is the case of finding one of your animals dead. Have no doubt about it, unless the animal was killed before your eyes and the heart is still pumping blood when you are ready to dress it, a dead animal is unfit for any type of food. Even if it is still warm, even if it was killed by lightning or some other injury just a little while ago, it won't be safe to eat. This is because the bacteria from the intestinal tract invade the blood vessels and the entire body within a short time and will cause spoilage or food poisoning.

Now, let's proceed with the antemortem inspection of an animal you wish to slaughter. Even though it looks healthy, take its temperature with a rectal thermometer to be sure it isn't coming down with an illness. Hogs are unfit for food if their temperature is over 106°F (41.1°C) and other livestock if 105°F (40.6°C) or above. If you are preparing to slaughter an animal and find its temperature above these critical marks, wait and see what is developing. Do not slaughter this individual until its temperature is back to normal and it seems healthy.

Never slaughter an animal with signs of rabies, tetanus(lockjaw) or other nervous system abnormalities. An animal that staggers, wanders aimlessly, walks in circles, bumps into solid objects, or has any other central nervous system signs may have one of the illnesses that show no postmortem signs and they should not be used for food unless they recover.

Occasionally you may have one of your livestock so seriously injured that you cannot save it. Hopefully, you can salvage it by using it for animal or human food so it is not wasted. Probably the most common situation will be a broken bone or a deep wound where you cannot get veterinary assistance or the value of the animal does not warrant professional care. The deciding factors in this situation are whether or not the wound is infected and the animal is feverish. If the injury is fresh, or in case of broken bones, the bones didn't break through the skin, go ahead and slaughter immediately. However, if a wound is over a day old, it is surely infected. If the animal has a fever, the infection is spreading and you cannot take a chance on using it. If the animal is not feverish, then you must make a judgement based on the location and condition of the injury. If it is full of pus, don't take a chance on it. If it is localized and the animal's temperature and condition are good, you should be able to slaughter it and trim out the damaged area. If the injury or wound is quite severe or widespread, such as a severe burn from a barn fire or a non-fatal lightening strike or severe multiple wounds from attack by dogs or coyotes, the animal will probably be in shock. In this case its temperature may not be elevated even though bacteria and toxins are spreading from the intestines and the wounds throughout its system. Animals this severely injured must not be used for food unless they recover. These cases will usually be a total loss.

Another common situation will be the pregnant animal that begins to give birth but is unable to deliver. Occasionally, the unborn fetus is deformed or misshapen in such a way that it cannot fit through the birth canal. In other cases, the mother's birth canal is misshapen from a previous injury or is too small because she was bred too young. Difficulty in birth is called "dystocia". Your decision of whether you can salvage the animal for food will depend upon its condition. Of course, try to assist her and try to determine whether or not she has any hope of delivering the fetus.

If she has been in labor a long time when you find her and she has been having difficulty, the fetus will probably be dead and your only alternatives are to get the fetus out and try to save her or if the fetus can't be removed, whether or not to slaughter her immediately for food. If she is down and so weak she cannot rise and it appears that she is in shock, you cannot use her. But if you have a different case where you recognize the dystocia early, before the mother becomes weak and worn out and you are positive that the fetus cannot be delivered, slaughter immediately. If the animal is good breeding stock, have a veterinarian examine her as soon as you recognize the dystocia. If he cannot deliver the fetus, perhaps he can section it into pieces so that he can remove it and save the mother.

There are several other serious problems involved with pregnancy and birth. Sometimes you will have a mother animal that is a "downer" before or after birth, that is she is lying down and cannot rise. This can be due to an injury to her nerves or to imbalances in her metabolism of certain nutrients such as with ketosis and eclampsia(milk fever). You cannot slaughter such an animal for food while it is in   the downer condition. You also cannot use an animal for food that recently gave birth if it has a severe infection of the mammary glands or uterus. These infections generally cause a fever with circulating toxins and bacteria.

Another area of decision is the animal with a tumor or cancer. If you raise any white-faced herefords, you will probably see a case of "cancer-eye" sooner or later. This is a malignant cancer caused by sunlight on their non-pigmented eyelids. If you see a white skinned animal developing a raw cancerous-looking growth on its eyeball or eyelid, you should consider utilizing it for slaughter right away. If the cancer gets to the stage where it is eating into the bone or the lesion is full of pus or the cancer is spreading from the eye to another part of the body, you should not use it for food. Technically, cancers that are confined to a small area can be cut out and the carcass used but, esthetically, I would prefer not to eat food from an animal with any type of cancer. Technically, meat or dairy products from even a tuberculous animal are safe to eat if they are cooked so that all parts reach 170°F (76.7°C) for 30 minutes. However, I wouldn't want my family handling or eating food from a sick animal no matter how well it was cooked. There is too much risk. However, if you have a carcass that you are in doubt about using for human food, you may decide to cook it throughly and feed it to your livestock or dogs. But don't spread disease by feeding poorly cooked meat or offal. Don't take a gamble you cannot afford to lose. Use your best judgement whenever it comes to food and, if possible, ask for professional advice when you need it.

When preparing a domestic animal for slaughter, withhold solid food for 24 hours but provide water for them. If you have several animals together, give them plenty of room so they don't crowd and bruise each other. At slaughtering time, handle the animal quietly and gently so it doesn't get frightened and excited. If it gets terribly excited it won't bleed out properly and the meat won't keep as well.

After killing, the animal should be immediately hung up by the rear legs. Its throat area should be liberally sliced to open the jugular veins and allow it to bleed out. If the animal was properly killed by a blow or shot to the brain, the heart will remain beating and will pump out all the blood.

Skinning

The outside of an animal is quite dirty and smelly. The hair of most animals, especially wild game, will give meat a strong flavor if you allow the carcass to get hair on it during dressing. This hair will find its way to the inside of the meat during butchering. Wild animals have various scent glands which must be avoided and removed from the carcass. Even the dander from the skin can impart flavors. The first rule is to clean and disinfect your knives after opening and removing the skin. Of course, some livestock like hogs and poultry are dressed with the skin left on but these are plucked or scraped and then washed well. Consider that when you split the skin down the belly and the inside of the animal's legs, you are going through hair, mud, dirt, urine and dried manure. You know that you must get rid of this contamination before you can go any further. Packing houses handle this problem by sanitizing their tools and washing the carcasses after skinning. They have containers of boiling water scattered throughout the dressing floor. The workers must frequently wash their knives and saws and immerse them in boiling water. After skinning the carcasses, they hose them off with a high-pressure water sprayer. In the case of large animals, it will help to maintain cleanliness of the carcass if you cut off the hooves below the shanks (at the lowest joint) before skinning or eviscerating (removing internal organs). If you are going to use the head meat from a cow or other horned ruminant, saw off the horns before skinning. Also, cut out the tonsils during dressing if you are going to use the head meat. Hose out the nose and mouth cavities. In the case of a dairy animal, cut off the udder in one piece before skinning and do not spill any milk from the udder onto the carcass.

Small carcasses can be skinned and dressed on a clean table but your job of maintaining cleanliness will be much easier if you can hang it up once you get the skin off. Then you can proceed with cleaning and eviscerating more easily. Hanging the carcass is almost a necessity for large animals like cattle or hogs. A really experienced team can dress a cow or hog on a clean, slanted floor. Some packing houses still do it this way but most people would end up with hair and dirt throughout their meat.

Eviscerating

I don't want to go over the step-by-step processes of dressing each species because most people have a fair idea of the processes and because there are lots of books and articles available on the subject. I simply want to emphasize a couple of points so that I can proceed with meat inspection. The single most important principle is to avoid cutting into the digestive tract and contaminating your carcass with the juices and organisms of digestion. The next most important principle is to know what to do when you do cut or rip the guts and get gobs of food in various stages of digestion all over the inside of your lovingly-cared-for carcass. The critical stage of the process is the first cut you make into the mid-line of the belly to begin to open the abdomen. Since the animal is dead and limp, there is a lot of pressure from the internal organs against the wall of the abdomen. For the beginner, the initial cut will be less dangerous if the carcass is laying on its back rather than hanging up. Down the middle of the belly (after the carcass has been skinned) you will see a white line, which is the tendinous attachment between the abdominal muscles of the two sides. Cut gingerly through this white line, a little at a time, until you go through it, making a hole just large enough to get your fingers through. If you are lucky, there will be a pad of fat just inside your incision. If not, there will be internal organs including coils of intestines and stomach. Put two fingers through the small hole, place them just inside the abdomen so they hold the internal organs out of the way and enlarge the incision, moving your fingers with the knife. Open the abdomen all the way from the ribs to the pelvis. Now extend the incision forward through the cartilages of the ribs to one side of the midline, so that you can open the chest. If you are doing a large or old animal and the cartilages are quite hard, use a pair of strong, sharp pruning shears to cut each cartilage. You may have to use long-handled shears of the type used to prune trees.

Now hoist the carcass up by a pair of hooks or a strong stick, through the tendons along the back of the hind legs. As you raise the carcass the internal organs will begin to spill out. At this time you should tie off the gut at the rectum so that you don't get any manure in your carcass. Reach inside the pelvis and squeeze or "milk" the contents of the rectum inward. Then take some twine or string and tie it around the gut as far back as possible, tearing loose some of the attachment tissues to do so. After tying it off, you can now cut the rectum loose by carefully cutting around the outside of the external opening (the anus) under the tail and pulling it forward through the pelvis. If the urinary bladder is full, tie it off with a string and remove it intact, with the rectum. You don't want to splash urine on your carcass. If the animal was female, cut the reproductive tract loose and remove it. Now you can carefully cut and tear the tissues which attach the entire digestive tract to the inside of the carcass.

If you are dressing a small carcass, lay the internal organs out on a clean table or pan for inspection. If it is a large animal like a cow or mature hog, drop the organs into a clean tub or onto a clean floor or large table. Slaughter houses use a basin-shaped table. After you get the digestive tract cut loose and hanging out of the carcass, the stomach, or the four compartments in the case of a ruminant animal (cow, sheep, goat, deer, etc.), will still be closely attached at the diaphragm. At this point, I would recommend that you tie a strong twine around the esophagus just in front of the stomach. This is a hard job in large animals because of the weight and size of the organs but it may save you from spilling stomach contents inside the carcass when you cut the esophagus to remove the stomach.

Now suppose the worst happens and you do cut into the stomach or intestines. Ingesta and juices will immediately pour out. Grab the area and try to stop the flow or to direct it outside the carcass. If you can, tie off the incised area with string or plug it up. Carefully finish removing the organs and try not to get the ingesta and fluids on the carcass any more than you can help. After you get the internal organs out and the carcass hung up, you must clean the areas that were contaminated. If it is a small area, take a sharp, flexable knife and carefully cut off the surface layer in one piece, all around the dirty area. If you do this properly and don't cut into the dirty area, you will have removed all the contaminating material with a thin layer of meat and connective tissue. If you really blew it and got fluids all over the carcass, I would recommend that you wash the carcass well with a clean water spray and then trim it. Start by hosing it down gently so as not to splash and spread the contamination. Use a clean towel to help pick off any material that sticks to the carcass, then hose it off again. After you have it well washed, the meat will keep better and avoid off-flavors if you peel off the top layer of connective tissue or fat or meat where the carcass was contaminated. Use a very sharp knife and rinse it in boiling water between cuts.

Finish the evisceration by removing the heart, lungs, trachea, esophagus and diaphragm in one piece, called the "pluck". This may include the liver. Now you should have a clean carcass hanging by the hind legs and several piles of internal organs. Now is the time to perform your postmortem inspection, to inspect for any conditions that would make the meat unfit for food.

POSTMORTEM INSPECTION

Postmortem inspection consists of looking at, palpating (feeling) and incising certain parts of the carcass and organs. You are looking for evidence of any disease which might make part or the whole carcass unsafe for food. You are also looking for any diseases or parasites that are affecting your flocks or herds, which would indicate a need for treatment or improved management. Start by inspecting all exposed surfaces of the dressed carcass, the animal with the hide and internal organs removed. This is easier in the case of large animals like cattle or hogs after the carcass is split into two sides by chopping or sawing it down the backbone. The head is usually removed by this time. Look for bruises (purple areas), swellings, pockets of fluid or pus or inflamed (bright red) tissues. If the carcass is from a cow, take a sharp, clean knife and slice deeply into the muscles of the jaw (the masseter muscles) on the side of the head. Make several slices and examine the muscle for small white nodules or cysts full of fluid. Next, examine the lymph nodes of the carcass. These are the organs that filter the lymph (tissue fluid) before it returns to the blood vascular system. They are firm, round, oval or kidney-shaped organs, usually a brownish color on the outside. Various species of animals have different locations of the lymph nodes but generally there are some under the lower jaw, around the salivary glands and the throat, in the pits of the front and rear legs and along the vessels in the pelvis which lead to the hind legs. Find these nodes and incise them (cut them in two). Normal nodes have a smooth brownish-colored external layer around a whitish or yellowish, firm center. Look for nodes that are hemorrhagic (red or purple) or full of pus or are infiltrated with hard nodules or enlarged, hard swellings. These are abnormal. Now examine the tongue and palpate it. It should feel uniformly soft with no hard lumps, ulcers, or tumors.

Now go to the internal organs. You will probably have removed the windpipe, lungs and heart in one group, maybe with the liver and diaphragm attached. Palpate the lungs with your fingers. There should be no lumps, abscesses or cysts. If you find a suspicious lump, incise it to see its consistency. Healthy lungs should be uniformly soft, pink and "puffy." Open the windpipe along the top to inspect for parasites or abnormalities. When you get to where the windpipe divides to enter each lung, you should find several lymph nodes around the bifurcation. Most species also have lymph nodes in the connective tissues between the two sides of the lungs (the mediastinum). Incise and examine these nodes. Now incise the heart to open all four chambers. It should be cleaned at this point to get rid of clotted blood that was left in the chambers. Examine all the surfaces of the heart.

Cut the liver free of its attachments to any other organs and examine all its surfaces. Palpate it and incise any hard lumps or fluid-filled cysts. Look for discolored or soft, rotten or pus-filled areas in the liver. In the center of the liver, near the large veins and gallbladder, you should find some portal lymph nodes. Incise and examine these. Remove the gall bladder and bile duct by cutting away some liver tissue around them. Be careful not to cut into the gall bladder or get bile on the liver or other food products. Then, on a separate table, cut open the gall bladder and bile duct and inspect for flukes (leaf-shaped flatworms) or other abnormalities.

Now go to the other organs, the stomach, intestines, spleen, pancreas, kidneys and reproductive tract, which will probably be in a pile together, except maybe for the kidneys. Some people leave the kidneys hanging in the fat inside the carcass until after chilling it. In the case of swine, inspect the area around the kidneys and incise the kidneys to look for pus or other abnormalities. Palpate the spleen and incise it in several places. Look for nodules, tumors or cysts or an unusually soft, swollen spleen. Examine the pancreas, the light pink organ along the small intestine just behind the stomach. Now spread out the intestines and stomach on a clean surface. The thin connective tissues which held the stomach and intestines in place is called the mesentery. The mesentery contains the blood vessels to the stomach and intestines plus lots of lymph nodes. Sometimes the mysentery is full of fat, as well. Examine and palpate these lymph nodes. Incise any that look unusual. Then start at the esophagus and open the stomach to examine its internal surface and contents. Look for worms and look for ulcers, nodules or tumors along the internal and external surfaces. Unless you are going to use the intestines for sausage casings, continue the inspection by splitting the

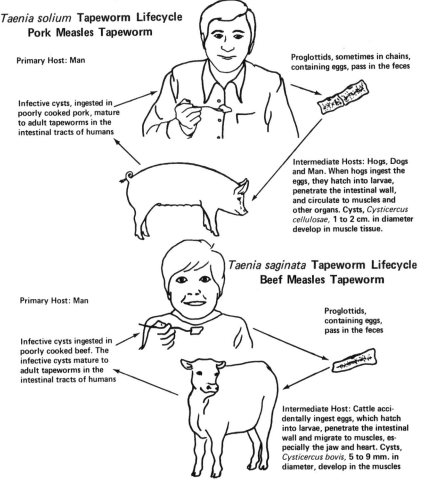

Taenia solium **Tapeworm Lifecycle**
Pork Measles Tapeworm

Primary Host: Man

Proglottids, sometimes in chains, containing eggs, pass in the feces

Infective cysts, ingested in poorly cooked pork, mature to adult tapeworms in the intestinal tracts of humans

Intermediate Hosts: Hogs, Dogs and Man. When hogs ingest the eggs, they hatch into larvae, penetrate the intestinal wall, and circulate to muscles and other organs. Cysts, *Cysticercus cellulosae*, 1 to 2 cm. in diameter develop in muscle tissue.

Taenia saginata **Tapeworm Lifecycle**
Beef Measles Tapeworm

Primary Host: Man

Proglottids, containing eggs, pass in the feces

Infective cysts ingested in poorly cooked beef. The infective cysts mature to adult tapeworms in the intestinal tracts of humans

Intermediate Host: Cattle accidentally ingest eggs, which hatch into larvae, penetrate the intestinal wall and migrate to muscles, especially the jaw and heart. Cysts, *Cysticercus bovis*, 5 to 9 mm. in diameter, develop in the muscles intestine along its entire length. Look for worms and look for lesions such as inflamed (red) areas, ulcers, nodules or tumors. If you wish to preserve the intestines for casings, cut them into the appropriate lengths, squeeze out the contents and turn the casing inside-out. Inspect the contents and lining for worms or abnormalities.

In the case of hogs, cut open all the lower joints of the legs and look for joints that are inflamed or full of pus.

In the case of poultry, open the entire digestive tract, starting from the back of the mouth. Then rinse and scrape the internal surfaces and any material there into a pan of water. Examine both the internal surfaces and the sediment in the pan. Use a magnifying glass if necessary. Look for small, thread-like worms partially buried in the mucosa (the internal surface). These are usually *Capillaria* species of worms. The proventriculus (the soft or glandular stomach)may show external bumps due to a worm that lives in the glands of this organ. The gizzard, the hard, clam-like digestive organ, should be opened and the horny lining removed to look for gizzard worms. The intestines, including the ceca, should be opened and scraped. Cecal worms move actively, often taking the shape of an "s." Capillaria threadworms, however, are very fine and inactive and hard to see. You may also see tapeworms and large roundworms in the small intestines. In hens, open the oviduct and look for inflammation and flukes (small, leaf-shaped flatworms). In geese, open the kidneys and look for flukes.

Besides looking for internal parasites, you should examine for all types of lesions or abnormalities in poultry just as in your other livestock. Be especially watchful for signs of avian tuberculosis, as discussed in the poultry chapter.

Disposition

After you have done your postmortem examination of the carcass and internal organs, you need to know what to do with any abnormalities you have found. In some cases, you must trim out the abnormal parts or throw away the affected organ. Other conditions require that you condemn the entire carcass. You may have to destroy it by burning or deep burial or you may be able to cook it for animal food. Let's start at the beginning of the postmortem inspection again and discuss the disposition of various conditions you may find.

Slicing the jaw muscles of a carcass from a cow is done to look for beef tapeworm cysts. If you find one cyst scar, the carcass is o.k. If you find extensive cysts or small white nodules, the carcass should be condemned. Moderate cysts require that you freeze the meat to 15°F (-9.4°C) continuously for ten days or cook it to at least 140°F (60°C) to be sure you don't give yourself tapeworms.

Examining the surfaces of the carcass, you should trim out any bruises or swellings. Don't try to cure a bruised ham, for it may spoil. If you found a small wound with pus in it, carefully trim out well around it. Trim off any area that gets pus on it. Then trim out the lymph node between the wound and the heart. If you happen to dress out an animal that was just coming down with a severe illness, producing a septicemia (bacteria in the blood), the tissues will appear inflamed. Hopefully, you will have eliminated this possibility by checking the animal's temperature on antemortem inspection but, of course, this isn't possible in the case of wild game. In any case, a carcass with generalized redness or widespread pockets of pus must be discarded, for it will cause food poisoning if used. If you dress a carcass from an animal that was ill and not eating or was starving, the carcass will be thin and the fat tissue will have a watery, "snotty" appearance. This is because the animal was using up its fat to live on. This condition is called "emaciation" or "cachexia" and the carcass should not be used. If you skin a hog and find the carcass is yellow, it may be due to peanut oil in the diet or to icterus. Icterus is an accumulation of bile pigments due to a liver or bile duct disease or obstruction. The color due to peanut oil in the diet will disappear after chilling the carcass, but the color from bile pigments will not. A carcass from any animal with icterus should be discarded. Cow and sheep carcasses often have a yellowish color to the fat, which is normal.

Hogs with generalized purple areas due to chronic erysipelas infection cannot be used. But if the hog appears recovered and after dressing, you find just a few localized purple areas, these can be trimmed out and the rest of the carcass used. Consult the swine chapter for further notes on erysipelas.

When you check the joints of the legs, you are looking for infectious arthritis, especially in hogs. If you find only one joint having pus in it, cut off that leg well above the joint and trim out the lymph nodes above it. If more than one joint is infected, the animal probably had a generalized infection with bacteria throughout the body, and the meat will not be safe to eat.

When looking over the lymph nodes of the carcass, a single lymph node that is full of pus indicates a local infection but several or all nodes affected indicates a generalized infection. Anytime you find a generalized lymph node abnormality, you should condemn the entire carcass. The most dangerous disease causing this condition is tuberculosis but there are several others. A single node that is enlarged with fluid, pus, hard or cheesy material in it may indicate infection or cancer of the part beyond the node. In general, I would discard that part up to and including the involved lymph node.

Examination of the lungs is important for they are indicators of many diseases and cancers. Any time the lungs are generally inflamed or reddened, or have diffuse abscesses or tumors (lumps) throughout, the carcass is not safe to eat. The same is true if only the covering of the lungs (pleura), the sac over the heart (pericardium), or the lining of the chest or abdomen is reddened. All these signs indicate infections that could cause food poisoning.

Ruminants (cattle, sheep, goats, deer, etc.) tend to get a condition called "traumatic pericarditis." This is an infection due to the migration of a sharp object like a nail or a piece of bailing wire through one of the stomachs, the diaphragm, and into the sac covering the heart. This condition causes the heart sac to be full of pus and requires condemnation of the carcass.

When you examine a carcass and find "tubercles" or nodules in the lungs that suggest tuberculosis, I would hope that you can take the sample to a veterinarian or a laboratory for testing before you use the meat. Tuberculosis can exist in a few tubercles, walled-off in the body. This does not make the meat dangerous but, of course, generalized tuberculosis is highly dangerous. If generalized, there will be tuberculous nodules, called "tubercles," throughout both lungs and, maybe, in the spleen, kidneys, bones, joints or sexual glands and in the lymph nodes. In the case of poultry, the tubercles will be along the digestive tract and associated lymph nodes and in the liver and sometimes in the spleen, bones and joints. Tubercles in poultry are generally soft and full of caseous (cheesy) material. Tubercles of other species of animals are usually knobby, hard nodules. When incised, they may "grate" due to calcium in the nodule, or they may be full of cheesy material or pus. These nodules are generally white or light-colored.

The liver is another blood "filtering" organ that is indicative of the health of the animal. If there are any abscesses (pockets or cysts full or pus), throw the liver away. Flukes are leaf-shaped flatworms that invade the liver from the digestive tract. They can cause the liver to have black, rotten areas or to be yellowish-green due to obstruction of the bile duct. If you see these conditions, or if you find a fluke in the gall bladder or bile duct, discard the liver.

Anytime you dress a carcass and find an abscess or pus-filled wound or sore in combination with a discolored, soft liver or a soft, swollen spleen or swollen, red kidneys or other signs of general illness such as generalized swelling of the lymph nodes or redness of the skin, the whole carcass is unsafe and must be discarded.

When dressing a young animal such as a suckling pig, lamb or kid, you may find one with an infection of the umbilical vessels. These are structures from the umbilical (navel) area of the belly to the liver and are remnants of the vessels from the fetus to its placenta. Infection with redness or pus in these structures makes the carcass unsafe due to the possibility of food poisoning.

In the case of a female animal that recently gave birth or was giving milk, any severe or pus-producing infection of the udder or uterus makes the carcass unsafe.

When examining the digestive tract, the presence of worms indicates the need for treatment and improved management of your herd. If you happen to get a carcass with a severe, gangrenous (rotten) infection anywhere on the body or severe, hemorrhaging ulceration in the stomach or intestines, the entire carcass must be discarded because it would be dangerous to use.

PROCESSING INSPECTION

Immediately after slaughtering and dressing, the carcass should be properly chilled. This requires that you hang the carcass at a temperature of 32° to 34° F (0 to 1.1° C). It should be hung in a clean place as sides or quarters, not wrapped, so it will chill rapidly and completely. It must not be allowed to freeze during this time as this will adversely affect meat quality. Don't hang it in a room with any stored vegetables or other items that might impart an off-flavor to the meat.

Pork and veal should be butchered and packaged for storage, curing or use immediately after complete chilling.

Beef, lamb, and chevon can be aged for flavor and tenderness or used or packaged immediately. They should be held at 34° to 38° F (1.1 to 3.3° C), hanging loosely in a clean cooler, not stacked or crowded together. Beef can be aged for 7 to 10 days, lamb for about 5 days. If you freeze the meat, however, aging is a waste of time. Aging is also a source of possible spoilage or off-flavors. The crystallization of freezing tenderizes the meat about as much as does aging.

LAMB CHART

RETAIL CUTS OF LAMB — WHERE THEY COME FROM AND HOW TO COOK THEM

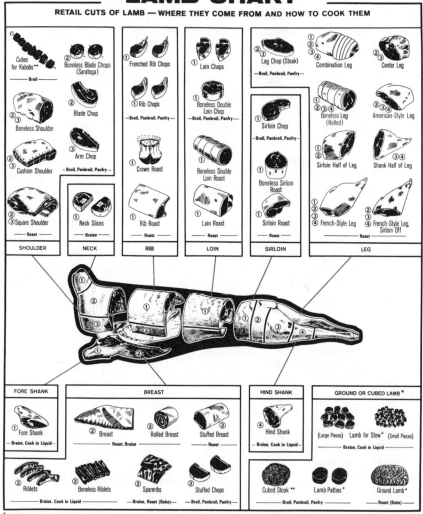

SHOULDER	NECK	RIB	LOIN	SIRLOIN	LEG

Cubes for Kabobs**

Boneless Blade Chops (Saratoga) ②

— Broil —

Boneless Shoulder ②③

Blade Chop ②

Arm Chop ③

Cushion Shoulder ②③

— Broil, Panbroil, Panfry —

Square Shoulder ②③

— Roast —

Neck Slices ①

— Braise —

Frenched Rib Chops ①

Rib Chops ①

— Broil, Panbroil, Panfry —

Crown Roast ①

Rib Roast ①

— Roast —

Loin Chops ①

Boneless Double Loin Chop ①

— Broil, Panbroil, Panfry —

Boneless Double Loin Roast ①

Loin Roast ①

— Roast —

Leg Chop (Steak) ②③

— Broil, Panbroil, Panfry —

Sirloin Chop ①

— Broil, Panbroil, Panfry —

Boneless Sirloin Roast ①

Sirloin Roast ①

— Roast —

Combination Leg ①②③④

Boneless Leg (Rolled) ①②③④

Sirloin Half of Leg ①②

French-Style Leg ①②③④

Center Leg ②③

American-Style Leg ②③④

Shank Half of Leg ③④

French-Style Leg, Sirloin Off ②③④

— Roast —

FORE SHANK	BREAST	HIND SHANK	GROUND OR CUBED LAMB*

Fore Shank ①

— Braise, Cook in Liquid —

Riblets ②

— Braise, Cook in Liquid —

Breast ②

— Roast, Braise —

Boneless Riblets ②

Rolled Breast ②

Spareribs ②

— Braise, Roast (Bake) —

Stuffed Breast ②

— Roast —

Stuffed Chops ②

— Broil, Panbroil, Panfry —

Hind Shank ④

— Braise, Cook in Liquid —

Cubed Steak **

— Broil, Panbroil, Panfry —

(Large Pieces) Lamb for Stew* (Small Pieces)

— Braise, Cook in Liquid —

Lamb Patties *

Ground Lamb*

— Roast (Bake) —

* Lamb for stew or grinding may be made from any cut.
**Kabobs or cube steaks may be made from any thick solid piece of boneless Lamb.

This chart approved by
National Live Stock and Meat Board

© National Live Stock and Meat Board

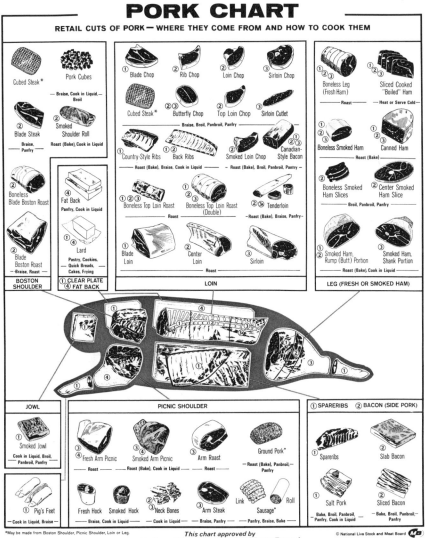

VEAL CHART

RETAIL CUTS OF VEAL — WHERE THEY COME FROM AND HOW TO COOK THEM

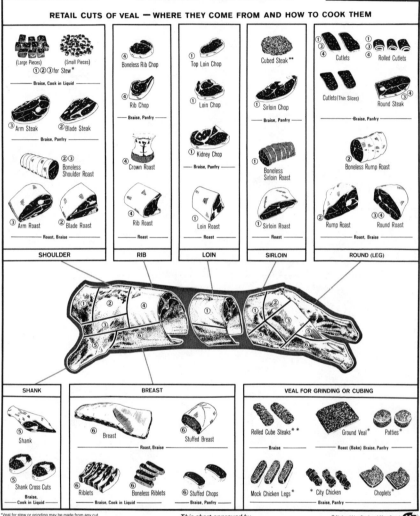

SHOULDER

(Large Pieces)   (Small Pieces)
①②③ for Stew*

— Braise, Cook in Liquid —

③ Arm Steak   ② Blade Steak

— Braise, Panfry —

②③ Boneless Shoulder Roast

③ Arm Roast   ② Blade Roast

— Roast, Braise —

RIB

④ Boneless Rib Chop

④ Rib Chop

— Braise, Panfry —

④ Crown Roast

Rib Roast

— Roast —

LOIN

① Top Loin Chop

① Loin Chop

— Braise, Panfry —

① Kidney Chop

— Braise, Panfry —

① Loin Roast

— Roast —

SIRLOIN

Cubed Steak **

① Sirloin Chop

— Braise, Panfry —

① Boneless Sirloin Roast

① Sirloin Roast

— Roast —

ROUND (LEG)

① Cutlets   ① Rolled Cutlets
③   ③
④   ④

Cutlets (Thin Slices)

③ Round Steak
④

— Braise, Panfry —

② Boneless Rump Roast

② Rump Roast   ③④ Round Roast

— Roast, Braise —

SHANK

⑤ Shank

⑤ Shank Cross Cuts

Braise, Cook in Liquid

BREAST

⑥ Breast

⑥ Stuffed Breast

— Roast, Braise —

⑥ Riblets   ⑥ Boneless Riblets   ⑥ Stuffed Chops

— Braise, Cook in Liquid —   — Braise, Panfry —

VEAL FOR GRINDING OR CUBING

Rolled Cube Steaks * *   Ground Veal*   Patties*

— Braise —   — Roast (Bake) Braise, Panfry —

Mock Chicken Legs*   * City Chicken   Choplets*

— Braise, Panfry —

*Veal for stew or grinding may be made from any cut.
**Cube steaks may be made from any thick solid
piece of boneless veal.

This chart approved by
National Live Stock and Meat Board

© National Live Stock and Meat Board

BEEF CHART

RETAIL CUTS OF BEEF — WHERE THEY COME FROM AND HOW TO COOK THEM

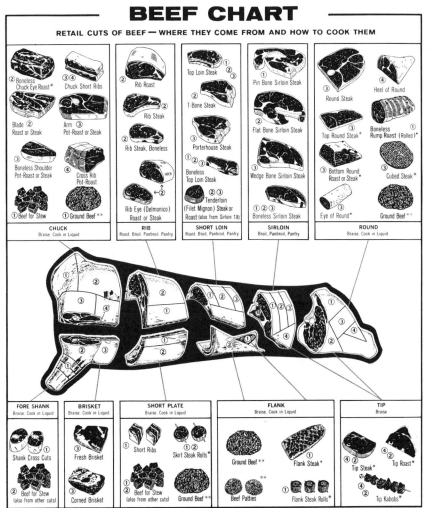

CHUCK
Braise, Cook in Liquid

RIB
Roast, Broil, Panbroil, Panfry

SHORT LOIN
Roast, Broil, Panbroil, Panfry

SIRLOIN
Broil, Panbroil, Panfry

ROUND
Braise, Cook in Liquid

FORE SHANK
Braise, Cook in Liquid

BRISKET
Braise, Cook in Liquid

SHORT PLATE
Braise, Cook in Liquid

FLANK
Braise, Cook in Liquid

TIP
Braise

*May be Roasted, Broiled, Panbroiled or Panfried from high quality beef.
**May be Roasted, (Baked), Broiled, Panbroiled or Panfried.

This chart approved by
National Live Stock and Meat Board

© National Live Stock and Meat Board

9
Dairy Goat Management and Veterinary Care

If you are on a small homestead or retreat, perhaps the most satisfying and most efficient creatures you could keep would be dairy goats. The rougher the country, the more the goats will thrive and the less likely dairy cattle will. If your place is in the deep woods or on the side of a mountain, then goats are your best choice for dairy animals. They are browsers, that is, they eat the leaves, tender shoots and bark from shrubs and bushes.

Dairy goats were among our first domestic animals. They were herded by nomadic tribes before men learned to stay in one place and cultivate the grasses which produce grains. In parts of the world, there are still nomads who herd goats between the valleys and mountains according to the seasons.

Fortunately, goats do well on many kinds of feed, even root crops. They are one of the most efficient food-converters of all our domestic animals. This trait is no doubt from their historic background of supporting poor people on poor land in all parts of the Old World. According to production records, good dairy goats produce more milk per pound of feed consumption than do most dairy cattle.

SELECTION OF DAIRY GOATS

For milk production, there are less differences between the breeds of goats than between individuals. Milk production is an inherited characteristic and dairy goats are bred for good milking qualities. Although there are many purebred breeds, crossbred and grade goats may be just as good. The main thing of interest when selecting a milk goat is her production records and the production records of her ancestors.

Goat breeders in the U.S. use these terms: female goats are does and males are bucks. A purebred is a goat with both parents of the same registered breed. A grade or unrecorded grade is an unregistered goat, often of unknown breeding. A recorded grade is a doe (female only) that is recorded by the American Dairy Goat Association according to her one known purebred parent.

An American is a recorded grade that has resulted from 3 successive generations of breeding recorded grade does to purebred sires of a single registered breed.

An unrecorded grade doe can be recorded as a Native on Performance if she produces at least 6 pounds of milk in 24 hours, or if she conforms to a specific breed type. A crossbred is a goat resulting

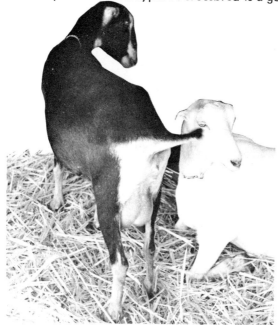

American LaMancha Does

from breeding parents of two different breeds. A crossbred can be recorded as an experimental animal.

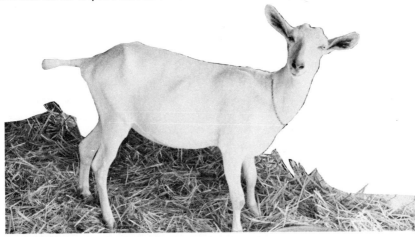

Saanen Doe

For the self-sufficient farm, you need not get purebreds unless you wish also to show them. If you plan to breed and sell goats, or if

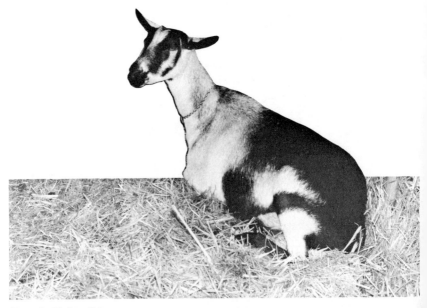

French Alpine Doe

there is any chance you may want to trade or hire out your buck, then you should stick to purebreds. Showing your livestock is the best advertising you can get, especially if you can win a few ribbons.

If you want them just for milk production, choose a breed or a breed-type of either grade or purebred that appeals to you. Find in-

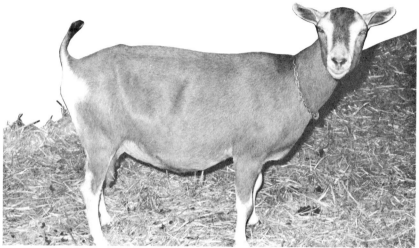

Toggenburg Doe

dividuals that are healthy and have a background of good milk production.

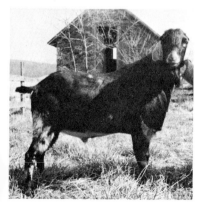
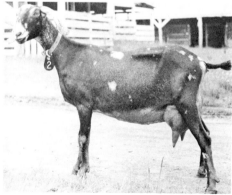

Nubian Buck   **Nubian Doe**
Courtesy Cherry Hill Farm, Purcellville, Va.

BREEDS:

Nubians are the most popular breed at present. They are large and have drooping or flopping ears and Roman noses. They may have a variety of colors and markings. Nubians usually average slightly higher butterfat and lower volume of milk produced than other breeds.

Saanens are white or cream color. The cream may reach a dark fawn but white is preferred. They are medium or large-sized with strong bone.

French Alpines are large goats with a variety of coat colors and patterns. The different recognized patterns have French names.

Toggenburgs are medium-sized goats with soft, fine hair, solid body colors and distinctive white markings. There are 2 white stripes down the face from eyes to muzzle, white ears with central dark-spots on each ear, white triangles on the sides of the tail, white spots on the neck near the wattles (fleshy appendages on the neck) and white lower legs.

American La Manchas are unusual because their ear flaps are very short or completely missing. Their faces are straight and their hair should be short and fine. They may be any color or pattern.

Angora goats grow a long coat which is made into Mohair. Angoras are not very common in the U.S.

The most important things to look for besides production background are soundness and conformation. Dairy goats should be thin, sleek, angular animals. Good dairy conformation is exactly opposite to good meat conformation. Their hipbones, pinbones and backbones will be prominent. Their bodies and necks are long and thin and their thighs are thin, not fat or meaty. The rib cage should be large enough that the front legs are not too close together and that you can lay a finger between the ribs. The backbone and topline should be rather straight and the rump fairly flat, rather than steep. The head, eyes and ears should appear alert and inquisitive, not dull or sluggish. The legs should be fairly straight and strong. The animal should be able to walk and move easily with no lameness. The feet should be straight and well cared-for. The dewclaws should not touch the ground due to weak pasterns.

The udders and teats are the most important factors in dairy conformation. The udder should be large, symmetrical and firmly attached to the body. Avoid goats with low-slung, pendulous udders because the suspensory ligaments may be torn loose and the udder will be injured by striking the feet or objects on the ground. Avoid goats with one teat or one side of the udder greatly larger or smaller than usual.

The udder should be moderately large and the teats fairly large and pointing slightly forward. After the dairy goat is milked, the udder should be soft and pliable. Examine the teats and udder by palpating them after milking. Feel for hard knots or lumps, indicating scars from mastitis or injuries. Avoid a goat with hard lumps or a firm, meaty udder. Examine the milk for clots, lumps, blood or strings of mucus which would indicate mastitis.

Always avoid a doe which leaks milk from the teat as she may be prone to mastitis. Avoid one that has extra teats or scars from having extra teats cut off or that has two holes in the end of the teat as these are very serious faults affecting production and heredity. Abnormal size, shape or direction of pointing of the teats are moderately important faults but they may be overlooked. Avoid one with an unusually small orifice (hole) in the teat as seen by the size of the stream of milk because she will be hard to milk.

Examine bucks that you breed to or purchase. Extra teats or the scars where they were cut off indicates a hereditary defect, as do teats with a double orifice. Avoid bucks with only one testicle or any abnormality of the testicles. Avoid ones with any other serious conformation defect, especially weak legs, low, weak pasterns, a crooked face, a navel hernia, blindness or any other serious defect.

Dairy goats are one of the few animals that I would consider buying as adults rather than as babies. The advantage of buying adult does is that you can find out their current production capabilities. The drawback is that you are more likely to bring home a disease problem. If you buy adults, insist on negative tuberculosis and brucellosis tests within the previous year as a condition of acceptance. Try to find out the production records of the goat's ancestors whether it is an adult or a kid, doe or buck.

Examine the mouth and teeth of any goat you consider. Goats and other ruminants have front teeth in only the lower jaw, with a dental pad for the uppers. Learn to tell the difference between the baby teeth of a young goat and the larger, adult teeth. The central pair of adult incisor teeth (2 front teeth) come in at one year of age. The next pair, one on either side of the centrals, come in at 2 years. The next, third or lateral pair come in at 3 to 4 years. The fourth or canine pair come in at 4 to 5 years. Avoid an older doe whose teeth are badly worn or missing. Her time is very limited.

Walk the goat to check for lameness and ease of handling. Pick up each foot and examine the hooves. Look for injuries, cracks or soft, rotten-smelling spots. Feel the neck and under the jaw for lumps or swellings which might indicate abscesses or other problems. Check the ears for sores or infection which would be indicated by pus or a rotten odor in the ears.

When you are considering the breed or type of goats to get, I would recommend that you choose the ones that are popular in your area. Even if you plan to be isolated in a remote area, I feel that you should cultivate an acquaintance with one or more old, established goat breeders. These people are always kind and helpful. You are sure to run into lots of unexpected problems and have lots of questions. Even if you have to ask questions long-distance, you need experienced people to help you get started. The other reason you need to keep in contact with established breeders is so that you can replace or add to your livestock if that becomes necessary.

HOUSING

Goats are hardy animals and can get by with minimum housing. They will be healthier and more productive if their housing suits your climate. Warm climates may need only a 3-sided shed to provide shelter from wind and rain. Cold climates require insulated, well-ventilated barns. I would recommend group housing, sometimes called open-housing or loafing pens, for your does, a separate box stall for does about to give birth, and another loafing pen for growing kids. Loafing pens are simply open pens which provide about 15 to 20 square feet of space per adult doe, somewhat less for kids. Bucks must be well-isolated from the does or, believe it or not, the milk will absorb the odor of the buck and acquire an off-flavor. Keep the bucks in a separate pen or barn, a good distance from the lactating does.

In colder climates, you will be keeping the goats indoors most of the winter, so your loafing pens should have floors of dirt or layers of gravel for good drainage. Build up your litter by regularly adding dry straw or other bedding. Be sure to check the bedding daily so that wet areas don't appear. The bedding must be kept dry by regular additions so that the goats will be warm and dry. This built-up litter method requires complete cleaning every 3 to 6 months, depending on its condition.

In cold climates, you absolutely must provide good ventilation in the winter, preferably as described in the chapter on housing. In winter, ventilate from the floor with a flue-type arrangement, providing at least one square foot of flue-cross-section per 24 head (or less) of goats. Your ventilation system should move about 20 cubic feet of air per minute per goat. This is easy to calculate only if you use electric fans. Hot weather requires ventilation near the ceiling to get rid of the hot, humid air.

In winter, regulate the ventilation, pen size and ceiling height to try to maintain no less than 50 to 55° F (10 to 12.8° C) in the pens. Your biggest enemy in cold weather is high humidity in the barn. Adjust your ventilation accordingly and be sure to prevent cold crossdrafts.

Loafing pens or loose housing allows the goats more freedom and exercise and, if they are bedded properly, keeps them warmer in cold weather. But, since the manure, urine and bedding build up, cleaning time can be quite a chore. If you have a tractor with a hydraulic loader, it will turn a backbreaking day of labor into a routine job. Of course, you must have a garage door or barn door opening into the loafing pens that will admit the tractor and loader. The fencing separating several loafing pens can be removed so that you can use the tractor from one pen to the next.

Any barn or shed that uses the built-up litter method must have the barn floor on a high spot and have proper drainage away from the barn. Otherwise, rainwater will enter the barn and ruin the bedding, making it damp, moldy and cold. This would be extremely unhealthy for the animals. Raingutters for the roof and drainage ditches may be necessary to keep water from running into the barn. Loafing pens require that all the goats be dehorned or polled (hornless by heredity). Otherwise you will have some severe injuries from goats horning each other. Never put a horned goat in with hornless ones.

Loafing pens are not the only way to keep goats. Commercial goat dairies often keep their does in some type of stanchion or individual stall arrangements called confinement housing. These are usually small, narrow stalls set side by side in a row with a gutter along the rear.

The floor may slope toward this gutter and the goats may stand on slatted platforms so that they stay cleaner. The goats are tied in the stalls or their heads are held in adjustable stanchions. The does are taken outdoors part of the day for exercise and pasture. This type of housing makes the barn cleaner because the manure and urine is all scraped into the gutter and shoveled out at least once a day. The gutter is often limed to keep it cleaner and to keep down odors. Large operations may even have automatic gutter cleaning devices and cesspools or digestion pits for the waste. These methods are all more costly and more work than are needed for a self-sufficient farm. Confinement housing also does not provide as much exercise for the does. However, you may wish to incorporate a partial method of confinement for feeding time. Many goat people use feeding mangers with locking head stanchions because of goats' tendency to pull hay out of a manger and trample on it. Once it is on the ground, they won't touch it. Often the manger has one or more spaces that are for the water buckets. The goats have to reach through for a drink and thus cannot easily contaminate the water.

For your pastures, I would recommend fences at least 4½ feet high for goats. I would not use a fence of barbed wire strands because goats always seem to get a lot of injuries from barbed wire. They can easily get cuts on their teats that go clear through to the milk cistern and require suturing.

Goats are very talented at opening latches, so design your fence gates to latch on the outside. I would never tether your goat on a long chain, as some people recommend. This may be a way to let her graze in an area that is not fenced but unless you plan to stand guard, you are taking too much of a chance that a stray dog or wild carnivore will attack her in this defenseless situation.

FEEDING:

Goats will eat quite a wide variety of feedstuffs. They are natural browsers, which means that they like to eat the tender new growth and bark of bushes, trees and shrubs. This is how they are able to survive on terribly poor soil and on mountainsides. For centuries, people of the Old World have managed to support themselves on rocky, infertile terrain with the help of their goats because goats can eat and digest plant cellulose and types of plants that otherwise could not have been utilized. Unfortunately, however, even goats cannot produce much milk on browse alone. You have to put nutrients into an animal in order to get nutrients out. In order to have healthy, productive dairy goats, you should feed them a variety of good, fresh feed. On the other hand, you must not over-feed them. Fat does are not as productive and over-feeding for record-breaking milk production usually leads to mastitis or other health problems. The types and amount of feed must depend on your climate— both for the amount of energy intake they need and for the types of feed you can grow. Your feeding also depends on the age and condition of the animals such as for bucks, kids, dry does, pregnant does and lactating (milking) does. I will give you some general guidelines for feeding goats and you can modify them for your needs. A cold, harsh climate may necessitate twice as much feed as a warm, tropical area just for maintenance. Your shelter and management will also make a big difference.

One of the most important sources of feed is your pasture. Many people let their goats browse in a woodlot but this can have its drawbacks. They are more likely to get into poisonous plants here so you must learn the dangerous plants of your locality and check the woodlot regularly. You can supply a large part of the nutrient requirements by growing legumes for their pasture and hay. Legumes are the alfalfa and clovers and the bean and pea crops. Legumes supply more protein than most other plants, as well as a good range of vitamins, minerals and energy.

Since goats are ruminants, they can make all their amino acids from any quality of protein but lactating does still need a high percentage of some type of protein in their diet in order to produce much milk. A doe in her early, highly productive period of lactation should have over 18% crude protein in her diet.

Legumes are one of the few types of plants that have this high a percentage of protein and legumes, as well as grasses, are usually higher in protein when young and tender. Both the protein and the total digestible nutrients (energy) fall as the plants become mature. Because of these facts, you may wish to set up your goats on a type of pasture called top-grazing. The idea of top-grazing, according to some recent research, is to set up 4 pastures or fenced areas, seed them with a mixture of legumes and grasses and rotate the animals to a new area every 4 days. If this system is set up properly so the number of animals fits the size of the areas, the animals will always be eating newly growing forage and the crude protein content of the forage will stay above 20%! The exact choice of plants depends on your locality. The legume portion might include such as alfalfa, ladino clover, alsike clover, red clover, soybean varieties, vetch or trefoil.

You may also include grasses such as bluegrass, orchardgrass, sudangrass, varieties of bermuda grass, millet, rye, oats or wheat. Sudan and millet are good in some areas with dry climate. Some new research has developed varieties of bermuda grass with extremely rapid growth. In moderate climates, alfalfa overseeded with ladino clover and top-grazed should last 3 years without reseeding and,being legumes, need no nitrogen fertilizer.

You must be very careful about turning your goats out onto a new, fresh pasture if they are not used to it. They can sometimes have digestive upsets from eating pasture that still has frost or dew on it as well. To prevent these problems, fill your goats with hay before turning them out onto a new pasture. Then bring them in after an hour or two for the first few days so their digestive organisms can get used to the change.

The carrying capacity of your pasture will, of course, vary with your climate. Warm, tropical climates may grow pasture almost year around. With plenty of water, an acre of top-grazed pasture might support 16 or more goats per acre. Dry climates will be lucky to support half this. And climates with cold winter will require that you grow a separate crop of hay for the winter. On an average, calculate 500 lbs. of hay per winter per goat if they are getting 6 months of pasture.

Goats will also eat silages, root crops like beets, mangels, carrots, cabbage, and others. Although I have heard cabbage recommended, I have also heard that it can affect the flavor of the milk, especially if fed within two hours before milking. Perhaps there are differences due to climate or varieties of cabbage. You will have to test this one out yourself. Strong roots like onion will, of course, cause off-flavored milk. The high-moisture feeds like roots and silage can be fed at a rate of 2 to 3 lbs. per day, taking the place of about a pound of hay. Don't feed silage or other strong-flavored feed within several hours before milking.

Silage can be made in anything from a barrel to a trench to a costly, automatic, glass-lined silo. But putting up good silage requires a lot of skill and experience. The moisture content of the plant matter must be within a narrow range, the silo must be air-tight and it must be used and handled properly to prevent spoilage. Goats which aren't used to it probably won't eat it at first. If you have a farm with good silo facilities and you don't know how to put up silage, don't try it by yourself. Get help from neighbors or the county agricultural agent. Silage is excellent for your cattle, as well as the goats, so it is well worth the effort if you can utilize it. You must also know that many people have died of asphyxiation from heavy gases after climbing down into a partially-filled silo.

Since you will be feeding high-quality pasture and hay, including legumes, with a high protein content, you will need concentrate (grain) mostly just for lactating does. For self-sufficiency, you must, in fact, utilize legumes so that you don't have to buy protein supplements to mix with your grains. With the top-grazing mentioned earlier, a plain mixture of home-grown grains should be more than adequate. But with old-fashioned pasture methods, or with poor-quality hay or all-grass hay, you should have a concentrate with 19 to 20% crude protein to supply sufficient protein for lactation. Of course, this will require the addition of protein supplements such as soybean oil meal from a feed mill.

If you are so isolated that you only have what you can grow, you can use excess milk or eggs in the ration for extra protein. Of course, goats have gotten along for centuries with minimal protein. They just produced less milk and were probably in poor condition while doing so. If you have access to a feed mill, you may find it convenient to simply purchase feed while you are getting started. In this case, I would recommend that you buy one of the pre-packaged grain rations for horses that contain a mixture of rolled or cracked grains and molasses. Don't get the ones that contain hay pellets and are a complete ration. Horse feeds are good because a good brand will have a consistent formula from one bag to the next and because the molasses makes it less dusty and more palatable for the goats.

Even if you are completely self-sufficient, you might consider shipping in bulk molasses. It can be purchased in large barrels and it keeps well. It is fed by many goat raisers for palatability, prevention of dust and prevention of ketosis in pregnant does.

If you are getting anything from a feed mill, I would also recommend that you keep a supply of wheat bran on hand. Bran is the best feedstuff for stabilizing the bowels. If your goats develop crumbly, dry or hard manure, simply add bran to the concentrate for bulk effect. Start with 10% of the concentrate and go, gradually, up to as high as 30% until the bowels become normal. On a regular basis, however, don't feed over about 10% bran because it is high in phosphorous and throws off the calcium-phosphorous balance.

The mixture of grains you use depends on your climate and milk production. Cold climates require more energy or calories (total digestible nutrients). Grain concentrates for cold climates can therefore be high in corn or sorghum grains, which are high in energy. These are lower in protein than wheat, oats and other grains. As a rule of thumb, I would recommend straight oats in moderate to warm climates and up to half corn and half oats in cold climates. Don't add more than about 20% wheat to the concentrate because of possible digestion difficulties. You can use a combination of most any grains that you can grow, such as millet, rye, wheat, oats, corn, milo, etc. The thing that you must always avoid, though, is a sudden change in the grain ration. Never change over from one grain mixture to another in one or two days' time nor put them on a full ration of grain when they aren't used to it. If you do, you will likely learn the hard way that this can cause severe colic or bloat. When you need to change rations, mix the new in with the old in increasing proportions over a week or more.

Now, let's consider concentrate requirements for the various goats according to their condition and pasture. A dry doe that is not pregnant should do well on pasture or hay alone. If root crops are available, you may wish to give her up to a pound of these a day. She will probably eat 2 to 2½ pounds of hay per day.

A dry doe that is pregnant should have a little grain, say ½ to 1 pound if she is on good hay or pasture. If she is on poor hay or pasture, her grain concentrate must contain added protein supplements. If she is on hay, root crops would be good for her, too. She will probably eat 2½ lbs. or more of hay per day.

A fresh doe (newly lactating) must have more concentrate according to her production and climate plus all the hay or pasture she wants. Under average conditions, she will need one pound of grain for each 3 pints of milk production. On good pasture such as legume topgrazing, she should need only a pound or less per 4 pints of milk. In very cold areas or with poor hay or pasture, she should get a pound of good-quality concentrate, with added protein supplement, for every 2 pints of milk produced. She may eat one to two pounds of roots or silage as well. She will probably eat 2½ to 3 pounds of hay per day.

As a rule of thumb, you can probably plan on needing 450 to 500 pounds of grain per year per doe.

Bucks should need no grain if they are on good quality pasture. If they are on poor hay or pasture, they may need 1 to 1½ lbs. of grain per day to maintain good body condition. During breeding season, you may need to increase the grain slightly so he doesn't lose weight.

All your goats should have free access to salt and calcium-phosphorus mineral supplements. Their salt should be crushed or granules, not blocks. They may not get enough salt off a block, especially when lactating. The mineral supplement is extremely important to the lactating does. Review the Nutrition chapter about types of mineral supplements and be careful of your choice. Remember that the supplement "comes through" in your milk. For planning ahead, you can probably figure 5 pounds of mineral per buck and 10 pounds of mineral per doe per year. I would recommend feeding them free-choice in separate feeding boxes. Some people mix the salt and mineral 50:50 but I would feed them separately so that heavily-producing does can take as much mineral supplement as they want, which they may not do if it is mixed with salt. It is imperative that the salt and mineral boxes be protected from rain and moisture. Check them regularly and clean them out if they become soiled or caked hard. Remember that goats won't usually touch any food that is contaminated with manure. If you are buying a pre-mixed ration, check the ingredients carefully. Don't buy feed that doesn't have a label telling the ingredients including the percentage of added salt or mineral. The formula can have up to 1% added salt and up to 2% added calcium-phosphorus mineral supplement. If you are mixing your own grain ration, I would recommend against mixing the salt or mineral in the ration because you will not be able to properly mix such a small quantity uniformly through the mixture by hand-mixing methods. Besides, some of the animals will require more of the supplement than others. If it is offered free-choice, they can take whatever they want. I would also recommend that you use a trace-mineralized or iodized, trace-mineralized salt, depending on the needs in your region.

Just for fun, let's calculate an average concentrate formula and see what it offers:

Feedstuff	Weight x Crude Protein %	= lb Crude Protein
Shelled Corn	35 lb. x 8.8%	= 3.080
Oats	40 lb. x 11.8%	= 4.720
Soybean Oil Meal	10 lb. x 45%	= 4.500
Wheat Bran	15 lb. x 14%	= 2.100
Totals	100 lb.	14.400 = 14.4%

Now, for minerals:

	Calcium% = lb. Ca		Phosphorus % = lb. P
Corn	35 x 0.03 = .0105		35 x 0.30 = .1050
Oats	40 x 0.10 = .0400		40 x 0.35 = .1400
SBOM	10 x 0.32 = .0320		10 x 0.67 = .0670
Bran	15 x 0.14 = .0201		15 x 1.20 = .1800
Totals	100 lb.	0.1035 lb. Ca	.4920 lb. P

This concentrate has 14.4% crude protein, 1/10% calcium and ½% phosphorus. It is therefore especially low in calcium and needs a mineral supplement, mostly calcium. It is sufficient for protein for lactation only if you are feeding a high-protein forage such as alfalfa or other legumes.

Goats are just like any other livestock in that they need a variety of good-quality feeds and they need to be fed by "eye." You need a little bit of planning and calculation to be sure they are getting adequate protein, energy, vitamins and minerals. Then you need to learn what a good goat is supposed to look like and feed your goats by eye to keep them in proper condition.

BREEDING

Goats have a fall breeding season. They come into heat about every 21 days from September through February. Their heat or estrus, when they will stand for breeding, may last one to three days. You may be able to detect this period by their activities. When a doe is in heat, she is usually restless and nervous, shaking her tail and bleating. She may get some swelling of the vulva and mucous discharge. She may mount the other does in her pen. It is usually best to separate her from the other does so she won't pester them. Breed her as soon as you detect her estrus. Turn the doe in with the buck and watch them to prevent injuries such as excessive kicking or butting, in case she is not receptive. After breeding, isolate the doe and try them again the next day. If the buck successfully covers the doe on the second day of estrus, this should be ideal. If she "settles" (becomes pregnant), she won't come into heat again that season. If she does come back into heat, breed her again. You do not need to skip the young doe's first fall season because of her small size. Tests have shown better lifetime fertility and milk production with does that are bred their first season. If you wish to breed her the first year do it toward the end of the breeding season.

The gestation period for kids is 150 days, plus or minus 5 days. Does average 2 kids but may have from 1 to 4. Mark the breeding date on your calendar. A week before her due date, put her in a private stall that is clean, dry and well-bedded.

Brush her daily and wash and clip her rear end as necessary to keep her clean for the upcoming delivery.

The udder will bag-up or enlarge 3 or 4 days before kidding. Some does will even begin to produce milk. Don't start milking her unless the udder becomes quite swollen and painful. Then only let off a little of the pressure to keep her comfortable until kidding. The last few days, add molasses and cut down her grain.

The first stage of labor is a period of uneasiness. The doe may bleat, paw the ground and seem very nervous. This stage may be extremely short or it may last for hours.

The second stage of labor begins with the actual contractions of the uterus. Usually some mucus passes from the vagina. Then the membranes surrounding the first kid may protrude and break, releasing a flood of "water." The first kid will usually be born within one hour. She will probably rest an hour or so between kids.

If the doe is in the second stage of labor, that is, she is having active contractions in the abdominal area that you can see and feel every few minutes, and she goes for over about 90 minutes without delivering, then she may be having difficulty. Difficult birth is called dystocia. There are several possible reasons for dystocia. The most common in goats is simply that the kid is not in the proper position for delivery. It may be turned sideways with its side or its back presented to the opening. It may have its head turned backwards or a foot twisted or poking in the wrong direction. The first thing to try for dystocia is to raise the doe's hindquarters, to move the kid forward by gravity, so the kid may turn to the proper presentation. Stand her on a ramp or put something under her rear end.

You should never enter the doe with your hand, except as a last resort. Get veterinary help if possible. If you feel that the doe cannot deliver naturally and you decide to enter her, first scrub her rear end and your hand and arm with surgical soap or iodine soap. Do it well! Then put sterile lubricant, a medical item, on your hand and arm. If possible, use a sterile rubber or plastic sleeve. Even then, scrub yourself in case the sleeve rips. Introduce your hand gently and feel for feet, legs and a nose or tail. If the kid is head first, you must get both front legs into the canal with the kid's chin resting on them. If one leg or head is turned backwards, you must repel the kid, gently, and pull the part into position. Then you can use gentle traction on the legs only when she presses with a labor contraction. If the hind end is first, get both hind legs into the canal. Once the legs are protruding from the doe's vagina, you may pull firmly in a direction out and downward toward the ground if she were standing. This is because the kid must arch his way through the canal so his shoulders and pelvis flex properly to fit through the mother's pelvis.

There are a few types of dystocia that you cannot help. Sometimes the kid is just too large. Sometimes it is deformed or some of

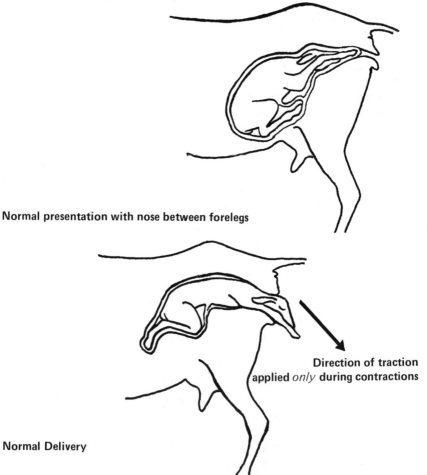

Normal presentation with nose between forelegs

Direction of traction applied *only* **during contractions**

Normal Delivery

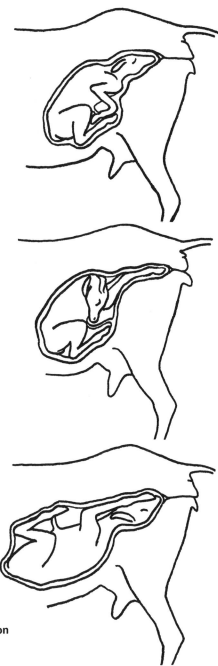

Foreleg Retracted

Head Retracted

Anterior Ventro-Spinal Presentation

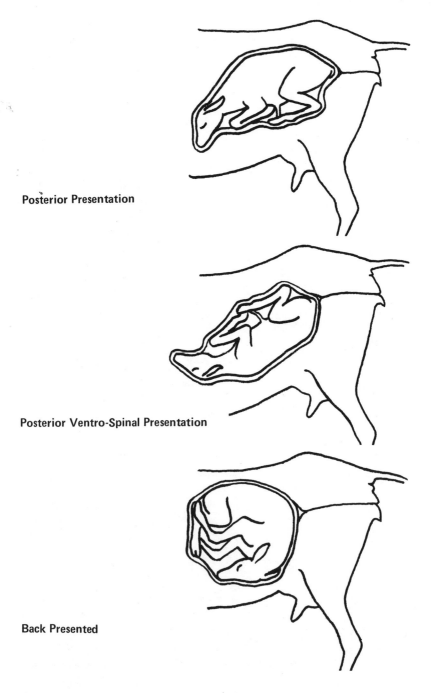

Posterior Presentation

Posterior Ventro-Spinal Presentation

Back Presented

its joints are stiff so that it won't fit through. Sometimes the twins are joined. If this type of situation occurs, you must get veterinary help or else you will lose the doe. If no help is available with an impossible birth and the doe becomes exhausted and weak, you should consider humanely killing her to prevent further suffering. Remember, only enter a doe if she has been actively laboring for over an hour and a half. Most does will kid very handily by themselves. In most cases, you are much better off to leave them alone and let them take care of it themselves.

As soon as each kid is born, remove it from the doe and put it in a small, well-bedded, warm box or stall. Clean the kid and dry it off well. After kidding, offer the dam a pan of warm water to drink to soothe her.

Watch closely for the afterbirth to pass. This is the placenta which surrounded the kid in the uterus. It should pass within 1 to 4 hours. If it does not pass within 6 hours, call a veterinarian. She may need medication to promote cleaning out. Within 1 or 2 hours after kidding, the doe should let down her milk, that is, you can get milk from her. The first milk after kidding is called colostrum. It is often very thick and contains many nutrients and antibodies which are needed by the kids. The antibodies are protective proteins which give the kid a temporary immunity to diseases until it has time to produce its own immunity. The kid can absorb these antibodies and utilize them only during the first few hours of its life, however. By the time it is 24 hours old, the kid will simply digest the antibodies like any other protein. Therefore, it is imperative that you save the colostrum and get some into the newborn kid as soon as you can. The colostrum also acts as a laxative to remove the sometimes hardened waste in the kid's digestive tract, called meconium.

The colostrum should be given warm. If the kid doesn't take it right after milking, it can be saved in the refrigerator and carefully rewarmed later. You must do this in a double boiler so that the colostrum isn't overheated. Heat will destroy the antibodies and nutrients. Warm the colostrum to 103° F (39.4° C) and feed before it drops below 100° F (37.8° C). Some breeders save colostrum by freezing it, in case they get an orphaned kid.

There are several ways to manage and feed new kids. Various breeders differ vehemently on the best methods. Let's discuss them so you can try them and pick the one which suits your situation. First there is the choice of leaving the kids with the mother to nurse naturally or taking them away immediately after birth. I have already recommended immediate separation but there are situations where natural nursing may be better. If you have other does that are milking and you don't need more milk at the present time, you may find it easier to let the latest kids stay with their mother and nurse. This may create a problem at weaning time, depending on how you handle it. I would only do this if you intend to leave the kids on the doe until they are eating enough solid foods for complete weaning from milk. Once the kids have begun to suckle the doe, you will probably never get them to drink milk from a milk-bottle or pan. They should be on sufficient solid food for weaning by 10 to 12 weeks of age, at which time they will be eating leafy hay and regular grain. Then the only trouble you may have is with the doe. Some does will resent hand-milking after they have been nursing their kids. This problem requires time, patience and gentle handling. Another situation where you might leave the kids on the doe is if the kids are males and you intend to slaughter them for meat, called "chevon," before 8 weeks of age.

Another problem with leaving the kids with the doe is that they may not nurse her out well. They may also nurse mostly from one side, producing a "lopsided" udder. You must then milk out the doe by hand.

For most people, it will be easier to separate the kids from the doe at birth and feed them by hand. You can feed them by nursing bottle or from a pan. Farm and ranch stores have rubber nipples (lamb nipples) that fit over a pop bottle. There is also a variety of commercial nursing bottles available, some with convenient racks for hanging the bottles while the kids nurse. But if you use bottles, you must clean them meticulously after every use and disinfect them with chlorox or some other disinfectant. The rubber nipples must be discarded as soon as they show cracks, which can harbor disease-carrying organisms. Kids are susceptible to scours (severe diarrhea) from poor sanitation. I would recommend that you start the kids right out on panfeeding. But to do this, you should give the first few meals by hand from a deep cup. If you offer a brand new kid a shallow pan of milk and stick her nose in it to get her started, she will shake her head and splash it all over. Start the kids with a cup of warm colostrum and gently put their noses in it to encourage them. The only disadvantage of nursing from a pan is that the kids may swallow a lot of air at first. But if the nursing bottle isn't working properly, they will get a lot of air that way, too. Once the kids learn to drink from the cup, you can feed them from pans. It is easy and convenient to build a small set of stanchions with pan-holders in front of them for the kids. The stanchions should have locking devices to keep their heads in. The pans should be held in place firmly. Build this kid stanchion so it will acommodate them while they grow and design it for the number of kids you envision having at the maximum. Then you can feed all the kids at once. The feeding pans must be scrubbed and disinfected after each use but pans are much easier than bottles and nipples.

Overfeeding kids is far worse than underfeeding. Overfeeding can cause diarrhea, which can become severe and can result in death. Underfeeding simply results in a hungry, thin kid. I would recommend starting new-born kids with 3 meals a day. You may decrease to 2 meals a day anywhere from 2 days to a week of age, depending on the weather and their condition. Start the kids with only about 6 ounces of milk per feeding and increase it with their appetites as long as they don't overeat. When they are quite young, you can offer them warm water after each meal to satisfy their appetites. I would give them straight goat's milk for the first week. After that, you can begin to add cow's milk or milk replacer if you want the goat's milk for yourself. You may use commercial calf or lamb milk replacer or powdered skim milk. Start by adding only a little of the replacer and slowly work up over several weeks' time. If they get scours, go back to goat's milk. Some milk replacers are good and others are very poor, almost invariably causing diarrhea.

After a week, start offering hay and grain to the kids. Pick out some fine, leafy hay and let them smell it. Put out some soft grain such as rolled oats. As soon as they start nibbling the grain, you can add the regular grain ration that you are feeding the does. Continue giving the kids about 2 pints of milk a day plus hay and grain. At about 10 weeks of age, start cutting down the milk ration and completely wean them within another week or so. By weaning them slowly, you give their digestive organisms time to adapt. This may avoid some digestive upsets. By this time, the kids will probably be eating a pound or so of grain each day.

You must decide right away what you will do with the buck kids (males). If you intend to slaughter them for food before 8 weeks of age, then you do not need to castrate them. If you intend to keep them over that age, you should castrate them young, between 2 and 10 days of age. At this age, it will be much less traumatic and less dangerous than when they are older and the gonads are more fully developed. Castration can be aided by a "key device" that is made of wire and shaped like an old-fashioned key-hole. Have one person hold the front of the kid upright while the other person scrubs the scrotum with surgical soap. Scrub it several times and rinse it until the area is clean. Use a sterile knife, make a cut through the skin over each testicle and pop the testicle out. If you have a "key" (sterilized) slip it over the testicle to help grip it. Hold firm pressure over the belly in front of the scrotum and firmly pull the testicle and cord out until it pulls loose. Then apply liquid or powder antibiotic. This method can be used on lambs and pigs but it cannot be used once the animals are more than a week or so old because it may cause fatal hemorrhage in an older male.

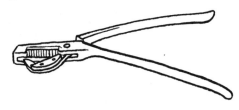

White's emasculator with crushing feature to prevent hemorrhage. For castration of older animals.

The only time you should leave a buck intact (uncastrated) is if you intend to replace your herd sire. After the intact buck is several months old, he should be separated from the doe kids. He will soon develop the typical odor and must be kept well away from the milking does. Then you can let him mature and decide if he is good enough to become the new herd sire.

An older buck should be castrated when he is not intended to be used as a sire. Put him in a stanchion such as a milking stand and feed him to help keep him occupied. Scrub the scrotum well to avoid infection. Use a sharp, sterile knife and cut along the rear and bottom of the scrotum over each testicle or simply cut off the bottom of the scrotum. Pull the testicle out, pushing the scrotum upward to expose the cord. Clamp the cord with a self-locking hemostatic forceps and cut below it. If you have one, you can use an emasculator that both cuts and crushes the cord. Leave the clamp on each cord for over one minute. When it is removed, you may get some temporary bleeding. If the bleeding comes in spurts, then you must get the clamp back on the cord and hold it awhile longer. Never castrate an animal during fly season.

doesn't develop the odor. He can then be slaughtered for food at any age.

I advise against using elastic band elastrators for dehorning, castration or tail docking of any species for several reasons. Elastrators are strong rubber bands that are applied with a special tool that spreads them open. The organ to be removed usually dries up and falls off over a period of several weeks, just like a big scab. But sometimes it begins to rot rather than dry up. If this occurs, the entire area may become gangrenous and you will probably lose the animal to infection. Another disaster can occur if the area around the elastrator becomes raw and is parasitized by fly maggots. Cases like these are quite a mess!

One of the things you must not neglect is dehorning the kids. Not all kids develop horns, depending on their genetic heritage. Check each kid carefully at several days of age for horn buds. These are hard nubs or bumps between the ears and forward on the forehead. There will usually be some curly hair, like a cow-lick, indicating the buds. If the skin over the location for horns moves freely, the kid will not develop horns. But if there are small bumps that do not move freely, these will develop into horns. Some goat breeders burn the horns off with an electric dehorning iron. This is like a large, old-fashioned soldering iron but the tip is round and concave instead of pointed. Other people use a caustic stick to burn off the horn buds.

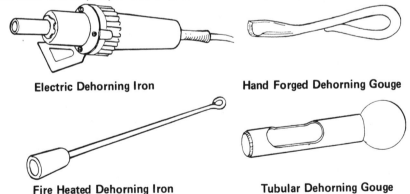

Electric Dehorning Iron   **Hand Forged Dehorning Gouge**

Fire Heated Dehorning Iron   **Tubular Dehorning Gouge**

For most people, I would recommend the electric iron to disbud kids. The main drawback is the initial cost of the iron. To get satisfactory results, though, you must do them young and you must do it properly. Buck kids, especially, should be done at no later than 2 days of age if you use an electric disbudding iron. Clip the hair over the top of the head and wash the area to remove dirt, which might cause infection. Turn the iron on and allow it to reach full heat. Apply it over the first horn bud and hold it there for a full 15 seconds. Allow the iron to heat up again before applying it to the other horn bud.

Disbudding can be done with an iron that is heated in a fire but this requires extra care. You should heat the iron until it just starts to turn dark cherry, let it cool to lose this color, then apply it to the horn bud. The problem here is knowing how long to hold it on. You must cauterize it enough to kill the horn-producing cells without damaging the underlying bone of the skull or the animal's brain! At the proper point, the skin will look well-burned, but not blackened. This takes experience.

Many goat raisers prefer to cauterize the horn buds with a caustic stick of sodium or potassium hydroxide. This works well if it is done properly but the caustic can accidentally spread to other parts of the kid's body, causing severe burns. The caustic stick must be handled very carefully so you don't burn your hands. It must be stored in a safe place because a child could burn his skin or blind himself by playing with it. Many people recommend that you put vaseline around the horn bud to keep the caustic from running out but I do not recommend this. I have known of cases where the caustic and the vaseline became liquefied and ran down the side of the kid's face. It could easily get in the eyes, as well, causing blindness. Some kids will use their rear foot to try to scratch their head and thus spread the caustic. For these reasons, I recommend that if you use a caustic chemical for dehorning, clean if off after the application, as I will explain. First, shave the hair all around the horn area. Wash the area well. Use a sodium or potassium hydroxide stick. Don't use silver nitrate, as it isn't as effective. It is important that the caustic stick be just moistened, not dripping wet. Apply the stick to the skin over and all the way around the horn bud. Rub it well into the skin with a twisting motion. Moisten the stick again and do the other horn bud. Wait about 2 minutes, holding onto the kid so it doesn't spread the caustic. Then blot off the excess caustic with a clean towel, paper towel or milk filter that has been wet and wrung out. Sponge the area but be sure you don't get caustic on your hands or spread it. Dry the area well. It helps to put an astringent on the area after cauterizing it. There are several types of astringents available, such as tannic acid in liquid or paste form. These seem to take away the pain. Again, don't get any astringent in the kid's eyes. After disbudding, feed the kid and put it in a separate stall or enclosure by itself.

After cauterizing by hot iron or caustic stick, scabs will form over each horn bud and later fall off. Watch these for infection, which would be indicated by pus under the scab. Infection should be treated by cleansing twice daily with warm water and mild soap and then applying antibiotic or antiseptic cream or ointment. A severe infection might require giving the kid antibiotics orally or by injection.

Another method of dehorning consists of cutting the horn bud out with a special tool. To make a dehorning gouge, take a short length of thin-walled pipe, about 3/4 inch in diameter. Fashion a handle or ball for one end of the pipe and grind the other end to a sharp edge all the way around. The best material to make this tool of would be stainless steel pipe so that it is easy to sterilize and doesn't rust. Clip the kid over the horn buds and wash the area with surgical soap. Then use the dehorning tool like a leather hole punch and twist it back and forth over the bud to cut through the skin. Then angle it and "scoop" the bud off. Apply pressure or styptic to stop the bleeding. Then put vaseline or antiseptic ointment on the wounds. This method actually causes less trauma to the animal than either burning or caustic, although most people don't like it because of the bleeding.

MILK PRODUCTION

After kidding, the doe may be very tired. Offer her some warm water to soothe her. Give her a smaller than normal amount of hay and grain for her first meal.

Often the doe's udder will swell greatly with milk and edema (tissue fluid) after kidding. Check her udder regularly for heat, hardness, and pain, indicating udder edema. For the first few days, you should check her 4 times a day so that you will recognize any problems before they become serious. Most does will have no problem with just twice-a-day milking but others will require milking 3 or 4 times a day until the udder edema subsides.

Goats or any other dairy animal should be milked at exactly the same time every day. Milking twice a day is best, although breeders may milk more often if they are trying to set a milking record. Most does will reach their peak of production by about 1 month into the lactation.

Most people prefer a raised milking stand so that it is more comfortable for them to milk the goats. This consists of a platform with a stanchion at one end. The platform is usually about 18" off the ground and it may include a ramp to walk the goat up onto the platform. Put some grain or hay in a box or pan on the front of the milking stand for her to eat while milking. Don't expect her to eat her entire ration during the short time it takes to milk her, though. You will need to provide a separate feeding manger to give her the rest of her grain plus all the hay she wants. After putting the doe in the stanchion, wipe her udder and teats clean of dirt and loose hair with a clean cloth and warm water. I would recommend clipping the entire udder and inside the legs regularly to decrease the likelihood of hair dropping into the milk. Get a commercial teat-dip disinfectant at a rural store and dip the teats before milking, using a cup. The purpose is to prevent mastitis and improve the keeping quality of the milk by destroying pathogenic bacteria on the teats. Dry the teats with a paper towel or unused, clean towel. Use a clean towel for each goat. A towel is not completely sanitary but it may be necessary to prevent chapped teats.

Disinfect your milk pail with chlorine solution just before using it. The chlorine will not leave any residue in the milk. I would recommend a stainless steel milk pail with the top partially covered to help keep out dirt. Wash your hands and dry them before milking.

It is common custom to milk the goats from the animal's right-hand side. You may sit on a stool with the pail between your knees or you may need to set the pail on the platform. When you become talented at it, you will be able to milk both teats at once by having one hand on each teat, alternately squirting them into the pail with great accuracy.

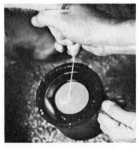

Squirt the first streams of milk into the strip cup.

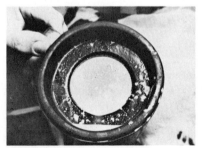

Flakes and curds from a gland with mastitis. Photos courtesy U.S.D.A.

Squirt the first stream of milk from each teat into a strip cup. This is a cup with either a fine screen or a piece of black plastic lying in it. If there are any lumps, clots, blood or strings of mucus in the milk, they will show up in the strip cup. These indicate mastitis, which we will discuss later.

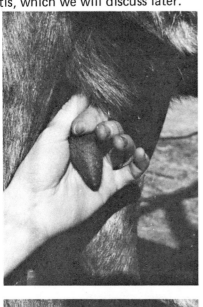
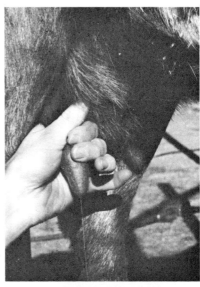
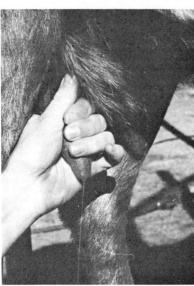
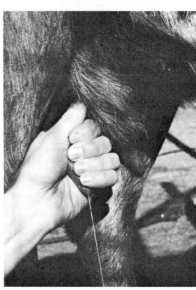

Milking should be done fairly gently but don't waste time. First, squeeze the thumb and forefinger at the top of the teat to close it off. This makes the milk go out the orifice, not back into the udder. Then, squeeze the full teat with the second, third, and little fingers, one at a time, in order. Then open that hand and repeat the procedure with the other hand on the other teat. This technique is awkward at first, but it must be done this way to avoid damage to the teats. You will soon learn to do it smoothly and quickly.

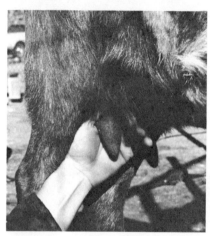

Nudge upward to see if she will let down more milk.

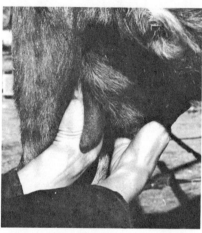

Gently massage the udder to get the last of the milk down.

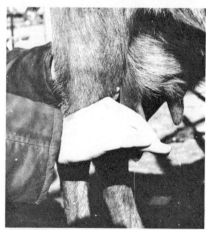

Support the udder like this while stripping out the teats.

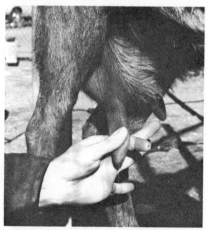

Don't strip the teats like this, without supporting the udder.

When the milk flow decreases until it almost stops, gently nudge upward to see if the doe will let down any more milk. At the end of milking, you need to strip the teats to get rid of the last of the milk so it doesn't sit there and grow bacteria. Take each teat between the thumb and forefinger, apply light pressure and run your hand down to the bottom tip of the teat, squirting out any milk. Only strip them a few times and do it gently so you don't bruise the teat. Milk let-down is under nervous system and hormonal control. The doe should be calm and quiet at milking time. Therefore, handle her gently and banish barking dogs and playing children from the area at milking time. If the doe is nervous or frightened, she won't release the hormones to let the milk down. Many dairies have piped-in music to soothe the animals at milking time.

After milking, you should strain and cool the milk immediately to between 40 and 45° F (4.4 to 7.2° C). The best way to do this is to put the milk pail into a bucket of ice water. Use a thermometer to tell when you've reached the proper temperature. Some people just put the milk in a clean, covered container in their refrigerator but rapid cooling seems to improve the flavor of the milk. Be sure to keep the milk bottle capped in the refrigerator to avoid absorbing flavors.

There are a number of things that can cause off-flavors. The most common might be having the buck close to the does. His bad odor is actually absorbed and passed in the milk. The doe's food is a common source of off-flavors. I have seen mention of turnips, cabbage, potato greens, onions, garlic and some wild plants causing flavor problems. Some people recommend feeding cabbage and turnips. However, I wouldn't feed these, or silage, within 2 or 3 hours before milking. If the milk is not cooled and stored properly, it will spoil, also causing off-flavors.

You can strain the milk in disposable paper strainers which are available at rural stores for this purpose. They will leave no taste as might a cloth strainer. Don't use metal screen strainers, as these are almost impossible to properly clean and sanitize.

Right after milking, you must wash the utensils you used. If you let the milk dry on them, cleaning will be very difficult. Wash first with cold water to remove the milk cells. Hot water would "set" the cells onto the surfaces. Then use hot water, detergent and a brush. Rinse them, sanitize them and set them on a drainer or clean rack, upside down. Never dry them with a rag, as this will only wipe bacteria all over them.

The soap or detergent you use should be an alkaline type to dissolve the milk residues. Home-made soap will, of course, be alkaline unless treated to neutralize it. Rural stores sell dairy detergents. However, milk-stone or mineral deposits may appear on the surfaces of your utensils after awhile. Commercial dairies use an acid (such as 4% phosphoric acid in water heated to 150°F (65.6°C) twice a week in place of the alkaline detergent to prevent mineral desposits. Never try to scrub mineral deposits off with steel wool, as this will just make more scratches for mineral deposits to accumulate in.

In most cases, your does will kid or freshen in the winter or spring and give milk well into the next breeding season in the fall. If you have several does, you should, of course, breed them at widely separate times so they will even-out the production of milk. Hopefully, this will allow you to avoid a period of no milk at all in the winter during the period of pregnancies. Of course, milk production is customarily "stored" by the making of cheese. It can also be frozen.

I don't recommend milking for record production. This is fine for breeders who wish to improve their stock or advertise good records, but it is not for the self-sufficient farmer. The reason is that record production requires maximum feeding and is a great physiological stress on the doe's entire system. She is then more likely to experience digestive upsets, mastitis or other infections or problems.

As lactation goes on, after the first month or so, milk production will usually gradually decrease. After breeding, most does will naturally dry up or stop giving milk. Some people dry up their does before breeding, but this is usually not necessary. If you wish to dry up a doe because she is giving too little milk, simply take her off grain, give her hay only, stop milking and watch the udder for hardness and pain. You may have to milk her a few times to give her relief. You can also dry her up gradually by skipping one milking a day, then milking every other day, then less until her production stops.

It is possible for a doe to continue at high levels of milk production for an extended period of time. If a doe is milking very well and you have other does, you may try skipping her breeding. She may continue milking throughout the next year. However, if you have only a few does, you shouldn't take a chance on her drying up in the summer when she won't come into heat to be bred. Some does will come in heat out of the normal season if kept close to a buck. Conceivably, you could stimulate her by controlling the daily periods of light and darkness to imitate fall and winter daylight. Seasonal breeding is thought to be controlled by the length of the days. Many people who milk goats prefer to drink their milk raw. They claim that pasteurization ruins the milk's flavor. I would never drink raw milk from any species unless I knew the animal had been tested negative for both tuberculosis and brucellosis, preferably within a year's time. Of course, commercial dairies must pasteurize their milk for public health reasons. Brucellosis causes Undulant Fever in humans. This is a severe and debilitating disease. Tuberculosis from milk can cause several forms of severe or fatal illnesses, including bone deformations in children, such as hunchback. Fortunately, brucellosis is rare in goats in the U.S. and T.B. is almost non-existent in our goats. Nevertheless, have all your dairy animals tested before you start giving raw milk to your family. A farm-animal veterinarian can do the tests for you.

Pasteurization of milk will destroy any pathogenic (disease-causing) organisms, especially T.B. It also helps the milk to keep longer. If it is done properly, it won't change the flavor very much. The easiest way to do it is to buy a home-sized automatic pasteurizer. If it is adjusted properly, it will take the milk just to the required temperature. The reasons for off-flavor are too hot a temperature and the use of utensils of the wrong material. Copper, iron or chipped enamel

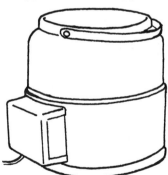

Electric milk pasteurizer

utensils will flavor the milk. You should use only glass or high-quality stainless steel. Use a floating dairy thermometer which is accurate. The fast or flash method of pasteurization is to heat the milk up to 161° F (71.7° C) and hold it exactly there for 20 seconds, then cool it rapidly to 60° F (15.5° C) or less. The slower, vat-type method calls for heating the milk to 145° F (62.8° C) and holding it there exactly for 30 minutes.

We can't leave the subject of goat's milk without mentioning that it comes naturally homogenized. The fat globules are quite small and this is why goat's milk is easier to digest than cow's milk. The only drawback is that this makes it harder to separate cream and make butter.

DISEASES AND PARASITES
Mastitis
Cause:

Mastitis refers to any inflammation of the udder. It can be due to physical trauma, such as the bruises from being kicked, or from the young nursing or it can be due to the swelling and lack of circulation from not milking her enough after kidding. The most common cause of mastitis is infection with bacteria which have entered the udder through the teat canal or through a wound.

Signs:

You may notice mastitis first by the doe's gait. She may be walking bowlegged due to pain. If she is not being milked out enough after kidding, the entire udder may be swollen and painful. If it is from a bruise, she may have a swollen, purple spot that is tender when touched. If, on the other hand, the mastitis is strictly a bacterial infection, the udder as well as the doe may vary from no obvious signs to severe illness and fever (over 104° F; 40° C) with a swollen, hot, tender udder. When you feel the udder, you may be able to feel hard lumps within it, especially after milking. In severe cases, there may be discolored purple or black areas on the udder which will slough and abscess. If you are using the strip cup before each milking, you should be able to catch a case of infectious mastitis at the very beginning. You will see anything from tiny, solid, white flakes to large curds, ropy mucus or blood-tinged milk in the first few streams from the affected side. The infection may be confined to a small area of one side of the udder or it may be widespread throughout both sides. A doe with mastitis often acts nervous and distressed due to pain.

Treatment:

Udder edema due to inadequate milking after kidding can get very severe. The best treatment here is prevention by checking the new mother 4 times a day to see if she is swollen. Obviously, more frequent milking is called for with udder edema but you must be very gentle. If you have let the udder become painfully swollen, you will probably need some diuretics from your veterinarian to help relieve the edema. Hot packing may help. Do this with a pail of clean, moderately hot water, a clean towel, and clean hands. Dip the towel in the water, partially wring it out, and hold it up around the udder. When it cools, re-wet it. You can use a saturated solution of epsom salts if you wish, but just don't use too-hot water. You can cause more harm than good by scalding her tender skin. After hot-packing dry the udder gently, milk it out and rub in lotion or camphorated oil. Massage it gently. Use the hot pack 4 to 6 times a day for 15 minutes each time. With infectious mastitis as seen by abnormal milk in the strip cup, you may also use the hot packs and frequent milking. You will also probably need antibiotics. Most of the cases are caused by *Streptococcus* or *Staphylococcus* species of organisms, although other species occasionally occur. Some of them will be sensitive to penicillin and streptomycin combinations but others will not. If possible, have a veterinarian culture the infection before you start antibiotic therapy. You see, the causative organism won't grow in the laboratory after you start her on antibiotics, even if the drug you used isn't curing the infection! So, if possible, get veterinary assistance for mastitis. If you use antibiotic ointments that you instill through the teat canal into the udder, be sure they are compatible with any other drugs you are using on the doe at the same time. Some antibiotics counteract each other completely. Never instill drugs into the teat canal until you have washed the teat with soap and warm water and disinfected it. Otherwise, you will just push dirt and bacteria up into the canal.

Prevention:

Prevent mastitis by preventing injuries and contamination. Eliminate sharp objects, high steps, mud wallows and manure from the does' environment so they won't injure themselves or get filth all over their teats. Whenever you have a doe with mastitis, milk her last and discard her milk as long as it is abnormal and for the required period after any drug use, according to the drug manufacturer's directions. After handling the diseased doe or her milk, never go back to a healthy one until you have washed and disinfected your hands and equipment. If possible, isolate the infected doe in separate quarters from the healthy ones. Disinfect the affected teats after milking, as well as before.

Obstructed Teat Canal

Cause:

Upon freshening, the teat canal may be obstructed, so that you can get little or no milk from that teat. It may be that the teat canal was never opened or formed, that it was too small or that it has closed due to scars from injuries to the tip of the teat. There may be a small polyp, or growth, that is growing inside the teat and it acts like a ball-valve.

Treatment:

This problem usually requires surgical care to open the canal or remove the polyp.

Leaking Teats

Cause:

Leaking teats are due to the production of more milk than is being removed, together with an abnormal formation of the teat canal. This is usually due to an injury to the tip of the teat or to inherited defects.

Treatment:

Defects of the orifice of the teat, whether from injury or inheritance, are difficult to correct surgically. A doe with this inherited defect should never be bred. If you have a doe with this problem, milk her more frequently. She is more likely to get mastitis as the leaking milk gets on her and everything else and draws bacteria-carrying flies. Some of these does will develop a habit of self-sucking.

Chapped Teats

Cause:

Teats and udders may become very chapped, dry, cracked and even raw and bleeding. The wind and dry air contribute to it but the biggest cause is frequent wetness, such as from not drying the udder gently after washing, or from milking with wet, rough hands.

Treatment:

Rub some lotion such as glycerine and water, olive oil or lanolin into the udder and teats several times a day until they improve. You may need an antiseptic or antibiotic ointment if they are exceptionally bad.

Ketosis

Cause:

This is a nutritional or metabolic disease or imbalance in carbohydrate metabolism in does near kidding time. It can occur in the last 3 weeks of pregnancy or within 3 or 4 weeks after kidding. Essentially, the doe becomes imbalanced, stops eating, gets low blood sugar and must metabolize her own body fat for energy.

Signs:

The doe with ketosis becomes depressed and stops eating. If it progresses for several days or more, she may go into convulsions or a coma and die. The doe's breath and urine will begin to smell like acetone because of her increased ketone level. Veterinarians have a simple test to check the urine for ketones, a sensitized strip similar to pH paper. Affected does may become unsteady and blind. They may grind their teeth and breathe hard. There may be a mucous nasal discharge, but they do not have fever.

Treatment:

The best treatment is intravenous medication, such as dextrose, given by a veterinarian. You can give the doe sources of energy such as brown sugar or molasses (1 to 1½ lbs. per day), or glycerol or propylene glycol (2 ounces twice a day), which ruminants can metabolize easily. Give these by drenching. That is, use a pop bottle to pour a little liquid at a time into the doe's mouth. Give her time to swallow and don't choke her with too large an amount at one time. Hold her head level or with her nose slightly high. Continue this daily until she is eating and no longer metabolizing her stored fat— that is, until the ketones disappear from the urine.

Prevention:

Prevention is the key to this problem because the actual physiology and cause of the imbalance is not completely understood. The mortality is high even if treated early; higher if not. Researchers think it can be caused by either underfeeding or overfeeding, feeding a poor-quality ration or making a sudden change in the ration. Also, lack of exercise, poor body condition, parasitism and multiple births seem to be associated with ketosis. A rapid change in weather, changing over 25° F (13.8° C) can throw even healthy animals into it. Your efforts must therefore be to prevent the conditions that contribute to it, except for multiple kids, which you can't control. In essence, you need to try to provide the best conditions to keep your animals healthy and strong, including exercise, sunshine, cleanliness, proper shelter and good, green, mixed legume pasture or hay and good grain. In cold climates, include milo or corn in the ration for extra calories. Don't make sudden changes in the diet. Feed at regular times every day. Toward the end of pregnancy, it may be helpful to cut down the grain a little and add bran to the diet so that about ¼ to 1/3 of the grain is bran. Check the does for parasites and worm them if necessary before breeding.

Milk Fever

Cause:

Milk fever is another metabolic and nutritional imbalance disease. It is a calcium deficiency that occurs near or after kidding. As milk production increases, sometimes the doe isn't getting enough calcium to support her own needs plus the requirements of milk production. Calcium is required in the blood stream for function of the heart and muscles. If a doe can't get enough from her diet and from her own skeleton, her blood level will fall.

Signs:

Signs usually occur after kidding, from a day or two to several weeks. The doe will lose her appetite and become nervous. Then she will begin to act excited. Her muscles and legs will tremble. As it progresses, she may stumble and fall many times until she can no longer rise. She will get convulsive stiffness of her body, then become comatose and die.

Treatment:

The doe must be kept upright and comfortable so she does not bloat. Blanket her in cold weather. Do not milk her! If she is showing severe signs, probably the only thing that will save her is intravenous calcium or combinations of calcium and other minerals, given by a veterinarian. Do not try to drench her, as her throat may be partially paralyzed and she may try to inhale the liquid. One of the original treatments was to pump air into the udder via the teats. This would stop production of milk by increasing pressure in the udder. In some stubborn cases that don't respond to medication or keep relapsing, this old-fashioned method is reverted to, sometimes with success. This is done with a tire pump and a sterilized inflating needle as used on footballs and basketballs. As she is recovering, try to take just enough milk so she doesn't dry up. If the case is severe, it would be better to dry her up than to lose her.

Prevention:

Prevention is the key to milk fever. Give your does free-choice access to mineral supplement at all times, especially during pregnancy and lactation. Offer the mineral in a separate box from the salt so that they can eat as much as they want. Give high-quality pasture or hay with legumes in it, from properly limed fields. Hay, especially legumes, is high in calcium, while grains are low in calcium.

Bloat

Cause:

Bloat is swelling with excess gas in the rumen, the first part of the forestomach. This may occur any time that the goat can't belch up its gases as it normally does. This may be due to choking, blockage of the esophagus with food such as pelleted feed, pieces of apples, crabapples, or corncobs. Or it may be due to the formation of excess gas and froth in the rumen which the goat can't eructate (belch up). This can be due to overeating on a new, lush pasture which the goats aren't used to. Sometimes it seems to be due to turning them onto a pasture that is very wet with dew when they are hungry. It can be due to a sudden change in ration, especially adding or increasing the grain portion suddenly.

Signs:
You will probably hear a bloated goat crying with distress before you notice the swelling. When you examine her, the upper left side of the abdomen will appear swollen behind the ribs. It may feel puffy and soft or it may even become hard and resounding like a drum. Goats seem to become very distressed, with difficulty breathing, with only a small amount of bloat. Look at her tongue and the color of her gums. It may become pale or even bluish. She may be getting up and down, slobbering and grunting or bleating. Sometimes they kick at their bellies.

Treatment:
This is an emergency situation! If veterinary help is close, take her in immediately, If not, you may be able to relieve the gas in her stomach by passing a tube down her throat. Improvise a stomach tube by cutting a short, 3-foot section from a small-diameter garden hose, smooth the edges on one end, lubricate it with vaseline and gently push it over her tongue and down her throat. Badly bloated goats may die at this time from the exertion. If it is successful, gas and foam will come out of the tube. This may have to be repeated. The old-fashioned method is to stab a trocar (sharp-pointed, small-diameter, hollow tube) into her side, into the rumen, to let the gas escape. The trocar is like a giant hypodermic needle. But this sometimes leads to peritonitis, infection of the abdomen, from contamination from the rumen, with fatal results. This is what is called a heroic measure, that is, a last-chance effort.

Prevention:
There are several steps that will usually prevent bloat. Feeding a mixture of grass and legume pasture, rather than straight legumes, will decrease the likelihood of bloat. Fill your goats up with hay in the morning before turning them onto a new, lush or wet pasture. Never run out of grain and then put them back on full grain a couple of days later. That is a sure-fire formula for indigestion or bloat. Make any changes in diet gradually, over several days' time. Make sure they can't accidentally get into a bin or sack of grain, especially corn. Keep them out of a wood lot that has old, dried-up fruits such

as apples on the trees or ground until you can clean it up.

Pinkeye or Contagious Ophthalmia

Cause:

This is an infection of the eyes and eyelids caused by a very contagious Rickettsia-type organism. It affects sheep and goats, occurs worldwide and is spread by direct contact by insects from an affected animal

Signs:

Signs occur 48 hours after exposure, with swelling of the eyelids and lots of watery discharge from the eyes. You will notice that the animals' faces are wet under the eyes. This discharge later becomes purulent. Both eyes may be affected at first or the second one may be affected several days after the first. The cornea (the clear part of the eye) becomes opaque, any color from grey to yellow to red. The cornea may ulcerate so badly it ruptures. The animals may lose weight because they can't see to eat or drink. This disease is seen more in young animals than adults.

Treatment:

Argyrol or 10% silver nitrate drops in the eyes is probably the best treatment. If you use this, be sure to wear rubber gloves, as it stains your skin black. Keep affected animals out of the sun and control flies. Antibiotics and vitamins may also be helpful but it pretty much must run its course.

Prevention:

Quarantine newly arrived sheep and goats. Never buy an animal with any signs of it nor with scars on the cornea, as it may be a carrier. Pink-eye of cattle is a different organism and you don't have to worry about cross-infections.

Sore-Mouth or Contagious Ecthyma

Cause:

This is a very contagious virus disease of sheep, goats, cattle, rabbits, and man. It is transmitted from one animal to another by direct contact.

Signs:

Signs appear after an incubation period of 7 to 10 days. It starts with inflammation (redness) at the corners of the mouth. Within a few hours there are red bumps, then small blisters after 24 hours. After another day, there are pustules (pimples). These rupture and form scabs with a red, ugly growth of tissue underneath. The lesions spread over the mouth and maybe over the whole muzzle. Secondary bacterial infection can make it much worse. Nursing youngsters will spread it to their mothers' udders. It occasionally spreads to the body or between the toes. The animals usually stop eating and become thin due to their sore mouths. Flies will attack the lesions, producing maggot infestations, fly strike. The outbreak usually lasts 1 to 4 weeks and may affect most of the young animals, less of the adults.

Treatment:

Treat the severe cases with gentle cleaning and an antiseptic such as carbolated vaseline or sulfa ointment. Don't remove the scabs. Control flies and remove any maggots. Use insecticide as necessary. If possible, have the rest of the herd vaccinated as soon as you get an outbreak.

Prevention:

Again, don't introduce it into your herd. There is a vaccine for this disease, which your veterinarian can get but you should concentrate on preventing any situation which would provide exposure to this type of problem. Vaccination introduces the live virus onto your land, so I would avoid it unless you are having a severe problem with it.

Foot Rot

Cause:

Foot rot in goats is uncommon, fortunately, but it is more common in sheep and can thus be brought onto your farm and transmitted to your goats. It is caused by bacteria carried by an infected carrier animal, together with wet bedding or wet barnyards so that the animals are constantly standing in wet filth. Poor foot care also predisposes.

Signs:

The animals will become lame. Their feet become swollen between the toes and they feel hot to the touch. The horn of the hooves will develop soft, rotten parts that stink with a characteristic odor. Later, the feet become deformed with long, rounded toes curling up in front, called "seedy toes." The animals become weak and emaciated because it is painful for them to get around to eat.

Treatment:

You must radically trim away all the soft, dead horn tissue with a knife and sharp trimmers. You must get rid of all the diseased tissue, even if you must cut into the quick and make it bleed. Otherwise, you won't be able to cure it. After trimming each animal, paint all the hooves with a solution of equal parts of full-strength formalin (37%) and glycerine. After trimming and painting, make all the goats (and sheep, if you have them) walk through a foot bath of 4% formaldehyde. This is made from 1 gallon of formalin (37%) mixed in 9 gallons of water. Put this mixture in a shallow trough in a narrow chute and force the animals to walk into it. Don't allow them to jump out. Each animal must stand in this foot bath for 4 minutes. Antibiotics may help get rid of it as well. Sheep raisers traditionally use copper sulfate (bluestone) as 20% solution by mixing 16 pounds of copper sulfate in 10 gallons of hot water but I do not recommend copper sulfate at all. I advise against it because it is so poisonous and corrosive. It corrodes any metal it touches and it stains everything, including the animals' skin, sheep wool and your hands. If an animal drinks any of it by accident, it is fatal. After you have used copper sulfate, you can't dump it on your ground or into a drain or stream because it is so poisonous. Formaldehyde is also to be respected. Because of its fumes, it should be used outdoors.

Prevention:

Foot rot is a herd problem. Prevent it by carefully inspecting prospective new sheep or goats. Once you bring it on your property, you contaminate the soil and it will be hard to get rid of. If you get it, after treating the entire herd, put them on clean ground. Clean up the pens and barnyards and establish drainage if necessary to keep them dry.

Goats' hooves should be trimmed regularly, whenever they become long or misshapen. On soft pastures, this may be required every month. On rocky ground, the hooves will wear down more. But they will also crack and be damaged by rocks so they still require attention. Trim them on a milking stand so they are easier to hold. Preferably, have a breeder show you what a normal hoof looks like and how to trim it. Use a sharp, short knife and a pair of sharp straight, short pruning shears. The outer horn or hoof wall usually grows the most. But if the bottom of the foot, the sole, isn't somewhat concave, it will need trimming, too. Cut around the outer hoof wall first so it is about parallel with the coronary band, which is the line where the hair stops and the hoof begins. If necessary, trim some of the sole. The softer sole at the back of the foot is the frog. If it is grown longer than the hoof wall, trim it carefully, a thin slice at a time, until it is level with the edge of the hoof wall.

Internal Parasites

Cause:

Goats are susceptible to a large number of species of internal parasitic worms. Most of the damaging ones belong to the type, roundworms. These parasites live in various parts of the gastro-intestinal tract and either suck blood or cause other damage or loss of nutrients.

Taenia ovis Tapeworm Lifecycle:

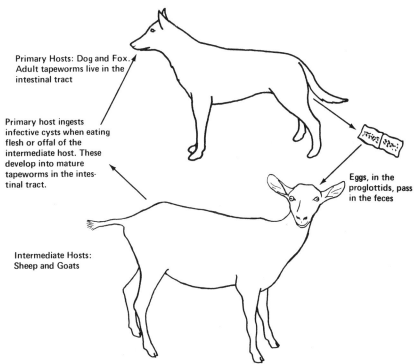

Primary Hosts: Dog and Fox. Adult tapeworms live in the intestinal tract

Primary host ingests infective cysts when eating flesh or offal of the intermediate host. These develop into mature tapeworms in the intestinal tract.

Eggs, in the proglottids, pass in the feces

Intermediate Hosts: Sheep and Goats

The intermediate host accidentally ingests eggs while grazing. The eggs hatch into embryos in the intestinal tract, burrow into the intestinal lining into blood vessels, and migrate to form cysts on the surfaces of the heart and diaphragm and in some other organs. The cysts are called *Cysticercus ovis*.

Signs:

Severe infestations cause greatly lowered production and lowered resistance to disease. They can be fatal, especially to young goats. The species of worms and the degree of infestation can be easily determined by a laboratory examination of a sample of feces. Worms usually make your goats look thin and unthrifty. Their hair may become dry, brittle and coarse-looking. Severe cases may develop diarrhea, loss of appetite and coughing. These are usually very anemic as seen by the pale color of their tongue, gums and the inside of their eyelids. The most severe ones may develop edema, swelling, under their jaws or elsewhere.

Treatment:
　　The safest drug that kills most of the species of goat parasites is thiabendazole. This is given by mouth with a dose syringe or drench bottle. It can be given on the grain as a powder if they will eat it but this method is not as reliable. It is given at the rate of 2-3 grams for adults and 1 gram for kids under 50 lbs. Phenothiazine can be used but it has slightly more chance of toxicity to the goats. It is given at the rate of 30 grams for adult goats and half this much or less for kids under 50 lbs. They should be over 2 months old. Again, it can be dosed, drenched or put on the feed. I do not recommend the older methods of worming with a mixture of copper sulfate and nicotine sulfate or with lead arsenate because these can be quite toxic. If you have problems with worms on your place, I would recommend that you worm the animals regularly, as often as every 3 months, until you get them cleaned up. Alternate the drugs so that the worms don't become immune to one. Each time you worm them, do them all at once and switch them to a new pasture that hasn't had any sheep or goats on it for at least several months.

Prevention:
　　The best prevention is to isolate your new stock until you can have their feces tested for worm eggs. I would worm them several times to be sure they were parasite-free before I turned them onto pasture or in with the other stock. The worms affecting sheep and goats can apparently transfer back and forth. Therefore, don't pasture goats in a field that has just had sheep on it or vice-versa. The best method of controlling internal parasites is regular pasture rotation so that the eggs are killed by drying and sunshine before the animals get back to that field. If you try the top-grazing pasture rotation method or some variation of it, you should not have much problem with worms. But, if you do have internal parasites in your herd, it will be a continuous problem and you should worm them faithfully at least twice a year, spring and fall. Don't drink the milk or use it for human consumption for 4 days after worming. Don't eat meat from these goats for 30 days after worming.

Lice

Cause
　　Goats commonly have lice which are small, 6-legged arthropods, insects that live on the skin. Some species of lice suck blood,

while others eat skin debris. Both types cause skin irritation and itching. Their damage may lead to skin infections or abscesses.

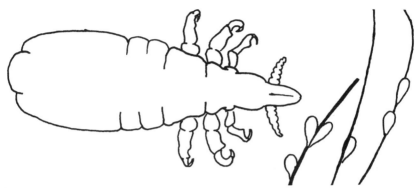

Long-nosed sucking louse of cattle and goats, *Linognathus vituli.* About 2 mm. long.

Nits, lice eggs, on the hair

Treatment:

Check new goats very carefully for lice by combing back the hair. The lice are small, only a millimeter or two, and may be white, grey, yellow, or red. They make egg cases or nits that are small, white, tear-shaped things attached to the hair shafts. This is usually what you will notice first. Get rid of the lice before bringing the goats onto your place. Lice can be killed by dusting or spraying with an insecticide. Use one that is labeled as safe for use on dairy animals, such as 5% rotenone. Once you get lice in your herd, on your place, you will have a hard time getting completely rid of them. You can repeat the insecticide whenever the goats begin to have problems with scratching or skin irritation caused by the lice. It is also helpful to brush your goats regularly to get rid of insects, dead hair and dandruff. Many people clip their goats down at the beginning of summer so they will be more comfortable. You can bathe them on a warm, sunny day.

Demodectic Mange and Abscesses

Cause:

Many species of animals are affected by *Demodex* species mange mites but goats get rather unusual symptoms. Mange is caused by mites, *Demodex caprae*, which are microscopic, 8-legged creatures that burrow into the hair follicles.

Signs:

Goats with Demodex develop abscesses in the skin, usually under the front legs in the armpits, or along the neck, face or flanks. These abscesses may grow to an inch or more in diameter and they can become infected with invading bacteria, producing large, dangerous abscesses. If the Demodex abscess breaks or is lanced, you can squeeze out a thick discharge. This discharge can be examined under a microscope for the typical, cigar-shaped, short-legged mites.

Treatment:

Each time a Demodex abscess appears, it should be scrubbed and then lanced with a sharp, sterile knife. The contents should be squeezed out, the wound cleaned and rinsed and the hole probed with a Q-tip dipped in strong 7% tincture of iodine or 4% formaldehyde. The tissues or cotton used on the wound should be burned to destroy mites and eggs. This is a herd problem and probably the mites are transferred from mother to kids. Then it takes a year or more for the mites to multiply sufficiently to start causing abscesses. Once you have Demodex in your herd, you will probably never be rid of it. Goats may continue getting Demodex abscesses until they are quite old. The Demodex lesions scar the skin, producing blemishes which will show if you make leather from it. The lesions themselves are not very serious but they may allow entrance for infections by dangerous bacteria.

Goats get abscesses from infection of the skin by bacteria. Pathogenic bacteria can enter through any cut, scratch, insect bite or other wound. In general, any abscess should be handled the same as a demodex lesion and it should be done early, before it becomes large and serious.

Constipation

Cause:

Kids may develop constipation after birth because the material, called meconium, that was in their digestive tracts during gestation can become rather hard. Adult goats often develop constipation if they are eating excessively dry, coarse feeds such as poor-quality hay with lots of stems. Confinement in the barn with little exercise contributes to the problem.

Signs:

Kids will strain to defecate. Maybe they can pass nothing or only a small amount. Adults will be passing dry, hard feces and perhaps straining.

Treatment:

Many people routinely give each new kid an enema right after birth. This should be done with a rubber syringe with a soft tip, not the kind with a hard, rigid tip. Instill about an ounce of warm, soapy water to loosen the meconium. This can also be done or repeated if the kid becomes constipated later. Adults should be treated by replacing part of their grain ration with bran, up to about half the grain, until the bowels become soft and moist. Then cut back to 10% or less of the grain ration as bran. Adults can be given warm, soapy enemas if the constipation becomes severe. Adults and kids can be given mineral oil as a laxative. It can be given as a drench but it must first be chilled, otherwise the goat won't feel it sliding down its throat and may inhale it. A kid can be given an ounce per day and an adult, 8 ounces or more per day until the bowels loosen. I would not recommend epsom salts laxative for kids, as it is too cathartic and may cause rapid dehydration and illness.

Prevention:

Enemas at birth usually prevent constipation in kids. Plenty of water, decent feed and plenty of exercise will prevent it in adults. If your stock have a problem, add bran to their ration on a regular basis.

10
Rabbit Management and Veterinary Care

SELECTION

Your selection of rabbit breeds will be based on their purpose. Retreaters interested in spinning wool for garments will probably be very interested in English or French Angoras. Their fine light wool makes the softest, most comfortable garments imaginable. For meat production, the medium-sized breeds, including the White New Zealand, Red New Zealand, and White Californian are probably most popular. Some people claim the White New Zealand is the best meat producer but there is probably more variation between individuals than between similar-sized breeds. There are several popular giant breeds, such as the Flemish Giant and Checkered Giant, but I would not recommend them for efficiency of meat production. The Giants mature later and eat more per pound of gain. For a small family, three medium sized does and one buck, producing nearly 400 pounds of live fryers a year, will supply plenty of rabbit meat for most tastes.

When you select your breeding stock, choose plump, meaty individuals. Feel the body and legs. You want them to feel firm, not fat. Be sure to choose healthy, alert-looking individuals. Healthy rabbits will keep themselves clean. They will look fluffy, with luster to their coats. Remember, the rabbits you breed will pass

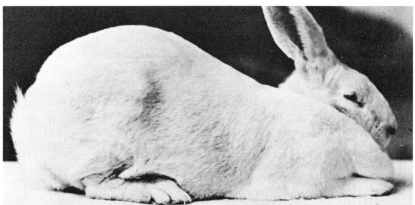

Flemish Giant Courtesy U.S.D.A.

their traits on to their offspring. When choosing which bunnies to keep for breeding replacement stock, choose only the best, strongest, meatiest individuals. Always try to upgrade your stock by purchasing the best breeding stock and choosing the best offspring to keep for breeding.

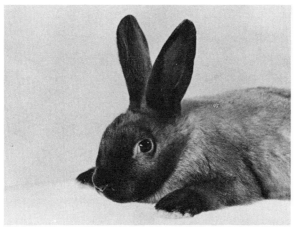

Black Silver Fox, Courtesy Joseph Laura, Jr., No. Middleboro, Mass.

BREEDING

Medium-sized breeds of rabbits become sexually mature at

seven months of age, giant breeds at nine to twelve months. For best fertility, you should have no more than ten does for each buck. Don't breed any one buck more than three times per week on a regular basis. Female rabbits or does do not have a detectable estrous cycle, but they become sexually receptive after being close to other rabbits for awhile. They will then allow a buck to mate with them and they ovulate after being inseminated. You should take the does to the buck's hutch for mating, not vice versa. If you mate them in the doe's hutch, she will tend to fight more the protect her territory. Her gestation period, from mating to birth, is 31 or 32 days. Birth or parturition in rabbits is called "kindling." Mark the date of mating on your calendar or records for the doe. Five or six days before her due date, give her a nesting box and some straw or other clean bedding. One design for a nesting box is 2 feet long, 1 foot wide and 1 foot high. The top is half-covered at the back and the front is cut down to six inches high.

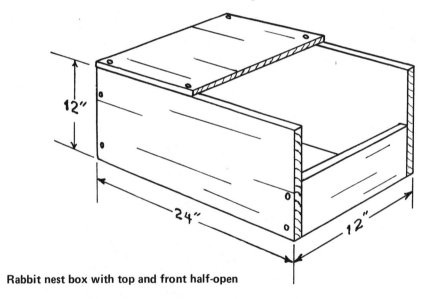

Rabbit nest box with top and front half-open

Five days before kindling, reduce her feed 25 or 30%. This procedure usually prevents ketosis. Leave the doe alone to make her nest. Don't disturb her any more than necessary. On the second or third day after kindling, carefully examine the bunnies for defects. Do this slowly and gently because if you get the doe frightened or excited she may hurt them. Destroy any defective bunnies. The doe would probably push the defective ones out of the nest or eat them anyway. At this time you can sex the bunnies. To do this, depress the genitalia, under the anal opening, to expose the pink mucus membrane. In the male it will protrude and form a circular bump. In the female it will lengthen into a slit.

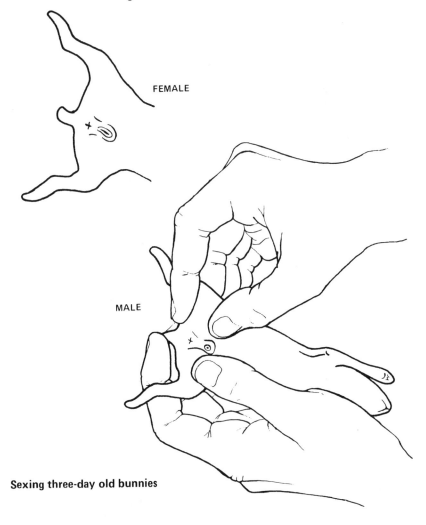

FEMALE

MALE

Sexing three-day old bunnies

Increase the doe's feed for lactation. The bunnies will nurse for 8 weeks and during this time they will begin to eat grain and fine leafy hay. Wean the bunnies at about 8 weeks of age. At this time they will be about 4 pounds and excellent for fryers. You can then re-breed the doe. Although you could breed the doe before you wean her bunnies, I do not recommend this practice. It takes too much out of the doe. By breeding at weaning time, each doe will produce four litters a year, with at least 8 bunnies per litter, or 32 bunnies per year. By this you can see that you don't need very many rabbits to produce a good supply of fryers. The number you decide to keep will depend on your family's taste for fryers. One word of caution: don't let the family make pets of the cuddly bunnies. They are friendly, tame, and become nice pets in a short time, following you around like a puppy. Keep them in their hutches and don't play with them or you won't be able to eat them. Remove the nest box after each litter and sanitize it.

HOUSING

The most important rule of housing is that you don't keep so many rabbits that they become crowded. They reproduce so fast that this can easily happen. Each rabbit needs its own separate hutch. Put together, they will fight or have false pregnancies. The hutch size depends on the breed. Medium-size breeds should have a hutch about 2½ feet deep, 4 to 6 feet long, and 2 feet high. Arrange the door so that you can reach all corners of the inside of the cage. The sides should be made of galvanized wire mesh or hardware cloth. Do not have wood sides or they will chew them up. The floor should be made of metal rods placed about ½ inch apart or of ½ to 5/8 inch square wire mesh galvanized hardware cloth. I do not recommend wood floors because the wood absorbs urine, rots and smells. It is then impossible to sanitize. Construct the hutch with the wire attached to the inside of the wood framing so they don't eat the wood and there are no ledges to collect manure or dirt. If the hutches are kept outdoors, put a solid roof on them and arrange them so you can attach solid sides to keep out wind and weather. In cold climates, you may wish to have permanent solid backs and sides with only the front open. Or you can keep the hutch inside a barn or shed. The hutches should still have solid sides in cold weather so the rabbits can warm the hutches with body heat. Don't close up the hutch so much that they get no ventilation. In hot weather, they need shade and plenty of ventilation. Rabbits are sensitive to the heat. You can help cool their hutch by hanging a wet burlap bag on one side of the hutch or let them out in a yard and wet down a sandy area in the shade for them to lie on.

The hutches should be raised three feet or more off the ground. Put galvanized metal sheeting around the legs to keep rats and mice from climbing up to the hutches. You could also use a circular shield or an inverted funnel on each leg. Otherwise rodents will get into the food and water and they may carry several serious diseases to your rabbits. Rats will bite the bunnies through the wire mesh, even chew off their feet. Some people keep their hutches

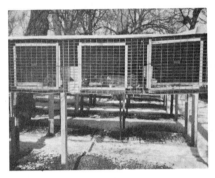 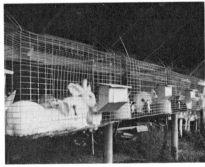

Wire cages covered on 3 sides for outdoor use. Rabbits have "setting" boards or carpet squares. Courtesy Doris Leibel

Wire cages hung by wire from ceiling. Courtesy Joseph Laura, Jr.

in a barn or shed and construct them completely of wire mesh put together with metal clips. They hang them from the ceiling with heavy wire. This keeps rodents from visiting the hutches and makes it easier to clean up the manure from under the hutches. These hutches are also much easier to clean. You should scrub the hutches thoroughly once a week to prevent buildup of dirt and resulting fungus and bacterial growth.

I would recommend that you allow the rabbits some outdoor exercise in a well-fenced yard so they can get regular sunshine and fresh growing greens. You must separate the bucks from each other and from the does. When they are in their yards, you must keep an eye on them so they don't dig out under the fence. Perhaps you could construct one or more small exercise yards and bury the bottom of the fence so they can't dig out.

The way you handle the manure under the hutches depends on the weather and your facilities. In most climates, you can let it pile up and compost under the hutches. Some people put earthworms in the piles to help compost it and let some bantam chickens roam around to eat fly maggots. If the hutches are on a concrete floor or if the weather is hot and the manure smells bad, it should be shoveled up daily.

FEEDING

Rabbits need a lot more water than you might imagine and they tend to tip it over or dirty it. Allow about one gallon of water per day for a doe with a litter. If you use small water dishes, you must check them frequently. You have to use heavy food and water containers or the rabbits will tip them over. Or you can attach the containers to the cage. Rabbit suppliers can sell you special watering nipples that dispense water automatically when the rabbits push on them. These are set up with a pipe to each hutch with the water from an elevated reservoir or pressure line. These automatic waterers prevent the spread and recycling of parasites through the water, as happens with water dishes. The only problem is that the system must be protected from freezing in the winter. If you can utilize these automatic waterers, I would recommend them as far superior to water dishes. Be sure to check the water supply several times a day, especially in freezing weather and in hot, humid weather. This is especially important with automatic waterers because there could

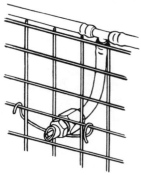

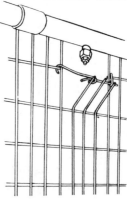

Automatic watering valve mounted inside the cage. Rabbits get water by moving the nipple.

Automatic watering valve mounted outside the cage. Rabbits reach through to drink from the nipple.

be a malfunction and it could go unnoticed for several days until the rabbits were quite ill. When you have an automatic device, you tend to take it for granted and assume that it will do your work for you, unlike the dishes that must be cleaned and filled regularly.

You should have no trouble feeding your rabbits an adequate diet on a self-sufficient farm. Rabbits eat all types of grains, vegetables, and forages. You should supplement their diet with free-choice trace-mineralized salt and mineral supplement. Dry does and bucks need about 12% crude protein, which you can supply with a good variety of grains and legume hay. Pregnant and lactating does and their growing bunnies need much more crude protein, preferably 17% to 20% of the ration. While many people have raised rabbits for many years on a lower protein diet, your rabbits will produce more and stay healthier if you give them the best in nutrition. Those people who have regular access to a feed mill can simply buy a prepared rabbit feed or add a protein supplement such as linseed meal, soybean oil meal or others. You can then calculate the amount of supplement to add as in the formulas in Chapter 3. But those of you on a truly self-sufficient place or an isolated homestead can add protein for the pregnant and lactating does and growing bunnies with surplus eggs and dairy products. Mix them with the grain and feed in a dish, not in a self-feeder, because the dish will have to be scrubbed daily. If you don't scrub the feeding container, the dairy or egg residues will spoil and cause scours or other problems. You can probably add these dairy and egg protein supplements up to about 15 or 20% of the concentrate portion of the ration.

The amount of feed you give your rabbits should be determined by the look and feel of each individual. In other words, feed your rabbits "by eye." This is because some does will eat too much if fed free choice. Then they become fat and are not fertile. On the other hand, pregnant and lactating does usually need to be fed all they will eat. They have a hard time keeping up with the requirements for themselves and their hungry babies. You need to supply enough nutrients so the bunnies grow and look healthy. The adults should maintain their condition, the feel of the flesh over their bodies and the appearance of the luster of their fur. When you are considering the amount of feed to grow for your rabbits, you can plan on the dry does and bucks eating about 4% of their body weight daily or about 160 lbs. of feed per year per 11-pound rabbit. This will probably consist of three-quarters grain and other concentrates such as dairy products, eggs and kitchen vegetable cuttings. The rest should consist of fine, leafy legume hay. Growing rabbits and pregnant and lactating does eat 6 to 7% or more of their body weight daily. This would amount to about 280 lbs. of concentrate and 80 to 100 lbs. of hay. You can figure feed for the bunnies if you consider them to have an average weight of 2 lbs. over an 8-week growing period. If each doe averages 8 bunnies and four litters per year, that's 32 two-pound bunnies fed for 8 weeks each. They will probably eat 4 or 5% of their weight per day in grain and hay, besides the mother's milk. That means 64 lbs. times 5% times 56 days. That is, all the bunnies produced by each doe will eat probably an additional 180 lbs. of feed in a year. This may consist of ¾ grain and ¼ hay.

I cannot give you concrete figures on the requirements, though, because of variations in climate and housing. You will just have to start out with a generous supply of feed and see how much your rabbits use for the first year or two.

If you are feeding dry grain, you can use a self-feeder made of galvanized sheet metal, available from country stores and rabbitry supply sources. These have a large storage bin that you fill occasionally and a smaller feeding trough that sticks into the hutch. The feed automatically runs into the feeding trough as the rabbits eat it. Make sure that the self-feeder you choose has a fine screen in the bottom to sift out fine dust. Otherwise the dust of the grain will build up in the feeder until it is excessive. Rabbits are very sensitive to this dust and will get sinus or respiratory problems from inhaling it.

Corn and similar hard-kernel grains should be cracked for your rabbits' ration. Oats and other hulled grains should be rolled or crimped. Wheat and similar small grains can be fed whole. Prepare your grains regularly so they are fresh. Cracking or rolling opens the protective shell or hull and allows oxidation and deterioration of the nutrients to begin.

When you calculate the amount of feed your rabbits will need per year, you can figure that they will consume about ½ to 1% of the total weight of their ration in salt and 1 to 2% in mineral, that is, calcium and phosphorus supplement. Be sure to plan for salt and mineral supplements and store these in a dry area, safe from rodent contamination. I recommend that you keep them in their original sacks in a steel drum or garbage can with a tight-fitting lid. Rodents will visit them and contaminate them with feces or urine if they are accessible. Remember that salt will speed corrosion of metal containers if it is taken out of the original sack. I would provide separate dishes or racks for the salt and mineral supplements so the rabbits can eat them free-choice.

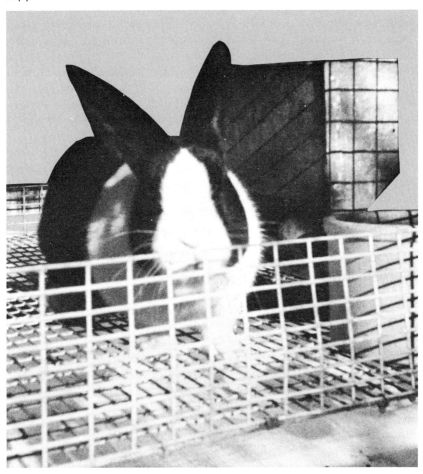

Dutch Rabbit. Note self-feeder behind the water dish, and "baby-saver" wire with narrower spaces at the bottom. **Courtesy Doris Leibel, Eagan, Minnesota**

Build a hay rack in each hutch. Some rabbitries have the hay racks between the hutches so that one rack serves two hutches. I would use mainly fine-stemmed, leafy legume hay. This is the early growth or the tops of the hay. The fine or early growth usually has the best protein content. Fine legume hay has much better protein than your grains, as seen in the Nutrients Table in Chapter 3.

When you start your rabbits on fresh greens, as in the spring of the year, start out slowly. Give them only a small amount the first few days or they will get diarrhea or bloat. Even when they are used to it, don't give more greens than they will eat in 20 or 30 minutes or they will over-eat. They will enjoy almost any garden vegetable, fruit or seeds. Dark green vegetable tops, roots such as carrots, beets, potatoes, etc., apples, pears and other fruits, sunflower seeds, almost anything from your garden or orchard makes happy munching for your rabbits. I wouldn't feed large amounts of lettuce, though, because of its scant food value. As with all your livestock, variety and freshness are the principles to follow to provide a good ration for your rabbits.

Rabbits have a mechanism called "pseudorumination." They normally eat part of their feces when unobserved. This provides them with B-vitamins and proteins which were formed in the rabbits' cecums and could not be absorbed by the large intestine. This mechanism makes them more efficient at digesting forages, since they are monogastric animals, that is, they have a simple stomach like man, pigs, and others.

DISEASES AND PARASITES

You can prevent most of the disease problems in rabbits by careful supervision and feeding and proper sanitation and housing. The biggest problem that many new rabbit raisers have is over-population. Rabbits reproduce so fast that their housing becomes overcrowded if you are not managing them properly. Overcrowding causes a rapid buildup of urine and manure and soiling of the feed and water. Then illnesses break out and spread rapidly. I would suggest some basic principles to prevent diseases and parasites, as follows: provide exercise space, preferably on a clean, grassy yard. Provide a separate hutch for every adult rabbit. Clean the feeding and watering devices as frequently as necessary. Some rabbits don't seem to be too bright about their personal sanitation, since they often urinate or defecate in their food or water. This problem is helped by giving them more space. Clean the hutches and nesting box litter as often as necessary for good sanitation. Quarantine ill rabbits far away from the others in clean, suitable quarters until they are well. Always scrub your hands after feeding or handling ill rabbits before returning to the other rabbits. Provide shade over your hutches if they are outdoors. Prevent wild rabbits from entering your hutch area. The wild rabbit tick *Haemaphysalis leporispalustris,* among other ticks, carries Rocky Mountain spotted fever, a disease dangerous to man. Therefore, you don't want wild rabbits attracted to your rabbitry.

I would like to explain some of the more common diseases and parasites in order to help you recognize and prevent them. Once you have your place set up and your breeding stock in residence, you probably won't have much problem with the infectious rabbit diseases but you should always be careful and follow good practices of preventive medicine. Your rabbits are always susceptible to physical illnesses even when they are on a well-isolated farm.

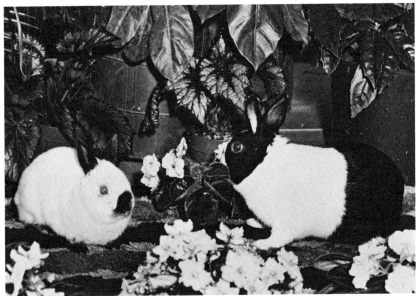

Left, Netherland Dwarf, Himalayan. Right, Dutch Rabbit. Courtesy Doris Leibel

Milkweed Poisoning
Cause:

The cause is ingestion of the wooly pod milkweed, *Asclepias eriocarpa,* in the hay. This weed is found only in the Pacific Southwest.
Signs:

The animals lose their muscular coordination. Their neck muscles become paralyzed and their heads droop.
Treatment:

Nurse the affected rabbits by holding their heads up to eat and hand-feeding food and water. Eliminate the contaminated hay. Give dark green vegetables and fruits for bulk and laxative effect.

Heat Exhaustion

Cause:

Heat exhaustion can occur on a hot, humid day if the rabbits have no shade, no ventilation, or are crowded together.

Signs:

On a hot day, you will find the rabbit lying on its side, panting. It is very weak, maybe in a coma. There may be a whole group of them affected.

Treatment:

Immediately immerse the affected rabbit in cool water up to its neck. Check the body temperature with a rectal thermometer. If the temperature is highly elevated, cool the animal in the water bath until its temperature is back to normal, 102.5°F (39.2° C). If you can, add ice to the water to cool it. If the temperature is not elevated, then remove the rabbit from the water bath and take it to a shady, cool spot. Stimulate it by squeezing its legs and toweling it dry. When it can drink, try to give it saline, which has 1 teaspoon of salt per quart of water.

Prevention:

Have water and free-choice salt always available. In the summer always shade the hutches. On hot days it may help to hang a wet burlap bag on the upwind side of the hutch to act as an evaporative cooler or let the rabbits lie on a spot of wet sandy ground in the shade. Be sure that you don't crowd your rabbits together on a hot day.

Wet Dewlap

Cause:

Some rabbits get the skin of their neck wet when they drink. This skin is loose and sometimes folded. The chronically wet skin becomes infected with bacteria and sometimes it is attacked by fly maggots after flies have laid their eggs on the wet, infected area.

Prevention and Treatment:

Change the position of the watering dish so the rabbit doesn't get its neck wet. The automatic watering nipples would be ideal or make a large-size version of the inverted bottle with a glass tube in the cork such as are used to water hamsters, etc. Clip the affected area of the neck to get off all the hair and dirty discharge. Wash the area gently with warm water and mild soap. Rinse the soap off well. Apply a soothing ointment or a drying powder, but not talc. Repeat the washing and medication daily until the area is healed.

Sore Hocks
Cause:

Rabbits easily get severe ulcerations of the pads and the backs of the feet of the hind legs when they are kept on rough or wet flooring or wet bedding.

Prevention and Treatment:

Change the bedding often and keep it dry. If they are on a rough, wet, wooden floor, build them something better. Wash their sore feet with warm water and mild soap. Rinse the soap off completely. Clip the fur over affected areas. If possible, put the rabbit out on a clean, dry, grassy yard in the sunshine. If you do this, you should use antiseptic powder on the sores. Don't use ointments because they would make dirt stick to the sores. When you put the rabbit back in a hutch, use wire or rod flooring and then coat the sores with an antiseptic ointment or cream. Clean the sores daily until healed.

Urine Burn
Cause:

This is similar to sore hocks, but the area of inflamation and infection is around the rabbit's vent. It is caused by sitting in urine-soaked bedding or on wet, rough, wooden floors. The skin becomes raw and infected with bacteria. In the process of licking the sores, the rabbit may spread the bacterial skin infection to its nose and lips. Then brown scabs and exudate form around the nose and lips as well as around the vent.

Prevention and Treatment:

Clean the litter frequently or put the rabbit on wire floors so the urine and manure fall through. Clean the rabbit's sore with warm water and soap and rinse well. Cover the sores with antiseptic or antibiotic ointment or cream. Repeat the cleaning and medication daily until the sores are healed.

Ketosis
Cause:

Ketosis is a metabolic imbalance with toxemia that occurs near kindling time. It is more common in fat does. Because of the imbalance, the doe rapidly breaks down her body fat, releasing toxic by-products faster than she can get rid of them.

Prevention:

Give your does exercise and fresh air and reduce their feed 25 or 30% about 5 to 7 days before their kindling due-date. Better yet, don't allow them to become fat in the first place.

Mucoid Enteritis, Bloat or Scours
Cause:

The exact cause is unknown but it can spread through a rabbitry, which suggests that it is caused by an infectious agent. It is one of the most important diseases of commercial rabbit raisers.

Signs:

It is usually seen in young rabbits, 5 to 7 weeks old. They become very depressed and sit huddled. Their ears droop, their eyes squint and they grind their teeth, probably from colic pain. They may either be constipated or have diarrhea but usually pass a profuse, jelly-like mucus. Their temperatures may be below normal. Affected young rabbits fail to do well and don't regain weight by weaning time.

Treatment:

Provide clean, warm, dry bedding. Force-feed lots of water and soft foods. Give them soft-curd cheese, fresh greens and vitamin supplements. Oral or injectable antibiotics are reported to help lower the mortality in young rabbits with this disease but apparently they don't always help. They probably just prevent secondary infections so I would recommend careful nursing care. If you have a severe epidemic of mucoid enteritis, get your veterinarian to give you medication for the diarrhea. I would suggest oral kaopectate or similar protectants to coat the intestines.

Colds
Cause:

Rabbits get infections of the nose and upper respiratory tract caused by various bacterial agents, probably aided by stress or lowered resistance due to wind, chilling, dampness, etc.

Signs:

The rabbits sneeze and rub their noses with their front feet. They have a watery mucus discharge from the nose which spreads over the fur of the front legs and feet. The disease is usually contagious and spreads through the rabbitry.

Treatment:

Immediately isolate any ill rabbit that you suspect has a cold because of the contagious nature of the illness. Check your rabbitry for drafts, dampness, inadequate water supply or other sources of stress. Keep all the rabbits, including the isolated ill ones, clean, warm, and dry. Clean the mucus discharge off their faces and front legs frequently. Use a washrag and warm water and then dry them well. Feed them fresh fruits and vegetables or fresh sprouts in the winter. Give vitamin supplements if possible. Be sure to wash your hands and change clothes after handling the ill ones.

Pneumonia

Cause:

Pneumonia may occur in adult or young rabbits. It is an infection of the lungs, usually by bacteria of the *Pasteurella* species but other species may be involved. It is usually brought on by stresses such as damp, cold or windy conditions, overcrowding, poor ventilation or other infections such as colds or mucoid enteritis together with poor care.

Signs:

An affected rabbit loses its appetite and sits huddled. It has difficulty breathing. You may see its chest and abdomen heaving in and out rapidly in an effort to breathe and you may be able to hear fluid sounds with the breathing. It often has diarrhea and a fever up to 104° F (40.0° C) or more.

Treatment:

Rabbits with pneumonia usually die unless given antibiotics and good nursing care. Penicillin-streptomycin injections twice a day or other antibiotics according to your veterinarian's instructions may save them. Remember that you cannot eat the meat for at least 30 days after injecting penicillin. Other antibiotics have various withholding times, which will be specified in the literature that comes with them. Provide warm, dry quarters and hand-feed water and soft foods.

Pasteurellosis

Cause:

This is an infection with the bacteria, *Pasteurella multocida.* It can be carried into your rabbitry by an apparently healthy new addition.

Signs:

There are three forms the disease can take: snuffles, abscesses and genital infections.

1. Snuffles: This is caused by *Pasteurella* infection of the lungs and air passages. An affected rabbit sneezes and coughs and has a discharge of mucus and pus from the eyes and nose. The discharges mat the fur of the front legs and become crusted around the face. In rabbitries with a *Pasteurella* carrier, the snuffles usually develop around kindling or other stress. Those that recover will usually be carriers. Many die of the infection.

2. Abscesses: Abscesses or pockets of infection full of pus develop under the skin. These usually develop from wounds on bucks after fighting. The organisms grow in the wound and create the abscesses. These may spread to a generalized, fatal infection.

3. Genital Pasteurella infections: This is a Pasteurella infection of the genital tracts of both does and bucks. It is passed at breeding. Does get a thick, yellow, purulent discharge from the vulva. Bucks may get swollen testicles or a discharge from the penis. Affected does often become sterile.

Action and Prevention:

If you have signs of this infection in your rabbits, take them in for culturing and identification of the organism if at all possible because it is such a tenacious and destructive organism. You should cull the affected rabbits and discard or sterilize all their housing and equipment. If the laboratory results are positive for *Pasteurella multocida,* you probably have a "normal" carrier in your rabbitry. This means that you should depopulate the whole herd and start over with clean breeding stock. If you begin having regular outbreaks of snuffles or problems with infertility, you will agree with me, though depopulation sounds radical. Antibiotics may cure the ill individuals but they apparently don't clear up the carrier state. If there is no way that you can get your suspected rabbits cultured, the least you should do is cull all the affected ones and sterilize their equipment and housing.

Pseudotuberculosis

Cause:

This is an infection with the dangerous organism *Pasteurella pseudotuberculosis.*

Signs:

An affected rabbit will become depressed, lose his appetite, lose weight and develop difficulty breathing. Affected rabbits usually die and it usually spreads to other rabbits in close contact with the sick ones.

Postmortem:

On postmortem examination of the carcass of a rabbit that has died of pseudotuberculosis, you will find hard, white nodules or bumps on the internal organs, usually the liver, lungs, spleen and the wall of the intestines. These nodules resemble the lesions of tuberculosis, hence the name.

Measures to take:

This organism can infect humans, so affected rabbits should

never be treated. The organism apparently spreads through contact with an affected rabbit or its urine or manure. Any time you open a carcass and find hard, white nodular growths on the internal organs, this is one of the diseases to suspect. If possible, take such a carcass in for culturing to identify the causative agent. If not, you should burn the carcass and destroy any hutch mates and any nearby rabbits that act ill. Burn all the carcasses and don't contaminate yourself. Wash and sterilize the hutches and equipment. Wooden hutches should be discarded or scorched with a blowtorch. Wash and disinfect your hands and clothing after handling such carcasses or their equipment. After you have had the illness in your rabbitry, remain watchful for lesions of the disease when dressing carcasses. If lesions show up again, continue culling or consider depopulation.

Myxomatosis

Cause:

This is a very contagious, usually fatal disease caused by a virus. The virus is spread by biting insects or by direct contact. It is seen mostly in California and Oregon coastal areas in the summer months.

Signs:

Affected rabbits become listless, lose their appetite and develop a fever up to 108° F. They develop swellings of the eyes, ears, nose and lips if they survive the first 48 hours of the illness. The swellings cause the ears to droop. They get a purulent discharge from the eyes and nose and have difficulty breathing. Those that live over a couple of weeks develop hard nodules on the nose, ears and forefeet, making this a cancer-causing virus. These rabbits usually die later.

Course of Action:

This disease is so contagious and destructive that you should destroy all ill rabbits immediately and burn the carcasses far from the others. Burn their bedding, nestboxes, and their feed. Quarantine for 3 weeks any rabbits that were exposed to the ill ones. They should be quarantined far from the others and their area should be screened from mosquitos. The virus is harbored by the California brush rabbit, so prevent wild rabbits from entering your hutch area. A commercial vaccine is available, so if you have trouble with this illness, consider vaccinating for myxomatosis.

Spirochetosis or Vent Disease
Cause:

This is a venereal disease caused by the bacterium *Treponema cuniculi.*

Signs:

Affected rabbits develop sores of the vent and sex organs with raw spots or scabs. They may develop enlarging masses under the sores. Because the rabbits lick themselves, the sores may be spread to the lips and eyelids.

Treatment and Prevention:

Always examine the genital regions of both bucks and does before breeding. Do not breed animals showing signs of spirochetosis. Penicillin injections, 50,000 units per day, are usually curative. The lesions will usually heal within two weeks and the recovered rabbits can then be bred without danger of spreading the disease. Be careful not to introduce this disease into your rabbitry. Don't breed to outside rabbits unless you are sure they are free of spirochetosis.

Coccidiosis
Cause:

This is a disease caused by an intestinal protozoan parasite passed from infected rabbits in the food, water or litter.

Signs:

The principle sign is diarrhea, which may be bloody. It usually is worse in young rabbits. They usually become depressed, lose weight, and sit huddled. Their fur becomes dull and they get a pot belly.

Postmortem:

Lesions are of two types, depending on where the coccidia infected the animal. With liver coccidiosis, the liver is covered and filled with small, greyish-white nodules that may be either milky or cheesy when incised. In intestinal coccidiosis, the intestinal walls are very thick and pale and the intestines are usually filled with fluid which may be bloody. This disease can be diagnosed by a veterinarian by a microscopic examination of the feces or samples of the affected liver.

Treatment and Prevention:

Commercial rabbit raisers often live with coccidiosis and simply try to prevent losses by good sanitation and feeding sulfa or other drugs in the feed or water. As a self-sufficient husbandryman, your best course of action is to avoid ever bringing it onto your farm. Quarantine new breeding stock or new arrivals for 3 weeks and have their stools tested for coccidia. Once you get it on your place, you will have recurring outbreaks unless you depopulate. Change yards, sterilize all the housing and equipment and get clean breeding stock because the older rabbits will carry and spread the parasite and it will remain viable in the soil.

Taenia pisiformis Tapeworm Lifecycle:

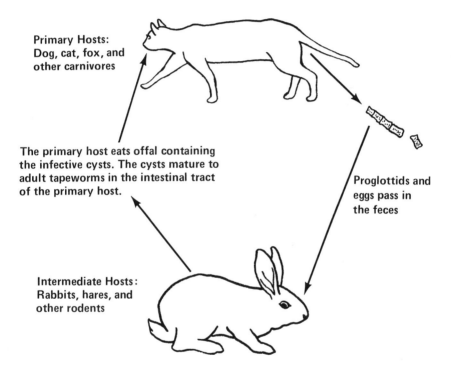

Primary Hosts:
Dog, cat, fox, and
other carnivores

The primary host eats offal containing the infective cysts. The cysts mature to adult tapeworms in the intestinal tract of the primary host.

Proglottids and
eggs pass in
the feces

Intermediate Hosts:
Rabbits, hares, and
other rodents

The intermediate host accidentally ingests eggs, which hatch in its intestinal tract into embryos. The embryos burrow into the intestinal lining, into the vessels, circulate to the liver, grow there, then burrow out of the liver into the peritoneal cavity, forming cysts on the abdominal organs, called *Cysticercus pisiformis*

Another species of tapeworm, *Taenia taeniaeformis*, has a similar lifecycle, but the primary hosts are mainly foxes and cats and related carnivores, and the cysts in the intermediate hosts develop only in the liver. Intermediate hosts are rabbits, mice, rats, and other rodents.

Tapeworms
Cause:

Rabbits are the intermediate hosts for the three species of dog and cat tapeworms, *Taenia pisiformis, Multiceps serialis* and *Taenia taeniaeformis.* These intestinal parasites require two different species of hosts to complete their life cycle. Adult tapeworms live within the intestinal tract of the dog or cat and produce eggs which pass with the feces. Rabbits then accidentally ingest the tapeworm eggs when foraging. The tapeworm eggs develop into larvae which invade the internal organs of the rabbits and develop there. Dogs and cats complete the cycle by eating the rabbit, thereby getting the larval stages, which then develop into adult tapeworms.

Signs:

The larval cysts are seen in or among the internal organs when dressing a rabbit carcass. They look like semi-transparent cysts, usually the size of a marble or smaller.

Prevention:

Tapeworms can be destructive to your rabbits and serious for your dogs and cats. The *Multiceps* tapeworm cyst can also infect humans and can be very dangerous, especially for children. Never feed uncooked wild or domestic rabbit entrails or organs to your dogs or cats. Keep dogs and cats out of your rabbit yards so they do not defecate there. When butchering a rabbit, do not cut open any of these cysts and let the fluid contaminate the meat. The fluid contains tiny infective larvae which may be infective for you if you accidentally ingest them. Cooking kills all stages of the parasite. Because a few species of tapeworm are dangerous to humans, I would recommend that you get your dog or cat wormed if you see the tapeworm segments in their stool. These look like small white pieces of rice or tissue that move. They are seen on freshly-passed manure, so don't confuse them with insect maggots which are seen on old manure. They may also be found clinging to the animal's rectum.

Ear Mites
Cause:

This is an infestation of the ears of rabbits by tiny mites. These are eight-legged creatures smaller than a pin-hole.

Signs:

Infested rabbits begin shaking their heads and scratching at their ears. The scratching may cause raw sores and scabs around the ears. The ears become filled with tan debris and crusts and maybe with dark dirt from the mites. The rabbits may damage their ears so much that they puff up with serum pockets which produce cauliflower ears if not drained and treated by a veterinarian. The mites can be seen with a magnifying glass on crusts from the ears.

Treatment:

Hold the affected rabbit tightly and fill the ear with mineral oil or sweet oil. Massage the ear canal gently and use cotton-tipped swabs to dislodge and remove the crusts. All the crusts and debris must be removed. Several types of ear mite insecticides are available. I would recommend one with rotenone rather than with lindane, since you are using the rabbits for food. The insecticide usually must be instilled into the ears 2 or 3 times weekly for 3 to 4 weeks to get rid of all the mites. You should clean and disinfect the hutch and equipment several times during the course of treatment to help eliminate the mites.

Ticks

Your rabbits will probably not get ticks, but I want to mention again that the wild rabbit tick, *Haemaphysalis leporispalustris,* among other species, carries Rocky Mountain spotted fever, a serious human disease. People get bitten by infective ticks while walking in the woods. People can also pick up the disease by removing ticks from wild rabbit carcasses when cleaning them and then accidentally ingesting the organisms by touching their dirty hands to their mouths. The ticks which carry Rocky Mountain spotted fever are fairly common throughout most of the U.S. but the disease is not terribly common in man. Take precautions by checking yourself often for ticks and removing them when you are in the woods. If you hunt rabbits, wash your hands well if you touch any ticks on them.

Rabbit Tick,
Haemaphysalis
leporispalustris

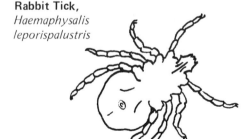

11
Hog Management and Veterinary Care

Hogs have a lot to offer for a self-sufficient farm. They are so vigorous when they root up the dirt, looking for edible matter, that they do an excellent job of breaking up the soil and bringing up the rocks in a rough field. Their manure adds good fertilizer and their rooting makes the field much easier to clean up and plow. They eat your kitchen scraps, surplus dairy and poultry products and cuttings from the garden and they can find a lot of edible grain in the droppings from cattle. Sows are very prolific, sometimes farrowing 12 or more piglets in one litter. Their meat and lard keeps well when handled properly. Many hunters add lard to their wild game meat when they make sausages and hamburgers, since some wild game is rather lean and dry.

The major diasvantages of swine are that they need especially good fencing to keep them in a field and they have a bad odor when not cared for properly. They don't need to have the objectionable odor that most commercial hog operations have. They have little odor when kept in a large, uncrowded field or when kept in a smaller pen, if the pen is cleaned properly and frequently.

SELECTION

You will need to know some swine husbandry terms before you go shopping. A sow is a mature female, after her first litter. A young, virgin female is called a gilt. A mature, breeding male is called a boar. A barrow is a male that was castrated young and a stag is a male that was castrated after he became sexually mature, usually when no longer wanted for breeding. A shoat is a weanling pig. A sow that is in heat is said to be "brimming." A seedy sow is one that has just weaned her litter and still has englarged mammary glands. There are other regional terms, as well, that you may hear when you talk to hog raisers.

When you start deciding which breed of hogs to raise, there are several factors you should consider. Hog breeds have changed greatly in this century. As the value of lard fell, hogs were bred for a meat-type conformation. The old lard hog type has been replaced by a lean, upstanding animal that is a pretty efficient feed converter. Hogs are monogastrics, that is, they have a simple stomach like ours so they need a higher quality of feed than cattle, sheep and goats. But they no longer need to produce the excessive fat that they used to. If you live in a hot, sunny climate, I would suggest that you stay away from white-skinned breeds because they are more sensitive to the sun. They have no pigment in the skin or hair to protect them and they get sunburned very easily. I would recommend that you look for hogs that are naturally good mothers and that are good grazers. Here are some of the common American breeds and some notes on each one:

Durocs are large meat-type hogs. They are very hardy and pro-lific and are excellent mothers. Durocs are red and have drooping ears. The boars average 900 lbs. and the sows 850. They are one of the most popular commercial breeds because of their prolificacy and fast gaining ability.

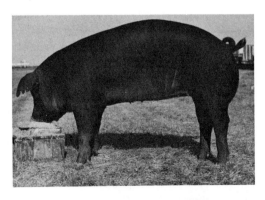

Duroc gilt

Hampshires are black with a white belt over their shoulders and forelegs and they have erect ears. They are a smaller, thinner type of hog. The breed was developed in Kentucky. Boars average 800 lbs., sows 650. They are hardy, prolific and good mothers. They probably produce the best carcasses except that some have light-weight hams. With their smaller size and other attributes, this breed would be a good choice for a small farm.

The **American Landrace** is a short-legged, medium-sized, long-bodied hog. They are white and have long, flop ears. They are from Landrace hogs imported from Scandanavia. They are not as rugged as some other breeds.

The **Berkshires** may have poor prolificacy and a short carcass, but the breed is being improved. The sows are good mothers. Berk-shires are black with white markings, usually with white feet, faces and tips of tails. They have a dished face and erect ears. This is one of the oldest English breeds of swine.

The **Chester Whites** are frequently too lardy. They are a large white breed developed in Pennsylvania. They are prolific, good mothers and fast gainers but I would not recommend them for their color and excess fat.

Yorkshires are a white-skinned breed. They are excellent mothers and are probably the best grazers. They have erect ears and a distinctive dished face. Yorkshires are the only white-skinned breed I would personally consider because of their other good qualities. They are a large breed with long, thin bodies, called the 'bacon-type' conformation.

The **Poland China** is an Ohio breed. It is one of the largest hogs. Poland Chinas are black with white on their faces, feet and tips of tails. They have flop ears. The breed is popular commercially but isn't as good for prolificacy or mothering as some other breeds.

The **Spotted Swine** or "Spots" are closely related to Poland Chinas but have more white spots. They are from 20% to 80% white.

The **Tamworth** is a very old breed from England derived from wild stock and they still look it. They have a long, narrow head and snout, erect ears, lean, bacon-type bodies and thin legs. They are of medium size and a red color. They are very active, good grazers, ex-tremely prolific and good mothers. This might be a good breed to consider for a small farm if you can locate some. They are not very numerous in the U.S.

There are a bunch of new hog breeds that have been developed from the other breeds, mainly at Agricultural Experiment Stations.

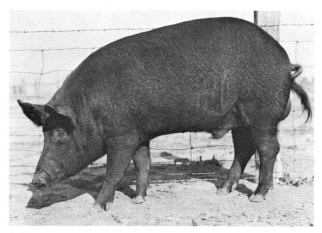

Tamworth boar

When you select your breeding stock, the individuals you choose are more important than the breed because there is a great deal of variation in type within each breed of hogs. You should select them for good health and conformation among other things. The type of hog you want is alert and active. It has a well-arched, smooth back with the highest point in the very middle, not at the rump or shoulder. It has smooth, full shoulders and hams and is wide at the hips. It has a high-set tail. Its legs are not too thin or crooked and it has a straight underline, not a fat, bulging belly. Both sows and boars should be checked for teats because they both pass on their traits for mammary glands. They should have at least twelve teats and these should be symmetrical, that is, evenly spaced, directly opposite each other on each side. Since most hogs are raised commercially and most operations have frequent opportunities for introducing disease, be sure to quarantine your new stock and have their stools checked for parasites. Worm them if necessary and have them vaccinated for the diseases that are predominant in your area. A local farm-animal veterinarian can advise you on this.

HOUSING AND EQUIPMENT

The housing and equipment you need for hogs depends on how intensively you wish to raise them. A few hogs of a hardy breed can spend the entire year on a small pasture in most climates. They can farrow, or give birth, and raise their pigs on pasture if they are bred so they farrow in mild weather such as late spring. Commericial swine-raising operations farrow their sows all year long and handle large numbers of sows with little labor. This is why they have elaborate, heated farrowing houses with automatic manure cleaners, fancy cesspools and, necessarily, rigid sanitation and disinfection procedures. The main things you need for handling just a few hogs are adequate shade in summer, a proper shelter for subfreezing weather and proper fencing.

Hogs become very uncomfortable in hot weather. You absolutely must provide shade in hot, sunny weather. In a treeless pasture, this can be simply a roof on posts. I would recommend that you build a summer shed on skids so that you can move it between pastures. The best would be a small shed with doors and hinged side panels so that you can open it up in hot weather and close it for wet, windy weather. It should have vents at the peaks for good ventilation. Allow at least 20 square feet of floor space per hog for summer sheds.

In cold climates you need to provide insulated winter housing. For only a few hogs, you could simply section off some space in your barn for them. Provide about 100 square feet of floor space for each adult hog and let them outdoors during the day. For subzero weather, their shelter should have insulated walls and not too high a ceiling so they can heat it with body heat. If your shelter is poorly insulated or damp, you will have to provide supplementary heat for them. The insulation should have a vapor barrier and it must be covered with substantial wood siding on the inside or they will eat the insulation. If you cover it with plywood, they will eat that, too. The most important factor of winter housing for hogs is ventilation. They are massive animals and they create a lot of humidity. This is their worst enemy for warmth and good health. Have the proper vertical ventilation as described in Chapter 1. You must provide plenty of dry, absorbant bedding for the winter housing. Add to it often enough that the surface stays dry. Clean it out as necessary to maintain a dry, odorless pen.

Fencing

Hogs require special fencing to keep them in a field. The fields that you intend to use for hogs need a strand of barbed wire along the *bottom* of the fence, strung about 4 inches above the ground. The regular fencing is placed with its bottom strand 4 inches above the barbed wire. The regular fencing should be 8 or 9 strand, 9 or 11 gauge wire. If you have electricity, two low strands of electric wire will work well. Many farmers just put logs along the inside of the fence for temporary pastures to keep hogs in. Commercial farmers put rings in the hogs' noses to keep them from rooting under the fences and elsewhere but this practice prevents one of the hogs' most useful functions, that of rooting up the soil. You should put hog fencing on three or more fields so that you can rotate their pastures every 6 weeks or so to prevent the build-up of internal parasites and to get rid of hog wallows.

Cooling

Hogs make wallows because they are hot, not because they are "dirty" creatures. Hogs cannot sweat adequately to cool themselves so they utilize any water they can find, which is usually a mud puddle around a watering trough or in a low spot in the field. In their efforts to wet themselves, they make a deep wallow. There are several ways to help your hogs tolerate hot weather and prevent wallows. One is to provide plenty of shade and put their watering trough on a concrete slab at the fence, sloped so the runoff goes outside the field. This way they cannot slop water out of the trough and make a wallow. Some commercial farmers build a pool or a shower for the hogs for hot weather. The pool is like a children's wading pool, shallow at one end, several feet deep at the other. These are made of concrete with a concrete "apron" sloping inward so they don't splash water out and make mud puddles. Don't build a sunshade over the pool or the hogs will never leave the water. If the pool is small, they will fight for its occupancy. A shower is made with a concrete slab which slopes to a drain or which drains outside the fence and with an overhead water pipe with tiny holes in it to emit a fine water spray. These facilities are certainly worth it if you have a lot of hogs because their wallowing can make some big, smelly mudholes. But if you have only a couple of hogs, your only big decision is whether to keep them in a little pen or on a field or pasture. I recommend running the hogs into the field. If you plant their pasture with some legumes and some root crops, they will "tend and harvest" their own crops. But if you keep hogs in a small pen, you must build a concrete slab or a wooden slatted floor because it will have to be cleaned daily and because they would dig big holes in the dirt floor of a small pen. If you are willing to go to this extra work, you can keep a few pigs in a very small area. This is fine for a small homestead but be sure to clean the pen often enough to keep down the odors. If you wish to try the slatted floor, build it up high or on a hill so you can clean the manure out from under it easily. I don't recommend the open cesspool or digester system directly under the floor of the pen. These seldom work right and usually stink to high heaven.

Troughs

Feeding and watering troughs for hogs must be very sturdy or the animals will mash them up. Troughs suitable for hogs can be cut from steel 30 or 55 gallon drums. Watering troughs definitely should be fastened down to a concrete slab or else they can be made of poured concrete. Half a steel drum mounted on posts is much better, though, because it can be arranged for cleaning. A trough that is not bolted down will be dumped by hogs and used as a toy. Remember that mature hogs weigh almost half a ton and they are quite strong. Also remember that if the hogs tip over their water in extra-hot weather, they may suffer from heat stroke before anybody notices. I would recommend a trough bolted down to a slab at the fence. Have a trickle of water running into the trough and have the runoff drain outside the fence to prevent wallows. If you can't pour a concrete slab, move the watering trough often enough that the hogs don't make a big mud wallow beside it. Provide a half a foot of watering trough space for each hog. For feeding troughs, I would privide at least 1½ feet of length of feeding space for each hog. Otherwise they will fight.

Use of snare and hobbles. Lariat could be used instead of snare.

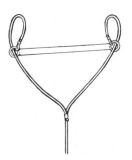

Swine hobbles, made of a 16'' piece of pipe with rings welded on ends.

Equipment

There are several handy pieces of equipment available to help you with your work when handling hogs. For trimming the tusks on a boar, you need a strong, stiff lariat rope, a good self-locking hog snare, and a pair of swine hobbles. The boar is caught with the lariat loop over his snout or first with a hog snare, which has a steel cable covered with neoprene or rubber. The snout of the boar is then tied snugly to a fence or post and the hobbles are placed on his hind

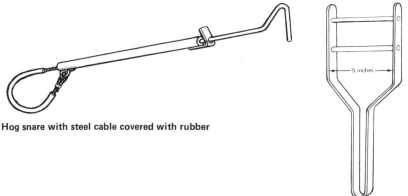

Hog snare with steel cable covered with rubber

5 inches

Mouth Speculum

legs. If you just used a loop of rope on his hind legs it would pull the legs together, maybe injuring him. The hobbles are placed and then he can be stretched out or dumped as you wish. The tusks are sawed off with a sharp hacksaw. You may wish to wear earplugs during this particular procedure. Between the boar's hollering and the sound of the hacksaw cutting enamel, it's enough to give you a headache along with the hog!

You might want a mouth speculum for examining the teeth of your hogs. This is to check for damaged or abnormally-positioned teeth or foreign objects when a pig is having trouble eating. It consists of a handle shaped like a slingshot with two horizontal rods between the posts. It is placed straight into the pig's mouth and then the handle is moved downward to pry the mouth open.

FEEDING

When it comes to feeding hogs, there is a ton of information and advice for you to choose from, much of it conflicting. There are several traditional and time-honored ways of feeding them. Hogs always used to be fed "swill," which was simply any available foodstuffs thrown into a barrel or kettle and soaked overnight or cooked. It was then "slopped" into the feeding trough. There is a lot to be said for this method if you do it right and are careful not to brew up a pot of ptomaine. If you are feeding hard grains, it aids the digestion to crack them and soak them. If you are feeding root crops, animal products or fibrous foods such as potatoes, field beans, beets, kitchen garbage or meat or fish offal or scraps, put them in a barrel or bucket with water and cook them. If you live near a feed mill, buy mill waste, a fine grain-processing byproduct, and throw some of it in. Be sure to let the swill cool off before feeding it. There are two reasons to cook the swill. The first is that hogs are monogastrics and cooking will aid their digestion. The second is that adequate cooking will destroy parasites and pathogenic organisms in any garbage or meat scraps. Even if you cook your hogfeed, however, never submit to the temptation to feed garbage from off your farm, even if it's free. The first rule of self-sufficient farming is to prevent the entrance of contagious diseases and feeding your hogs garbage from somewhere else is just too dangerous. Even if you are careful, you can bring on a serious outbreak of illness by just one little slip-up. The smallest amount of raw or inadequately cooked pork, if it is infected, might wipe out your hog operation.

Gleaning is the practice of turning the hogs into a field after harvesting a crop so they can clean up anything that has been left on the ground. This is an excellent reason to put up hog fencing on several of your fields. The hogs will make sure that none of the crop is wasted. Hogging down is a way of salvaging a crop that was blown down by a rainstorm or hailstorm before it could be harvested. Be sure to wait a few days until the ground is not too wet and soft, however. And be careful about turning them into a lush, green crop if they aren't used to it. Only let them in it for half an hour or so the first few days or the sudden change in their diet will give them indigestion and colic.

The most important point about feeding hogs is that they are not able to digest cellulose and poor quality protein like cattle, sheep and goats. You must give them a fairly good-quality, high-protein ration. They don't usually do well on forage alone, although some hogs can get along well if you plant their pasture in legumes and root crops such as beans, peas, alfalfa, beets, carrots, Jerusalem artichokes and others. The amount of supplemental grain and protein they need depends on the severity of your climate and the amount of calories they need. Some breeds are better at foraging than others.

If you live near a feed mill, you can purchase standard hog feeds prepared for various stages of their life cycle, such as weanlings, growing, pregnancy and lactation. But I would rather that you learn to feed them on a self-sufficient basis with your own grains, vegetables, and forages.

Supply free-choice mineral supplement and free-choice salt in feeding boxes that are protected from rain.

During pregnancy and lactation you will want to feed your best high-protein diet to your sow. Put her on a pasture that has some legumes, such as alfalfa, peas, beans, soybeans or peanuts. For extra protein, give her your surplus dairy products, including whey, skim milk and buttermilk, perhaps a gallon or more per day. Give her excess eggs, but don't feed old, cracked eggs because they might carry *Salmonella* species organisms from the chickens which would cause enteritis or a digestive upset. For most climates you will probably want to give a pregnant sow about 1 pound of grain for each 100 pounds of her body weight per day. This can be a mixture of the grains you grow, mostly corn or milo. Preferably the grains should be cracked or crimped. The last 3 weeks of pregnancy, you should go to about 50% oats in the grain and perhaps it would help to add an ounce of laxative oil such as cod liver oil. During lactation, especially if the litter is large, you should increase the grain and protein supplements about 50% to help the sow keep up with her energy requirements. She should be getting at least 18% crude protein during pregnancy and lactation. Feed by "eye," and give her enough feed that she doesn't lose condition.

Manage your pastures by rotating them often enough that the hogs don't eat everything to the ground and trample it bare. Keep the forage over 4 inches high so that the hogs will pick up fewer parasite eggs and because the top growth of forage is more nutritious.

When you are fattening your pigs for butchering, there are several things to avoid. Don't feed high proportions of high-oil feeds such as soybeans or peanuts. The unsaturated vegetable oils will produce a very undesirable soft pork fat. Don't feed much fish scraps or any aromatic foods such as garlic or onions or they will flavor the pork. If you have good pasture for your hogs, you will not have to set aside very much grain for them. Just enough for pregnancy and lactation and for fattening the pigs for slaughter. If you give a 600-pound sow 6 pounds of grain a day during a 114-day pregnancy and 9 pounds of grain a day during an 8-week lactation until the pigs are weaned, that amounts to 1188 pounds of grain for one sow. If it

were 75% corn and 25% oats, this might require around 0.16 A corn
and 0.18 A oats:

900 lb. Corn ÷ 56 lb./bu. = 16 bu ÷ 100 bu/Acre = 0.16 Acres.
300 lb. Oats ÷ 32 lb./bu. = 9.4 bu ÷ 50 bu/Acre = 0.18 Acres

————————   ————————
1200 lb. grain   0.34 Acres

Add a little to this for fattening the pigs and for a small amout of
grain for the boar and non-pregnant sows if necessary to keep them
in good condition. As you can see, it won't take much to support a
few hogs in high style and in most climates they won't need this
much if you provide good pasture.

BREEDING

The way that you go into your hog breeding operation
depends upon how intensively you want to raise them, that is, the
number of sows per laborer on the farm and the type of facilities
you want. Commercial operators have intensified their hog raising
operations to the point that they resemble factories. In order to
raise more hogs, they have built year-round farrowing houses. They
buy their feed rather than raise it themselves and with today's rising
cost of feeds, together with the mortgage payments on the fancy
farrowing houses, commercial hog raisers' margin of profit has nearly
disappeared.

The average boar reaches puberty at 4 to 7 months of age.
They can be used for breeding after this time but should not be used
very often until they are over a year of age. Boars maintain good
breeding capacity until about 5 years. Some farmers keep a male
pig out of the litter, use him for his first breeding season and then
castrate him. This way they do not have to keep a large, mature
boar on their place. A boar castrated after maturity like this is called
a stag. You must wait a month or two after castrating him before
you can slaughter him for food so that his meat will be acceptable.
Uncastrated boars have a terribly strong odor and flavor to the meat.
Most people wouldn't be able to stand cooking it or eating it. I
would recommend this method of keeping only young boars because
older, full-grown boars are so large and, sometimes, so ill-tempered.
When they go into a rutting season, they run or pace up and down
the fence, snapping and slobbering. At this time they will bite and a
large, mature boar can inflict severe wounds. A boar acting this way
is said to be "ranting."

Sows reach puberty at 4 to 5 months of age. You should allow them to reach 250 pounds or so before breeding them. They will still be growing while they are developing their fetuses.

Sows are more difficult than most livestock to detect when they are in heat. Fortunately, the boar knows! This fact makes artificial insemination in hogs less practical than with cattle. The only problem with natural mating of hogs is that they are so big and clumsy that the sow may not be able to support the weight of the boar during mating. You can improve their efficiency by helping them along. Bring the sow in and tie her head to a post or put her in a stanchion or head gate. Put bales of hay or similar supports on either side of her to help support her and the boar during mating. Commercial hog breeders build special chutes with headgates at one end for this purpose. These have ledges on either side for the boar's front feet to rest on. You can detect the sow's heat period if she is in the field when you see her standing still for the boar to mount her. Some sows show other signs of heat by mounting other sows, urinating more often, and maybe having a discharge from the vulva or female opening. Sometimes the vulva will be swollen. Breed them twice on two consecutive days. Her heat period will last 2 to 3 days. Her entire estrous cycle from one heat to the next, is 21 days. Sows cycle pretty much all year-around.

Gestation is 113 to 114 days in most breeds. This is easier to remember as 3 months, 3 weeks, and 3 days.

For the self-sufficient farmer, I recommend that you breed your hogs only at a time of year when the weather will be moderate at farrowing time and that you let them farrow in the pasture. For most climates this means farrowing in late spring or early summer but in places with exceptionally hot summers you should farrow earlier. In warm climates you can farrow your sows twice a year if you can use that much pork or if you can sell it for a profit. Farrowing in a clean, grassy pasture in nice weather is certainly far healthier for sows and pigs than in a dirty, dark, damp barn. Sows with poor mothering ability may lie on some of the piglets, so you may lose a few with pasture farrowing but not as many as if you farrow them in a poorly-kept farrowing house. There, you may lose them all, including the sow, to disease and infection.

For pasture farrowing, provide a small, three-sided or partially open shed for the sow to make a "nest" in. The main requirements are that the shed must have a waterproof roof and be on raised ground so rainwater won't soak the ground under it. Put some straw in the shed or just in front of it and the sow will make her own nest as she wishes. Sows with good mothering ability will raise most of their piglets very well in a natural setting such as this. But when you confine them to a small pen in a barn, they invariably lie on some of the piglets unless you put them in a farrowing crate.

Posts must be sunk in ground or extended to roof and braced to prevent sow from breaking the pen up.

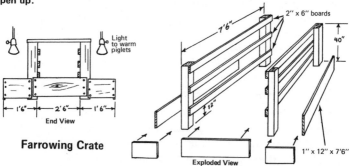

Farrowing Crate

If farrowing time is getting near and the weather is really lousy, you may wish to farrow her indoors. Indoor farrowing should be done in a shelter with a concrete floor for proper cleaning. The temperature should be adjusted to around 65° F (18.3° C) but a range of 40° to 80° F (4.4° to 26.7° C) is acceptable. The floor should be slightly sloping. You will have acceptable results with indoor farrowing only if you build a farrowing crate for the sow. This is a narrow pen just large enough for the sow to lie down in. It has openings at the bottom for the piglets to get out so that they can stay out of the way of the sow. Without a farrowing crate and the sow confined to an indoor area, she will accidentally lie on baby pigs which are against a wall or under the straw. A good farrowing pen is 2½ to 3 feet wide and about 7½ feet long, so there is just room for the sow to lie in but not enough room to turn around. The bottom boards on each side of the pen are 12" above the ground so the baby pigs can get out. There is then a small enclosure on each side to keep the baby pigs confined. Hang heat lamps over the baby pig areas so that the temperature of the floor is about 85° F (29.4° C) for the first few days, then reduce it gradually to ambient temperature over a week's time. Thoroughly disinfect the pen and floor before putting the sow in it. Be sure to provide good ventilation because cold, damp conditions are highly fatal to newborn pigs.

Right after farrowing, inspect all the piglets for defects and wolf-teeth. Most people recommend swabbing the umbilical cords with a 50:50 mixture of glycerine and 7% tincture of iodine. This probably isn't beneficial but it may help dry the cords sooner and therefore prevent infections. Cut off the wolf teeth, the sharp corner incisors, with a sharp, clean pair of nippers or wire cutters. If the teeth aren't erupted yet, inspect them daily and keep them trimmed back. Otherwise the piglets will lacerate the sow's teats when nursing.

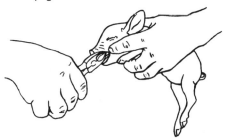

Cutting the sharp milk teeth. Don't leave any sharp fragments showing.

Keep the indoor farrowing pen clean and dry and lightly-bedded with soft, absorbent bedding such as straw. You will probably have to clean it 2 or 3 times a day. If the weather allows, return the sow and her litter to pasture in a week or as soon as possible. Put a shovelful of clean dirt in the baby pigs' pen so they can get nutritional iron. They are not born with much iron reserves and soon become anemic when kept indoors on concrete floors.

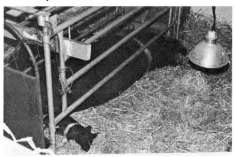

Sow and pigs in farrowing crate

Castrate the male pigs at 2 to 4 weeks of age. This is a simple process but you need to have a veterinarian or an experienced person show you how to do it so that you don't kill too many pigs. In general, you make an incision over each testicle, pull the testicle out and cut or pull out the cord. The operator should have scrubbed his hands and should use a sterile knife. His helper should hold the pigs upside down by the two hind legs, with the front end of the pig between his knees. I would put an antiseptic solution on the area before the operation and maybe antiseptic or antibiotic solution or powder on the wounds afterwards.

There are several devices on the market to hold the pigs so one man can do the castrating, but you will probably have more injuries to the pigs than if someone holds them for you. Don't let them get too big before castration or you will have more problems, especially with bleeding as well as the physical effort of holding them. A pig with a hernia or large bulge in the scrotum or sac holding the testicles is called "busted." Don't castrate one of these yourself or you will have intestines trailing out all over the ground. Have a veterinarian repair the hernia, or if it is not worth the price, or you are too isolated, use it for roast suckling pig, quite a treat!

Wean the pigs at 6 to 8 weeks of age, or at no less than 25 pounds of weight. You can leave them with the sow longer if you wish. Two days before weaning, decrease the sow's ration 20% or just eliminate supplemental feeds if she is on good pasture. This is to reduce her milk production. Move the sow to another end of the farm so the sow and pigs can't hear each other. This will reduce much of the trauma of the weaning procedure. Leave the weanlings on the same pasture and put the sow on something similar so they don't develop digestive upsets from a change of ration. You can start the pigs out on a mixture of cracked or ground corn and oats or another home-grown grain combination. Feed them by "eye" to fatten them to your liking. More grain and dairy products in the ration will make them gain more weight. Ideally, pigs under 25 pounds (sucklings) should get 22% crude protein, 25 to 75 pound pigs 16% C.P., and over 75 pounds, 13%. This is easily within your abilities on a good farm with little more than legumes, grain, and surplus dairy products. Understand that you don't have to fatten the pigs until shortly before slaughtering time. If you wish to raise a barrow to full size for slaughter, feed him on pasture, vegetable trimmings, and other farm waste just to keep him growing. He will be lean during this time. Then fatten him for a month or two.

DISEASES AND PARASITES OF SWINE
Metritis—Mastitis—Agalactia Complex
Cause:

Infection in the uterus and/or mammary glands due to bacteria, commonly *Streptococcus* or *Staphylococcus species* or others, together with such stresses as poor nutrition, too much feed near farrowing time, physical injury to the mammary glands, prolonged or difficult labor, retained placentas or exposure to severe weather. They can also carry an infection which they got from the boar at breeding time.

Signs:

The sow may be depressed, have no appetite and be shivering. She will usually have a fever, usually 105° to 107° F (40.6° - 41.7° C), the higher with gangrenous mastitis. Agalactia means lack of milk. This may be due to mammary gland infection, uterus infection or other stresses. With mastitis (mammary gland infection) she has little milk and the udders are hot and painful when touched. An udder is discolored purple and cool to the touch if it is gangrenous. The piglets act nervous and are noisy because they are hungry. The sow will have a purulent (creamy pus) discharge from her vulva with metritis (uterus infection) or she will have a clear reddish discharge with retained placentas.

Treatment:

The specific problem must be diagnosed and treated. If the sow has dead fetuses inside, she needs surgery or medical treatment by a veterinarian. If the sow is in labor for over 8 hours, it is likely that the pigs will be born dead or will be retained. If the sow has mastitis or metritis, again, she needs treatment, including antibiotics. If no veterinary services are available to you, you need to be especially careful to prevent this farrowing-associated disease complex.

Prevention:

Use your own healthy boar and avoid bringing infections onto your farm by breeding to outside hogs. Give your sows plenty of exercise and good nutrition. This disease complex is most common in sows kept indoors or confined in a very small pen. Prevent stresses such as chilling or overheating. Provide the proper shelter so it is available when the hogs need it. If you should lose a sow you can make up a formula and hand-feed the pigs with nursing bottles. Mix one quart of milk with 7 ounces of cream and 2 ounces or Karo-type syrup. Give each pig 1½ ounces every 2 hours at first, decreasing the frequency and increasing the amount as you go along. If they develop diarrhea, add limewater, thin the milk with water and decrease the amount fed for awhile.

Baby Pig Diarrhea or Nutritional Scours

Cause:

Eating too much milk or supplemental feed together with stresses such as chilling will cause diarrhea in young pigs.

Signs:

The pigs will develop loose, yellow stools with a sour odor. You will usually notice this because the fecal material becomes spread all over the pigs' tails and rear ends. Often the sow's udders will be inflamed (reddened) at the same time. This usually occurs from 1 to 4 weeks after birth and has up to a 25% death rate.

Treatment:

Decrease the sow's feed in order to decrease her milk production. Clean up the pen to get rid of contaminated bedding and eliminate any sources of drafts, chilling or dampness that are putting stress on the pigs. Give the pigs kaopectate or other soothing protectants orally. This can be done with a rubber ear or bulb-syringe by putting the tip in their mouths and giving it slowly. It would help to give them extra water or saline, as well, to fight dehydration.

Salt Poisoning

Cause:

Pigs will accidentally ingest too much salt when their salt box is dumped into a puddle or is rained on, producing a strong brine.

Signs:

The pigs rapidly develop diarrhea and nervous symptoms. They stumble and wander aimlessly. They may fall over, kick their feet and go into severe convulsions. The problem is diagnosed by inspecting the salt box area because the signs and post-mortem findings are not diagnostic.

Treatment:

Those that are not in convulsions can be given water, slowly. Clean up the source of salt and try to prevent a reoccurrence.

Hog Cholera

Cause:

This is a super-contagious, fatal disease of hogs caused by a virus. The disease is reportable to authorities for eradication regulations in most countries. The U.S. has almost eradicated hog cholera but it still poses a very big threat. U.S. hogs are no longer vaccinated so a widespread epidemic would be very destructive.

Signs:

When hog cholera strikes a herd, most of the pigs stop eating, develop diarrhea and get a fever of 105° to 106° F (40.6° to 41.1° C). They develop an eye discharge which is watery at first but then changes to pus. The hogs are very weak and depressed, and they lie around. Most of the hogs in the herd die within a few days. You may notice reddish to purplish hemorrhages in the skin.

Postmortem Signs:

The dead hogs will have hemorrhages in the urinary bladder, kidneys, lymph nodes, spleen and maybe elsewhere.

Transmission:

The hog cholera virus is transmitted in any tissue from an infected hog. Wild and domestic animals can carry it mechanically from one farm to another. Possibly there are carrier pigs, as well.

Prevention:

Get only healthy pigs. If your locale is still vaccinating for hog cholera, be sure your hogs have been vaccinated before you buy them. Stay away from livestock auctions and don't visit commercial hog farms. Disinfect your footwear and change clothes after visiting another farm that has hogs. Never, but absolutely never, feed any garbage from off your farm.

Erysipelas

Cause:

This is a disease of hogs, turkeys and man caused by a bacteria, *Erysipelothrix insidiosa.*

Signs:

This disease takes one of 3 forms: a) in the acute form several hogs in a herd develop a severe fever of 107° to 108° F (41.7° - 42.2° C). It is more common in young pigs. These affected ones become severely depressed. If one is aroused, it will run and then flex its legs as if the joints are sore. Then it will lie down carefully. Young affected pigs may have diarrhea and older ones have constipation. Some may have edema (swelling) of the nose, ears and limbs; b) in the subacute form, the affected animals become depressed, lose their appetites and develop a fever of 106° F (41.1° C) or more. Some may show lameness; c) in the chronic form, hogs develop severe arthritis and lameness with swelling of the joints after having the acute or subacute form. Often they develop patches of cyanosis of the skin with purple blotches over their bodies. These spots later die and slough off in pieces. Parts of the ears and tail may also slough off.

Treatment:

Intramuscular injections of penicillin will reduce the high fevers within 24 hours and prevent deaths or further spread of the disease. This is the way erysipelas is differentiated clinically from hog cholera.

Brucellosis

Cause :

This is a disease affecting swine, man, and other animals caused by a bacteria, *Brucella suis.*

Signs:

Usually the first signs of this disease in your herd are abortions, stillbirths and infertility. You may notice swelling and soreness of the testicles of your boar. Sometimes you will see lameness or ever paralysis in your hogs. You need professional advice and blood tests if you suspect brucellosis in your herd. I would recommend brucella blood testing whenever you have lameness, abortion, or infertility problems. Usually, two blood tests 30 to 60 days apart are done because hogs tend to have false-negative tests.

Prevention and Procedures:

This is such a dangerous and destructive disease that you should cull the entire herd if you have positive test results. Start over with clean hogs on a different field. Be very careful when handling aborted piglets because of the danger of brucellosis to you. Don't touch aborted tissues or pigs if you have a cut on your hand. Use plastic or rubber gloves and burn or bury all aborted tissues. Get your hogs blood-tested right away if you start having abortions. Always scrub your hands well after handling any after-birth tissues.

Leptospirosis

Cause:

There are many different species of *Leptospira* bacteria which affect hogs, cattle, horses, dogs, man, wild animals and rodents.

Signs:

This disease usually shows up in a swine herd by causing abortions, stillbirths, or mummified (dried, dead) fetuses. Live newborn pigs will be weak and squealing. Sows may become weak, feverish and lose their appetites. They will develop uterus infections. It usually spreads slowly in a herd. Affected hogs may have icterus, which is a yellow color to their pink membranes such as the gums and inner eyelids. Often sterility follows infection with leptospirosis. This is a disease that requires professional advice and blood testing to diagnose.

Treatment and Prevention:

This organism is passed in the urine and can spread to humans and to other livestock. Be careful when handling aborted pigs or tissues. Have the herd blood tested if abortions start and, if they are positive for leptospirosis, have the herd treated with antibiotics to try to eliminate any carriers. Then vaccinate for lepto before each breeding. Since rodents can carry and spread it, practice good rodent control. Protect feeds from rodent contamination.

Anthrax

Cause:

Anthrax is a severe and dangerous infection with the bacteria *Bacillus anthracis.* This bacteria can lay dormant in the soil as a spore and can be washed to the surface or onto your farm by floodwaters. It is a common sequel to severe floods. It affects virtually all animals and man.

Signs:

Anthrax appears as a herd outbreak with sudden deaths. Affected animals may be ill for several days, stop eating, lie around, and then develop bleeding from the nose and bloody diarrhea. The discharged blood does not clot well. Affected animals may develop swelling of the throat and difficulty breathing. They have a fever of 105° to 106° F (40.6° to 41.1° C). Animals dead of anthrax are cyanotic, that is, their skin is a dark bluish color.

Treatment and Prevention:

You need professional help for diagnosis and disposition of animals with suspected anthrax. Never cut open a cyanotic-looking carcass yourself. Anthrax is very dangerous to humans and opening the carcass exposes the organisms to air and causes them to form resistant spores. Ill pigs respond to intramuscular injections of penicillin, usually 10 million units per day for 4 or 5 days. Dead carcasses must be burned completely until nothing remains but ash. Don't just bury carcasses if you suspect anthrax. After an anthrax outbreak disinfect all housing and equipment with hot lye. Never use unsterilized meat scraps or bone meal from off your farm as this is a possible source of anthrax spores.

Tuberculosis

Cause:

Swine are susceptible to avian (chickens), human, and bovine (cattle) varieties of the bacillus, *Mycobacterium tuberculosis.*

Signs:

Usually the only signs of T.B. you will see in swine are the lesions that you find in the organs while slaughtering. These lesions usually consist of hard nodules or swellings along the intestinal tract and in the lymph nodes associated with the alimentary tract, including the lymph nodes under the jaw. The lymph nodes of swine with human or avian type T.B. are hard and fibrous but not calcified. if the hog was infected with bovine T.B., it may have nodules throughout the internal organs. These will be swollen areas full of cheesy or liquid material.

Prevention:

Any time you open a carcass for slaughter and find, on the

internal organs, nodules that are hard or filled with cheese or liquid, do not use the carcass for food. If possible, have the affected organs seen by a veterinarian and sent to a lab for positive diagnosis. If the nodules are not a dangerous disease, you can go ahead and use the carcass. If you cannot get the lesions checked, do not take the chance of exposing your family or the other livestock. Burn or deeply bury the carcass. The organisms from a T.B. lesion are extremely dangerous to the person butchering the carcass and the family using it. Prevent active T.B. in your swine herd by slaughtering the older sows and boars (after castrating) and keeping only young hogs for breeding.

Sunburn

White hogs or those with white patches are most susceptible to sunburn. In rare cases, certain plants under certain conditions can sensitize them, making them extremely sensitive to any exposure to the sun.

Treatment and Prevention:

Bring them off pasture and keep them in a barn until the skin is healed. Use soothing lotion or medicated powder on the skin. After the sunburn is healed, put them on a different pasture than before in case there were some photo-sensitizing plants and provide them with adequate sun shades.

Heatstroke

Cause:

Hot weather, no shade, insufficient water or salt and excess exercise, such as with vaccinating or castrating on a hot afternoon, can cause heatstroke.

Signs:

Affected hogs begin to pant excessively, stagger and fall over. Their pink membranes may become pale or cyanotic (bluish-gray color). Some may go into a coma and die.

Treatment:

Cool an affected hog slowly to avoid further shock by putting cool water on its head and legs first, then on its body. If it is a small pig, immerse it slowly in cool water. Continue cooling until the animal's rectal temperature is down to normal (102° F; 38.9° C). Do not do any castrating or other procedures that require chasing the pigs around on a hot day.

Lice

Lice are common external parasites of swine. They are small, light colored, six-legged creatures found on the skin. They lay eggs on the hogs' hairs. The eggs look like little white hardened drops and are called nits.

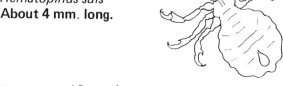

Sucking louse of hogs,
Hematopinus suis
About 4 mm. long.

Treatment and Prevention:
Try to avoid bringing them onto the farm by dusting new hogs with mild insecticide while they are in quarantine. If you have lice on your hogs, use insecticide powder or make an oiler of burlap tied on a chain strung up so they can walk under it and rub against it. Oil it with a non-detergent oil or mineral or vegetable oil. This will discourage louse infestation.

Ascarids or Roundworms
Cause:
This is usually the most destructive internal parasite of hogs. It is a large, long, round, white worm, from 6 to 16 inches long, that lives in the small intestines. There can be so many of these in one hog that they block the intestines or bile duct and cause death. Always check the inside of the intestines when slaughtering to see if you have worm infestations. When bringing new hogs onto your farm, have stool samples checked for parasite eggs. If you have round-

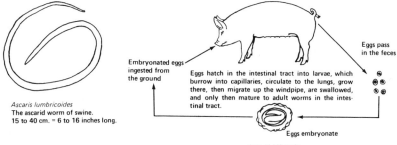

Ascaris lumbricoides
The ascarid worm of swine.
15 to 40 cm. = 6 to 16 inches long.

Embryonated eggs ingested from the ground

Eggs hatch in the intestinal tract into larvae, which burrow into capillaries, circulate to the lungs, grow there, then migrate up the windpipe, are swallowed, and only then mature to adult worms in the intestinal tract.

Eggs pass in the feces

Eggs embryonate

Ascarid Lifecycle
Adult worms live in the intestinal tract.

worms, the hogs can be treated with piperazine, 10 grams per 100 pounds of body weight. If you have ascarids in your herd, they will multiply and become a severe problem. The worm eggs are passed in the bowel movements and the hogs reinfest themselves by eating the eggs.

Be sure to check and treat sows before breeding. Commercial hog raisers use the "MacLean County Swine Sanitation Program" to control ascarids because they become such a problem on commercial swine farms. The System includes worming every sow before breeding her, disinfecting farrowing pens before use, washing each sow with disinfectant before putting her in the farrowing pen, moving the sows with their new litters to pasture in a truck or wagon rather than letting them walk over contaminated barnyards, rotating pastures every 6 months or less and avoiding crowding on pastures. This full system may not be necessary on a small farm but I would recommend rotating pastures. In fact, I would prepare three or more small pastures and rotate them every 6 weeks or even sooner if the hogs eat the forage low to the ground. These same sanitation measures should control stomach worms and coccidia, which are other internal parasites.

Trichinosis
Cause:

Trichinosis is caused by a tiny roundworm parasite that will infest most mammals including man. It is acquired by ingesting infected, poorly cooked or raw meat. Pigs commonly get it by eating dead rats or other wild carnivores which they find in their pen. The rats pass it among themselves by eating the dead members of their own species.

Signs:

Hogs usually show no signs of infection. If signs occur in hogs or other species, the classic signs go by stages. The intestinal stage occurs during the first week with diarrhea, fever, abdominal pain, nausea and vomiting. It can be fatal here. Humans are known to die after eating poorly cooked infected meat, such as when hunting bear or wild hog. The second systemic stage includes loss of appetite, muscular pains, difficult breathing, edema, or fluid in the limbs and low fever. The muscles of respiration, chewing and swallowing are sore and maybe swollen. These signs last from the second week to the fourth or fifth week after exposure. The third, encystation stage usually has no signs unless the infection is severe. The severity of the disease is dependent on the numbers of worm larva ingested with the infested meat. Third stage signs may include muscular stiffness, nervous disorders, heart weakness and breathing difficulty.

Trichinosis occurs only by eating raw or poorly cooked infested meat from carnivores or omnivores such as hogs. Never feed garbage that includes raw meat or offal, even from your own farm. Never throw raw carcasses of dead animals to the hogs. Control rodent habitation on the farm. Cook your ham before eating, even if it was cured and smoked. Destroying the organisms requires thorough cooking so every part of the meat reaches 137° F (58.3° C), or boiling at 212° F (100° C) for 30 minutes or freezing for a prolonged time. Freezing at 5° F (-15° C) requires 20 days to kill the larvae. Thiabendazole, a commercial worm medicine, is specific for the infestation in valuable animals.

Tapeworm Cysts
Cause:

Swine can become infested with the intermediate cyst stage of several species of tapeworms. The species are *Taenia hydatigena,* the tapeworm of dogs, cats and other animals, which produces cysts in the liver and abdominal cavity; *Echinococcus granulosus,* of dogs and others, which produce cysts in the liver, lungs and other tissues; and the human tapeworm, *Taenia solium,* which produce small cysts in the connective tissues of the muscles and nervous system. The latter is called "pork measles" for the cysts, 6 to 10mm by 5 to 10mm in size, in the muscle tissue of pork. *Taenia solium* and *Echinococcus granulosus* are extremely dangerous to get on your farm because people, especially children by their unsanitary habits, can become the intermediate hosts and develop tapeworm cysts in their own internal organs.

Prevention:

Never let dogs or any other carnivores defecate in the hog pen or pasture. The same goes for farm laborers. Tapeworm is common among migrant laborers and contributes greatly to "pork measles" which is found at commercial packing houses. Always trim out areas of meat that have small clear or whitish cysts. Cook meat well. Never eat raw or poorly-cooked meat. Never feed raw meat or offal to your dogs, cats or hogs.

12
Poultry Management and Veterinary Care

SELECTION OF CHICKENS

There is a great deal of variation among breeds of chickens. Some breeds are tremendous egg-layers but lousy mothers while other breeds are good meat producers but poor layers. The commercial poultry industry has bred the White Leghorn breed for specialization. The hens are small, and therefore eat less food, yet they lay hundreds of eggs per year, averaging sometimes almost one per day. Commercially, these breeds are usually kept in small cages in huge batteries. Their life is so artificial that they seldom live over a few years. The White Leghorns have become such poor mothers that they can only be raised by incubating the eggs and brooding the chicks artificially. A White Leghorn hen won't set a clutch of eggs consistently enough to even hatch them. I doubt if this is the type of chicken you would be interested in for a self-sufficient farm or homestead, no matter how many eggs they lay. There are three types of breeds: layers, meat producers, and general-purpose chickens that produce both eggs and meat reasonably well. White Leghorns are layers. They produce a great number of medium-sized white eggs. Mature hens average around 3 pounds and are flighty, nervous and poor mothers. They are also poor at foraging food for themselves. Minorcas are another breed of layers. There are White, Black and Buff Minorcas. They lay extra-large white eggs but not as many as Leghorns. Minorcas are also poor mothers. Plymouth Rocks are a general purpose breed. There are White and Barred varieties. Barred Plymouth Rocks have fine black and white stripes resembling bars. Mature hens average 8 pounds. They lay brown eggs. Rhode Island Reds are a slightly smaller general purpose breed. Mature hens average 7 pounds but they lay larger eggs than Plymouths, also brown. New Hampshires are a good early-maturing, early-laying general purpose breed. The meat type breeds are very poor layers so you will not be interested in them but they cross well with the other breeds. If you have several breeds together on your farm, you will get crossbred chickens. If you cross Cornish birds or other meat-type breeds with layers or general-purpose breeds, you will often get some very good general-purpose chickens. Cross-bred birds are often hardy and self-sufficient because of hybrid vigor.

There are many "fancy" breeds of chickens. These are chickens that are raised mainly for exhibition because of their fancy colors or feathering. One of these breeds, the Araucana, is very well-suited for a small farm. This breed lays eggs of various bright colors. Breeders call them "Easter egg chickens". But besides this unusual characteristic, Araucanas are one of the most independent self-sufficient breeds. They forage very well for themselves and so require less feed.

We can't neglect to mention Bantams. Almost every family farm I have been on has a few Bantam chickens. We always call them "Banties". They are very self-sufficient birds but they won't provide much meat or eggs because they are very small. They are great to have around a manure pile or under the rabbit hutches because they will eat all the fly maggots and other pests. The one point that I would make about Banties, though, is that you should keep them separated from your other chickens. Keep your meat and egg birds in an enclosure and let the Banties roam free but don't let them "socialize" with your meat and laying birds. This is because your Banties will live longer and maybe develop tuberculosis or carry parasites.

I would recommend that you set up your poultry operation for minimum work on your part and maximum health and self-sufficiency for the chickens. Don't bother with a high-production laying breed that you have to incubate and brood by hand. Take the time to set up proper housing and fencing for their health and safety and then get chickens that take care of themselves and raise their own chicks. After all, chickens that are foraging and getting a good variety of nutrients, fresh air and sunshine will he healthier and raise healthy chicks. Hens that are good mothers have a better hatching percentage and reproduction rate than you can get with artificial incubating and brooding.

There are several ways that you can get into the poultry business and your method of doing so may be critical to your success. You can get fertilized eggs, day-old chicks, started chicks, or ready-to-lay pullets, all from a commercial hatchery. Some people buy culls or aged hens from a commercial poultry farm. I feel that it is extremely important for you to start out right, get disease-free birds, and put them on land that has not had poultry on it for a number of years. Therefore, I recommend that you not bring culls or even started chicks onto your farm. They will too often carry diseases or parasites. I would get fertilized eggs or day-old chicks from a reputable hatchery or from a private farm. You will then have to brood the chicks or incubate and brood the eggs yourself but this is a small price to pay in order to get disease-free chickens on your farm.

The only time you really need to incubate and brood poultry is when you are bringing new birds onto your farm or starting a new flock. Be sure that your eggs or day-old chicks are from a source that guarantees them to be pullorum-free. Pullorum is a disease we will discuss later. It is extremely destructive and you don't want it on your farm, ever! If you buy day-old chicks, you can get either pullets or straight-run chicks. The pullets will be female chicks that the hatchery has picked out or "sexed." Because chicks are difficult to tell the sex, you will still get 5 to 10% cockerels (males). If you order straight-run, unsexed chicks, you will usually get a little over 50% males, the normal ratio, unless the hatchery is disreputable and sends you extra males. I would recommend that you get straight-run chicks because they will have been handled less and therefore have less chance of carrying parasites or diseases. Since you will have lots of cockerels, you will have an excellent supply of poultry meat within a few weeks and from then on. The pullets won't usually begin to lay for 5 or 6 months but you will get edible cockerels, 2 to 3 pounds each, at only 8 to 12 weeks of age. They are then very tender broilers. There is no other species of livestock that could give you edible meat in such a short time unless you bought pregnant rabbits or a fattened calf or pig ready to slaughter. Because of the high quality of the protein in their meat and eggs and the ease of keeping them, I think most people will definitely want poultry on their place.

HOUSING AND EQUIPMENT

Housing and pasture management are just as important with poultry as they are with other species of livestock although you wouldn't think it to see the arrangement most farmers have. The fact that poultry survive what most people do to them just means that they are tough and do well in spite of their owners.

Housing requirements for poultry are just common sense needs like shelter from wind and precipitation, good ventilation and sanitation or regular cleaning, but poultry have a few problems that make managing them more difficult. They are very dusty creatures and their food tends to be dusty and their manure makes a great deal of ammonia. You can actually cause blindness by putting them in a small building with no ventilation. The ammonia fumes get so strong that their eyes absorb it and become cloudy. But there are ways to arrange your poultry housing so it is comfortable for the birds and nearly labor-free.

First, consider where you will locate your chickens. I would put the poultry area near your house because you will be visiting it at least 3 times a day. Put it downwind of the house on high or sloping ground. If you have shade trees in that direction, put the hen house where it will get afternoon summer shade. If you have a large number of chickens, you can set them up in a garage, a large hen house or part of your barn, but if you have a small number, I would recommend that you build a small hen house.

Design your hen house so it has at least 2½ square feet of floor space per chicken. If it's too small they will be crowded and develop health problems. If it's too big they won't be able to keep it warm with their own body heat in cold weather. You must have windows that you can open for ventilation and for hot weather. These must have window screens to keep out bugs and wild birds. Then put a Sheringham ventilation window at the ceiling and a small hole at the floor, also screened and covered with hardware cloth, for vertical ventilation and to let the ammonia escape. Ammonia is heavier than air and stays near the floor.

Accumulated poultry manure is very objectionable for several reasons. It is very compact and therefore very heavy to shovel. One

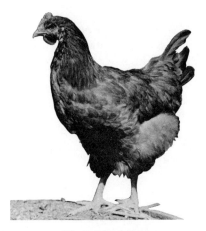

Rhode Island Red hen

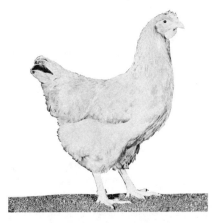

New Hampshire Red hen

hen will deposit about 120 pounds of manure per year. After it has accumulated for awhile it becomes dry and dusty. In some parts of the midwestern U.S., poultry can carry Histoplasmosis which they catch from wild birds. A person shoveling manure from these infected chickens may catch the disease himself. There is nothing dustier and dirtier than shoveling poultry manure out of a small, unventilated hen house. You need to wear a bandana or facemask.

There are several ways to get around this problem and I highly recommend you adopt one of them or think up a better one of your own. The ways are to have a door large enough to use a tractor with a hydraulic loader, to use built-up litter methods or to have the henhouse on skids so it can be pulled off the built-up manure. Another factor in your planning is that you need to have roosts, which are just horizontal poles, in the henhouse. The birds sleep on the roosts and deposit most of their manure under them. If you have a large number of chickens and keep them in a garage or barn, I would put the roosts in front of a large door in bleacher-like fashion. Then you can clean under the roosts by opening the big door and maybe using a tractor with a front-loader. When you want to clean out the entire house, just move the roosts. If you have a small number of chickens and a correspondingly small henhouse, you should still build the roosts like bleachers and have a low, wide door behind them for cleaning. If you wish to put a small-size henhouse on skids for moving, you should install a floor of strong heavy-guage hardware cloth or wire mesh. This will allow the manure to drop through but will keep out small predatory animals like rats, weasels foxes, etc. If you don't have some type of concrete foundation or heavy wire mesh floor, you will lose a lot of chickens and eggs because the predators will burrow into the henhouse. If you build the house on skids, when the manure builds up, pry up the skids with a bar or pole to break them lose from the ground and move the whole house with a tractor or horses. In warm climates, some people put the poultry house up on poles. I wouldn't do this in a cold climate because this type of housing isn't as warm. If you do put it on poles, be sure to install a covering of galvanized sheet metal around each pole so the rodents can't climb up to the henhouse.

No matter what the size of the henhouse, I would recommend that you use the bleacher-style roosts with a large door behind them for easy cleaning and then use the built-up litter method for the rest of the house. Put chicken wire around the sides of the roosts and directly under the poles so the chickens can't get underneath it.

The built-up or deep litter method is a rediscovery of a natural way to handle manure. Commercial operations evolved over

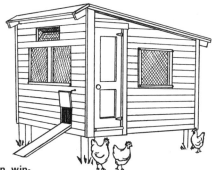

Chicken house. Note top ventilation window, window screens and plenty of ventilation.

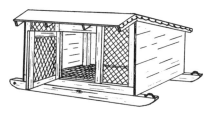

Small poultry house on skids. Wire floor for sanitation. Small chicken entry and nest box doors in rear.

the years to the point of keeping chickens in wire cages and scraping the manure out from under them with automatic,timed scrapers. Now we have come full circle and found that chickens are healthier in a natural environment, scratching around in properly-managed deep litter. This is a deep layer of litter or "mulch" and manure which you build up over a period of time. The mixture "works" or composts by natural bacterial action. If it is working properly, it has little odor or dust and the pathogenic bacteria and parasite eggs from the chickens become inactivated. Start the deep litter by putting down 4 to 6 inches of suitable clean litter material such as straw, ground corn cobs, wood shavings, peanut hulls or bark chips on a clean henhouse floor. When you put the chickens on the new litter, add a thin topping of more clean litter every few days for 3 to 4 weeks. Then just top-dress it weekly or more, whenever the manure begins to be evident. Stir the litter occasionally to keep it dry. The deep litter should be cleaned out and started new about twice a year. However, if an area of the litter becomes soaked with spilled water or too much manure, it "spoils" or becomes anaerobic and smells. This section should then be cleaned out. The only drawback to this litter method is that when it comes time to clean it out, there is a lot of material to move. If you have power equipment, though, it has a great advantage. Even if you don't, most farmers would rather make a big job of it and work like mad to clean out a barn twice a year than to have to shovel out a piddling amount every few days. This is what you are faced with if you use the "clean-floor" method of putting down just a little bit of litter to absorb the moisture. Then, if you don't clean it several times a week, it becomes a stinking,heavy mass. And if you let this go long enough, the bottom layers become packed into a concrete-like slab. In an old neglected poultry house the manure almost has to be chipped out. The idea of the built-up litter is to keep it fluffy and dry on top.

Even with the built-up litter method you will probably need to clean regularly under the roosts. The chickens will often deposit more manure under the roosts than your built-up litter can handle. If so, put chicken wire under the roost poles and around the sides of the roosts to keep them out of this accumulation and clean it out as needed. If you have plenty of roost-space, though, try just adding extra litter under the roosts.

I would recommend that your henhouse have a full-size door for your convenience but a miniature door for the chickens.

Their door should be only large enough for them to enter. It can have a ramp up to it and a secure hinged door. Keep the large door closed and then if you forget to close the small door, no large dogs can get inside the henhouse. Foxes and other small predators could still enter, though, so you should always secure all the doors at night.

If you have severe rodent problems, put the henhouse on a concrete slab and nail sheetmetal flashing all around the walls at the foundation and around the bottoms of the doors and doorjams. Rats can chew out the corner of a door in one night's time.

You should provide range (pasture) space for your chickens. Many homesteaders just let the chickens run loose on the farm and forage most of their food for themselves. I don't recommend this casual an attitude because of natural predators. Neighborhood dogs and cats, even your own, and all the local wild carnivorous animals and birds just love to dine on fresh chicken or baby chicks. Owls and hawks will take a great toll in most areas of the country. The only way that free ranging your chickens will work is if your farm has lots of trees and bushes so the chickens have plenty of natural cover. Even then you will lose some to foxes, hawks, cats and other predators. If owls and hawks are a problem in your area, your outdoor ranges must be covered with chicken wire on top. I have even heard of owls landing on top of the wire, frightening the birds until they fly into the air and then biting off any chicken heads that are unlucky enough to poke through the wire. People with this problem must then construct chicken pens with double ceilings of two layers of chicken wire 4 inches apart. This is done by putting horizontal 2" X 4" supports over the top of the pen and tacking a layer of chicken wire to the tops and a second layer to the bottoms of the supports. If you don't need to put tops on your chicken pens, then set up two or three large yards or ranges for them. Fence them with wire that is fine enough to keep out predators. If the predators burrow under the fences, you can dig a trench around the range, set the fence in the trench and back-fill it so the bottom 6 inches or so are underground. If this still doesn't foil the diggers, then try again laying about 6 to 12 inches of the fence wire horizontally in the bottom of the trench, outside of the vertical portion of the fence. When the varmints try to dig under the fence, they will run into the horizontal portion of fencing.

The reason to provide two or three ranges instead of one is for rotation, to allow the vegetation to grow and parasite eggs to dry out and die. Turn the chickens into one pen or range at a time and let them dig and chew it up. When they have worn that one down a little, rotate them to another one for awhile. Plant a variety of grasses or vegetables or whatever you have and water it if needed for good growth. If the chickens are able to reduce all the ranges to bare ground before the first one has re-grown, then you need more range space. This is the criterion for how large to make your ranges or pens.

If you have fenced ranges instead of pens with tops, you may have trouble with chickens flying over the fence. Some breeds of chickens are better flyers than others. The way to ground them and keep them at home is to clip their wings. Whatever you do, don't clip both wings on each bird. You can clip them down to the nubs and the bird will still fly -- they just have to work harder at it. The way to do it properly is to clip the flight feathers on one wing only. This puts them off-balance and they will stay on the ground.

If you have fenced ranges there are several ways to rotate them. For a large operation with lots of chickens and a big hen-house, place the fences so they form four ranges around the house, with the fences attached to the sides of the house. Place a miniature door in each side of the henhouse, one leading into each range. Then you can control the range rotation by whichever door you open for them. If you have a small operation with a small henhouse, put the house on skids and pull it to a new location when you want to rotate ranges. If you have small covered pens, you can have an alleyway or separate doors to the pens to control the chickens' access to them. If you are really lazy and just let the chickens roam free, coax them into the henhouse each evening with food and water and lock them in so they will be safe from predators at night.

Your poultry equipment can be as simple or as fancy as you wish to make it. I would advise against using open pans or buckets for feed and water because of their habits of contaminating everything with manure. Poultry waterers are very inexpensive and simple. They usually consist of a jar turned upside down in a shallow pan. Water automatically re-fills the pan as it is used. This provides a constant source of clean water. You can devise an automatic watering system with any airtight container that feeds into a pan. Water won't run into the pan until the water level is low enough to allow some air up into the container, which relieves some of the vacuum and lets some water out. But you should have some type of cover above the water so the birds don't walk in it or stand on the edge of the pan and defecate in it. The easiest way to feed is to just scatter it on the ground and let them peck around but this is also rather wasteful. I would recommend a trough which is covered with parallel wire rods or with hardware cloth (wire mesh) with holes about 1" square. The wire prevents the birds from slinging the food out of the trough while they are pecking through it looking for their favorite grain. Poultry troughs or food hoppers should have a rotating dowel or cover above them so the birds can't sit on the trough and foul it. Another method of feeding chickens is to hang up a bucket that has small holes drilled in the bottom of it. The holes must be the right size for the grain you are feeding so the chickens can peck it out of the holes but it won't run out by itself. Cover the bucket and hang it just high enough that the chickens reach up for the food. You can feed millet and similar grains without threshing by hanging them by the stalks just off the floor.

Roosts should be made of 2" by 4" boards with the thin side up or of well-cured, not green, limbs or saplings. I would set them up so the poles are 12" apart and each one is 6" higher than the one in front of it, so they are arranged like bleachers. Allow at least 12" of roosting space per bird. I would recommend that you provide extra space so they can huddle together near the ceiling in cold weather or spread out for comfort in hot weather. Enclose the roost area to keep chickens out from under it because of the large accumulation of manure. Arrange the roost so you can move it or remove the poles so you can get under or behind it for easy cleaning.

Nest boxes are where the hens lay their eggs (you hope) and brood their chicks. Make them in a row by building a long box with partitions and a slanted roof. The box is usually 2 ft wide and the partitions are placed every 12 inches so each nest box is 1' by 2'. The partitions should be 8 to 10 inches high and the open front of the nest box about 6 inches high. The roof is placed 18 to 24 inches above the nest boxes and is slanted steeply so chickens won't roost on top of it. Put the nest boxes 2½ to 3 feet above the floor and put a walk or roost pole in front of the nests. I would recommend that you have hinged doors in the back of the nest boxes so you can approach them and remove eggs without disturbing the chickens in the nests. The nest boxes could be placed on the henhouse wall and the access doors could be opened from the outside so you don't even have to enter the henhouse to gather eggs. Keep clean, fresh litter such as straw in the nest boxes. Provide at least one nest box for

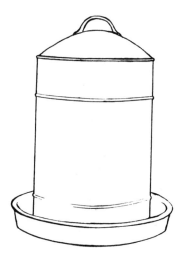

Large galvanized waterer

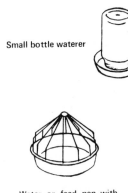

Small bottle waterer

Water or feed pan with
wire roost-guard

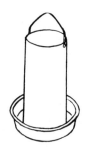

Hanging feeder. Keep a top on it..

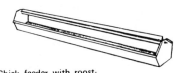

Chick feeder with roost-
guard roller across the top

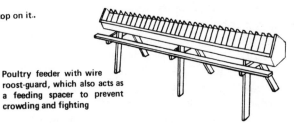

Poultry feeder with wire
roost-guard, which also acts as
a feeding spacer to prevent
crowding and fighting

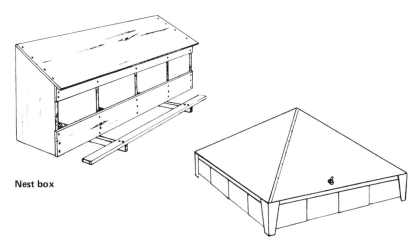

Nest box

Electric brooder with curtains

every 3 or 4 hens. Keep plenty of clean, dry litter in the nest boxes to prevent broken or dirty eggs and egg-eating by the chickens.

CHICKEN FEED

Poultry need a variety of feedstuffs with a high quality of protein. Commercial feeds have of course evolved to a high degree of complication. In general the commercial feeds are of the "all-mash" types or the "mash and scratch" types. In the all-mash formulas, the computer-selected feedstuffs, chosen for nutrition and cost, are all ground finely and mixed. The ration may be put up in small pellets to prevent dust and waste. Some people feed both the ground mash and the pelleted form. In the mash and scratch formulas, the mash is a finely-ground variety of feeds, mostly high-protein concentrates, and the scratch is a mixture of whole or cracked grains. Together, the mash and scratch provide a complete formula. Obviously you must purchase matched formulas of mash and scratch from the same company so they will be nutritionally complete. Since the chickens will prefer the grain scratch to the dusty, powdery mash, the mash is left out in feeders all the time but the scratch is fed in measured quantities.

Remember when studying the literature available on feeding poultry that commercial feeds are designed for pushing birds to maximum production in crowded, unhealthy conditions. These same birds are usually on constant antibiotics and coccidiostats to hold down disease and parasites.

For the purposes of self-sufficiency, you should never be pushing for maximum production,although you will probably get excellent results if you raise your livestock in a healthy environment. Also, for self-sufficiency,you need to produce your own home-grown poultry ration. This should consist of a variety of grains, fresh, growing greens, calcium-phosphorus supplement, salt, grit, and constantly-available fresh water. Since your birds will be scratching around in the dirt rather than being confined in tiny wire cages, they should get plenty of grit on their own unless your soil has no coarse sand. I would recommend that you stockpile just under a pound of salt per bird per year and maybe 3 pounds of calcium supplement per hen per year. This can be ground oyster shells or any of the regular calcium-phosphorus supplements. You should re-feed all your egg shells by drying them in the oven and mashing them.

You need to plan on several types of rations. For young birds I recommend both mash and scratch. Scratch is the whole or coarsely-ground grains. Chickens have their preferences for food so they will eat the grains they like best and leave the others. Their preferences may keep them from getting a balanced ration unless you feed mash. This is a finely ground and well-mixed, balanced variety of grains and supplements. Since the birds can't pick their favorite items out of the mash, they get a better balance. You must limit the amount of scratch you give them and leave the mash out all the time to get them to eat it. A chick-and-growing mash is very finely ground so the little chicks can eat it. For most climates,for chick-and-growing mash you can mix equal parts of yellow corn meal (white corn has little vitamin A), ground wheat and ground oats. These can be ground in a home flour mill. If available, add 10% fish meal, meat meal, alfalfa meal, dried milk solids,or some other protein supplement. Add 2% calcium supplement such as bonemeal. Add salt equal to 1% of the ration and mix it *very* well. Other supplements that could be used, if available, would be such as 1 or 2% brewer's yeast, 1 or 2% wheat germ, 1% kelp,and cod liver oil in small amounts. When you feed mash, keep it in a clean trough or feeder and check it daily for wet or moldy spots by stirring it. Whenever you have a molded spot, empty the trough, scrub it and dry it before using.

Chick scratch consists of finely cracked grains such as cracked yellow corn, cracked wheat, ground oats, pinheat oats or other cracked grains. Growing scratch is more coarse, such as medium cracked corn, cracked wheat and oats. The grains you use can vary with your area, but try to formulate a ration as high in protein as you can without using more than about a third wheat.

Laying hens can be fed both mash and scratch or, if they are good at foraging and have a large, productive range, just feed scratch because it is simpler and they should be able to get their own protein supplements from forage and from the worms and grubs they dig up. Their scratch is coarsely ground or whole grains. Hard grains like corn or milo should be cracked. Small or soft grains like oats and wheat can be whole or crushed. The calcium supplement can be mixed in the mash at the rate of about 4% of the total ration for layers or 1% for growing birds but it will work out better if you just let them eat it free-choice out of protected self-feeders. The same with the salt at 1% of the ration. If your growing or laying chickens aren't getting enough protein and are doing poorly, that is, gaining poorly and laying poorly, you can add protein to their diet with protein supplements or with surplus dairy products. The only problem here is one of sanitation. Any feeder in which you put a milk product must be thoroughly scrubbed out later that same day.

You can plan that your chickens will eat about 90 to 100 pounds of feed per adult bird per year. Therefore you can plan on your needs for grain. If you figured that they would get at least 20% from foraging, that would leave 80 lbs. per bird. For forty chicken, you would then need 3200 pounds per year. If you calculated that as half corn, a quarter wheat and a quarter oats, you would need approximately:

1600 lb corn	÷	56 lb/bu	=	28½	bu	÷	100 bu/A	=	0.29 A corn
800 lb oats	÷	32 lb/bu	=	25	bu	÷	50 bu/A	=	0.50 A oats
800 lb wheat	÷	60 lb/bu	=	13-1/3 bu		÷	30 bu/A	=	0.44 A wheat
									1.23 Acres

This is just an example but it is very liberal and yet it doesn't require very much acreage. For your own purposes, you must use the data for yields and requirements for your local area.

There are lots of things you can feed your chickens for extra variety. You can grow some millet. Harvest it leaving the stalks on the heads and tie them in small bundles. Hang a bundle or two in the henhouse so the birds can reach it but it is off the floor. Grow sunflower seeds and feed them whole. Feed kitchen scraps such as bread and vegetable trimmings. You could even feed dry, grated meat scraps. In the winter, I would recommend that you sprout seeds and feed the sprouts or else put the sprouts in the sun and grow greens for the poultry. One thing to avoid is barley grain because they may choke on the coarse "beard." Barley must be processed (de-bearded) before being fed to chickens.

In conclusion, I would set up a chicken operation so that the birds have lots of room and a variety of feedstuffs, including forage. Cultivate, lime and water their ranges. Then let them get their own grit and protein supplements. Don't try to push them for maximum production. The harder you try to push their diet and control their production, the more problems you will probably have.

MANAGEMENT AND CULLING OF LAYERS

Even though I recommend letting your chickens forage for themselves and live in a natural environment and social order, that does not mean I have casual attitudes toward management. Proper management of your hens is imperative or you won't be satisfied with your poultry operation. Fortunately there are just a few important points of management of layers. These are feeding, confinement for egg-gathering, breeding, culling and depopulation. I recommend that you become familiar with the natural life cycle of chickens and then follow a few basic principles of flock management.

Most hens will start to lay at around 5 to 7 months of age. It is important that you have nest boxes available when they first start because each hen will develop a habit of laying her eggs in the same place each time, even if it is in a dirty corner of the house or under a bush somewhere. Line the nest boxes with clean litter of a type that is fluffy and soft. Straw or dry grass is preferable to something like sawdust or shavings because the hens can shape the nest to their liking. It might help if you try to put each young hen in a nest box just to acquaint her with it before they start laying. They will of course jump right out but that is no problem. Their curiosity will bring them back later. Once they start laying you should inspect all the nest boxes daily. Change the litter in them whenever it becomes dirty or at least every few weeks.

One of the main reasons to confine your chickens in a hen house each night is to make egg-gathering easier, as well as to protect them from predators. Visit the henhouse very early each morning and gather eggs but don't let the   hens out then. Open the windows if the weather will be warm. Some of the hens will lay quite early and others will wait until almost noon. Return to the henhouse around noon, gather the rest of the morning's eggs and then let the chickens out to forage the rest of the day. This method will allow you to easily gather most of the eggs your hens produce. It is much easier than hunting all over the field or barnyard and it prevents the misfortune of gathering an old, spoiled egg and cracking it into a bowl of other ingredients. Speaking of which, I would recommend that you always crack each egg into a bowl or saucer by itself rather than directly into the pot. This enables you to inspect it for abnormalities so you can dispose of it if it doesn't suit you. Some of your family members may balk at eating an egg with a blood-spot on the yolk (fertilized). There is nothing wrong with a fertilized egg unless you plan to store it. Fertilized eggs store poorly over a long period of time. You can easily "candle" your eggs, as described later, if you are putting them in cold storage for several months. Be sure you don't store your eggs near onions, garlic or other strong or aromatic items.

There are many types of abnormalities of eggs, some of which can be diagnosed and corrected. Odd-shaped eggs are usually due to heredity or are seen at the very beginning of a hen's production or when she is getting old. Thin, soft-shelled eggs may be due to old age of the hen, heredity, extremely hot weather, inadequate dietary calcium, phosphorus, manganese or vitamin D or excess phosphorus. This can also occur when the hen was terribly frightened the night before she laid the thin-shelled egg. Exceptionally rough shells can be hereditary or from excess dietary calcium. High levels of certain drugs can also cause it.

When you crack an egg into a saucer, the white should remain close and thick around the yolk, not spread out thin and watery. This is one of the major criteria of grading eggs. Thin egg albumen (whites) can be caused by extremely hot weather, high levels of ammonia fumes in the hen house, heredity, old hens, prolonged storage or storage at the wrong temperature and humidity. Blood in the whites can be hereditary or due to hemorrhage in the oviduct for some reason. Blood spots on or in the yolks are due to fertilization of the egg, hereditary characteristics, vitamin A deficiency, old hens, or maybe severe fright. Exceptionally dark yolks are usually due to pigments in the diet. Brownish green yolks may be due to one of the worm medicines, piperazine, or due to the chemical, gossypol, from cottonseed oil meal in their diet. Gossypol may also cause pink, colored whites and mottled yolks. Mottled yolks may also be due to excess ammonia fumes or certain chemicals in the diet.

Off-flavored eggs may be due to feeding fish meal in the diet or from storing the eggs near melons, onions, apples, or other foods with special odors.

If you wish to get maximum production from your hens, you will probably become interested in controlling their lighting. Laying decreases in winter with the shorter period of daylight. You can provide artificial "daylight" by simply lighting the henhouse. This fools the chickens' natural control system and stimulates them to lay more. For this program, you need to use 40-watt bulbs, placed about 7 feet from the floor, with one bulb per 200 square feet of floorspace. You must keep the bulbs clean so they provide the necessary light and you must have them on so the artificial day is 14 hours long. Timer switches are available to accomplish the proper lighting intervals. These are available from poultry supply sources.

The most important and most difficult part of poultry management is proper culling. In general, you want to cull the unhealthy ones, the poor layers and the excess cockerels, but it will take a long time and lots of experience to learn to be efficient at culling. The unhealthy, poor layers will usually appear thin and "dull." They have narrower heads and beaks. When you pick them up and feel them, they have narrower backs and breasts and less meat on their bones. Their combs tend to be pale colored, dull, and maybe somewhat shriveled. Their eyes may be rather dull and sunken. Their feathers appear more dull and unkempt and these birds are less active. They are called "boarders" and should be culled. Another type of boarder is the pullet that never begins to lay. These are harder to detect. They usually appear more immature, with a brighter yellow color to their beaks and feet. They have small, dry, puckered vents while an active layer has a round, moist vent. If you cannot detect any differences in the appearances of your chickens, you should confine them to separate areas or pens until you determine which ones are laying. This will help you learn to recognize the differences.

Chickens moult or shed their feathers and grow new ones in the fall. When they moult, they usually stop laying. The hens which moult first, early in the season, should be culled because they aren't as economical to keep over for another season. The first laying season is their best and the ones which moult early, especially before September, will have the poorest long-run egg production. These should go to the roasting pan or stew pot. They are too old and tough for frying.

Another management problem you may have is that of a good

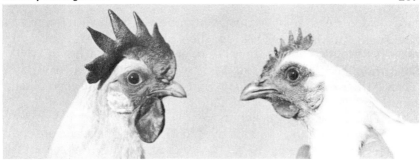

Good producer on the left compared to non-layer on the right, White Leghorn hens.

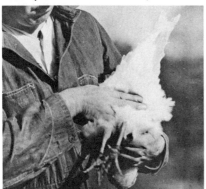 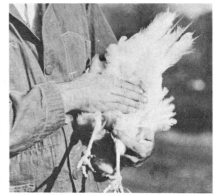

The pelvic bones and pelvic inlet are narrow in the non-laying hen and wide in the laying hen.

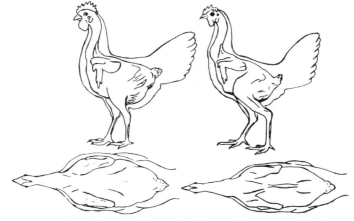

If you had X-ray vision, culling would be easier. The good layers, as well as the good meat bird, should have a body that is deep, broad, and well-developed. The back should be broad and flat, the sternum or keel should be long and full with a full breast. Eyes should be alert, not sunken and dull. You must examine the bird by feeling it to detect these characteristics.

layer which stops laying in the fall but doesn't moult with the rest of the flock. This is serious because she won't begin to lay again until after her moult. You can force her to moult by putting her in a darkened room and fasting her by giving water but not food for 3 days. Then let her out and feed bland food like oats. She will then usually moult and begin laying again.

Of course, the cockerels are the other birds that you cull. Cockerels reach 2 to 3 pounds by 8 to 12 weeks of age and are good broilers, very tender. By 12 to 14 weeks of age they average 3 to 4 pounds or more and are good fryers. From 14 weeks to 6 months of age, or over 4 pounds, they are roasters. Over 6 months, they become tough and are stew-pot meat. The most important point about culling cockerels is to save the best, healthiest, strongest ones for breeding. Don't cook up your best breeding stock, whatever you do. Save at least 1 rooster for every 10 or 12 hens.

The guiding principle of breeding all your livestock is to constantly upgrade your herd or flock by always choosing the best producers, the healthiest, most sound individuals and the ones with the desired characteristics for breeding. You will be accomplishing this if you regularly cull the poor individuals and use them for food and allow the best roosters and hens to socialize in a natural way. Your only problem is if you allow yourself to keep too many roosters or if you get too many "broody" hens. Broody hens are those that want to set continuously. They do a fine job of raising chicks but they stop laying while they are brooding. You can either let a broody hen build up a clutch of up to 15 eggs and hatch them out or you can try to break her. If she isn't laying, you can slip some other hens' eggs under her and hope they are fertile. If you wish to break a brooding hen, put her in a wire cage in the middle of the hen house. Give her food and water but keep her confined for several days. This may break her for awhile.

Natural breeding and brooding has it all over artificial incubation and brooding of chicks. If you do an excellent job of operating an incubator you still won't get as good a hatching percentage as an average mother hen. You will usually lose more chicks during the brooding period than the hens do, too. However, there are several situations where you should do your own incubating and brooding. The first, as mentioned before, was when you buy your first batch of day-old chicks or fertilized eggs to start your poultry operation. The other situation is the occasional de-population of the flock. De-population is done for the control of dangerous diseases and parasites.

Killing off an entire flock and starting a completely separate, new flock may seem cruel to some people and just a lot of extra work to others but I will tell you later why it is necessary. When we discuss poultry diseases you will see that there are many parasites and diseases that build up in a flock and their environment. Some of these diseases are dangerous to your other livestock and to your family, such as avian tuberculosis. Most of these diseases are caught from wild birds or other animals then they build up in your flock over a period of a few years. Even the diseases and parasites that are not dangerous to you or your other livestock will build up in a flock of chickens until they become very unthrifty and unproductive. Eventually you will become very dissatisfied with your flock and you will be quite ready to depopulate them. But if you wait until this time, your dairy animals and hogs may have contracted t.b. because of its concentration in the flock. You must realize that throughout the history of man, his production and the production of livestock has been severely hampered by diseases and parasites. In just the last few decades modern technology has conquered most of these. Now, commercial producers are able to concentrate their livestock, but they often over-do it by relying on drugs and chemicals. The self-sufficient farmer must avoid both the natural diseases and the man-made problems of crowded livestock production. I would recommend that you depopulate your chicken flock every 3 years at least. Start this by rounding up a large batch of fertilized eggs. If you have some chickens that are better producers, isolate them from the others, put the roosters with them and collect their eggs. Collect at least 2 times as many eggs as the number of chickens you want in the new flock. Remember that over 50% will be cockerels and many will be infertile or the chicks will die. Clean each egg with warm water and a soft cloth to remove all dirt and discharges. Put the eggs in the incubator in an area isolated from the rest of the chickens. From now on, the new "flock" will have no contact or contamination from the old. Wash your hands well before handling the incubator or eggs. Sterilize any equipment that will be used for brooding the new chicks. After you have hatched a satisfactory number of new chicks, brood them somewhere apart from the old chickens and where no other chickens have been for several years. While you are raising your new flock to laying age, you must steadily kill off the old flock for the table. When the old flock is gone, carefully sterilize all their equipment and disinfect their housing. If possible, use new housing for the new flock. The new flock should be put on ranges that weren't used for chickens for several years. If you have access to a good hatchery, you may wish to purchase another batch of day-old chicks rather than incubate your own.

INCUBATOR MANAGEMENT

Incubating your own eggs requires regular supervision and attention to details but it's not difficult. In fact, it's really a lot of fun to keep track of their development and then be rewarded as they hatch out. You can purchase a commercially made incubator or make your own. They are available in all sizes and prices from poultry supply sources. You can make a better one with more capacity than the cheaper commercial ones. If you purchase yours, get one with a thermostatically controlled heating source. There are commercial incubators made to use kerosene, as well as electricity, for heating. If you make you own, make a square or round container, like a big box. Have an access door, preferably on one side instead of the top. The door should be large enough so you can reach in easily to handle the eggs. I don't recommend opening the whole top because that will cool the interior too much and too rapidly. You will want a window in the top or side so you can view them without opening the door. For the heat source, you can use a heating element, 3 or 4 small lightbulbs, or whatever you can devise but it should be thermostatically controlled if at all possible. Don't use a single lightbulb because if it burns out and the embryos chill before you notice it, you will lose them. If you use several lightbulbs, space them out in the top of the incubator. Use ceramic sockets for safety. If you can't make a thermostatic system, have the heat source suspended through a hole in the top of the incubator. Then you can raise or lower the heat source to adjust the temperature inside. Place the bulb of the thermometer or the thermostat at the level of the top of the eggs and shade it from direct heat. Adjust the temperature so it reads at 101.5 to 102°F (38.6 to 38.9°C) for still-air incubators. If you use a ventilating fan, keep the temperature at 99.5°F (37.5°C).

You will need a small hygrometer to measure the humidity inside the incubator. I would recommend that you get the old-fashioned kind, with 2 thermometers, one that has the bulb covered with a wet wick from a water reservoir. These have a chart which tells the relative humidity based on the difference between the temperatures on the wet and dry thermometers. These are much more reliable than the new dial types. You can never be sure the dial-type hygrometer is registering properly. Your humidity should be kept around 55% for the first 18 days, then at 65% until hatching for chicken eggs, higher for duck and goose eggs. In fact, you should sprinkle water on duck and goose eggs every day to keep them moist, whether you incubate them artificially or under a broody hen. To maintain the humidity, put open cups or pans of water in the corners of the incubator or under the tray that holds the eggs. Vary the surface area of the water to vary the humidity. You should check it daily and adjust it as necessary because the humidity of incoming air varies with the weather. In particularly dry weather, you may have to hang pieces of cloth or place sponges in the cups to increase evaporative surface area. Capillary action will keep the cloths wet. Just don't drape the pieces of cloth over the side of the cup or the water will siphon out and dampen the bedding.

You need to provide good ventilation in the incubator to bring in fresh oxygen and remove waste gases which the chicks pass through the pores of the shells. Put several holes around the bottom of the incubator and at the top. Air will circulate through the incubator by convection because the warm air inside will rise out the upper holes and draw fresh air in at the bottom. Put swiveling covers on the holes and then you can adjust them to get the proper balance of temperature, humidity and ventilation.

If you build a large incubator for a large number of eggs, put the eggs on removable trays. Have a door like a refrigerator and have a small electric fan inside to circulate air and keep the temperature even throughout. The biggest problem you must solve with any home-built incubator is the variation of temperature in different parts of it. Even from the top to the bottom of the egg it may vary several degrees. The more even you can keep the temperature the better your results should be.

Place the eggs on sheet cotton or soft cloths or other clean bedding. Some recent research showed that if incubating eggs are touching each other, the developing chicks hatch more nearly at the same time than if they are placed far apart. This suggests some type of communication or regulation mechanism that allows naturally-reared chicks to be about the same age. This is of benefit both to the hen and the chicks. The only problem with placing the eggs close together is that if one dies, the poisonous gases from the spoiling egg can kill the other embryos. Avoid this disaster by candling your eggs every so often. Make an egg candler out of a closed box with a light source inside and a round hole in one side a little smaller than the size of your eggs. Candle the eggs in a darkened room by holding each egg over the lighted hole. As you turn the egg you can see the internal structures. You should see the yolk in the center and an air sac attached to the shell at the large end. By 72 hours of incubation you can see a spidery area of thin blood vessels on the yolks of fertile eggs. By 5 to 7 days you should see a "blood spot", the developing embryo, on the outer surface of the yolk. By the end of the second week you should see a moving, pulsing embryo. Take the eggs out of the incubator only long enough to candle them and immediately replace them. Regularly throw out non-fertile eggs.

If you wish to hatch out a large batch of chicks but you only have a few good laying hens, you can save up fertile eggs in the refrigerator. Collect the fertile (hopefully) eggs three or four times a day so they don't start to develop. Let them cool for a few minutes at room temperature and then place them in a clean container, small ends down. Put them in a place in the refrigerator that registers 55° F (12.8° C). The humidity should be about 70%. Turn each egg every day. Most of the eggs should still be fertile at the end of a week. Take them out of the refrigerator and let them warm to room temperature for a while. Then put them in the incubator and warm it up to proper temperature. This method should produce a batch of chicks that all hatch out at about the same time. If you hatch chicks at different times so some are several days older than others, the older ones will beat up on the younger ones. If you buy hatching eggs by mail order or at a feed store, cool them in the refrigerator at 45° to 55°F (7.2° to 12.8°C) for 24 hours to improve hatchability after shipment.

Place your eggs in the incubator with the large ends up, the long axis of each egg at 50° to 60° from horizontal. As each chick develops, its head moves to the top near the air cell. It will open the top of the shell when it hatches. Turn each egg at least 4 times a day to move the embryo so it doesn't stick to the shell. You can stop turning them the last 2 or 3 days before hatching.

Chicken eggs will take 20 to 21 days to hatch, turkeys 28 to 30, ducks 28, geese 30 to 32, and most wild game birds around 22 to 23 days. After your chicks hatch out, let them dry off in the incubator before removing them. Have the brooder warmed up and give each chick a drink of water when you transfer it. Pick it up and dip its beak in some warm water to get it started.

BROODER MANAGEMENT

The requirements for brooding chicks are mostly common sense with just a few specifics. They need ample space, clean water, proper feed and you must keep their manure cleaned up and keep them warm. You can purchase a variety of brooders from the most simple to the most fancy using several types of heat sources. Any large clean box will do but a round structure will be much better so the chicks don't crowd their mates into a corner and smother one or two. Most of the brooders look like a round washtub turned upside down with short legs holding it off the ground so the chicks can run in and out. Install a heat source in the top of the brooder. Again, don't depend on a single lightbulb since it could burn out. Several bulbs or infra-red lamps are commonly used.

The heat source must be adjustable so you can change the temperature during the brooding period. If you are using bulbs, have a hole in the top of the brooder so the bulbs can be raised or lowered through it. You must be able to change from incubator temperature clear down to outdoor temperature while the chicks are growing. The easiest, of course, would be a thermostatically controlled heater. If you place the brooder in a barn or henhouse, install a curtain around the bottom of it to keep out drafts.

Provide ventilation by having holes in the top of the brooder. Put a thermometer inside so it measures the temperature 2 inches above the floor.

Design your brooder so it provides 8 to 10 square inches of floor space per chick. Cover the floor with a deep layer of fine litter such as ground corncobs, sawdust, peanut hulls, or something similar but it must not be dirty or dusty. The litter should be several inches thick. Now cover the litter with a layer of paper which will stay on for the first few days so the chicks won't eat the litter. Put a low circular solid fence or brooder guard around the outside of the brooder to keep the chicks from wandering too far and getting chilled. A circular fence keeps them from getting crowded into a corner. It can be removed in a few weeks.

Set the temperature at 95°F (35°C) and put the new hatchlings under the brooder. Provide a gallon's worth of watering devices for each 50 chicks. Start them on chick mash in saucers or paper plates. Sprinkle a little fine sand over the mash to provide grit. Try to show each chick the food and water. This may be difficult with a large number, but it is worth the effort to get them started right. Pick up each chick, dip its beak into warm water, then into the mash.

Try to get it to eat some. This is really more fun than work.

Decrease the temperature in the brooder a little each day so it decreases about 5°F (3°C) per week. Scrub the watering devices and feeding dishes or troughs at least once a day. On the second day, clean the litter paper or replace it. Add finely cracked yellow corn as their chick scratch. Give it to them twice a day. After 6 or 7 days you should be able to remove the litter paper. Hopefully the chicks won't fill up on the litter by then.

Make a miniature poultry feeding trough, or purchase one, with sides about 2" high and a roller on top so they won't stand in it. Provide about 2 inches of trough space per chick. Put mash with a little grit in the trough and check it regularly for wet spots. Increase the finely cracked corn scratch. Start giving them some finely cut dark greens such as vegetable cuttings or freshly grown greens or seed sprouts from oats, wheat or alfalfa. Only give them a little at first, what they will eat in 15 or 20 minutes.

Stir through the litter daily and scoop out any wet spots. Clean up the manure as much as possible to keep it clean and dry.

By about the end of the second week you can change to medium cracked corn for the scratch. Be sure to add more water capacity as needed. Feed more greens, say, enough to last 30 minutes or so. If the weather is decent you can take them outdoors for a romp every day, on a clean, dry, grassy yard. Let them learn to scratch around in the grass and dirt and begin to forage.

By the 4th week you need to increase their floor space. Enlarge the circular fence to provide about ¾ square foot of space per chick. Increase the feeding and watering facilities to provide 3 inches of feeding trough per chick and 2½ gallons of waterers per 50 chicks. Continue the chick mash with sand, the medium cracked grain scratch and the greens. Be sure to keep the litter clean.

By about the 8th week you will probably have the brooder down to ambient temperature. Whenever you reach this stage, turn off the brooder heat. Add a separate feeder with oyster shell and grit. Now you can start increasing the scratch, or cracked grains, and decreasing the mash feed. At this time you can change over slowly to a coarse scratch, consisting of a variety of coarse cracked and whole grains. The chicks should now be quite large and about fully feathered. If so, you can begin letting them out all day unless the weather is bad. Start opening the chicken house windows in the daytime and remove the brooder. The young chickens will probably have abandoned the brooder and be using the roosts by now anyway. During this time you can be adding litter to the floor to get the built-up litter going.

There are lots of different ways to raise chicks. All you really have to do is provide their basic necessities and use common sense. Some people prefer to start the chicks on a platform of wire mesh instead of litter so that the manure drops through. For this method, build a frame large enough for the entire brooder area and stretch wire mesh over it. Another idea is to put just the feeders and waterers on wire mesh platforms.

After you have raised some chicks you will be able to tell their general condition just by listening to them. Healthy, comfortable chicks peep "cheerfully". Shrill chirping means that something is wrong. They are probably too hot, too cold, suffering from a draft, or coming down with an illness. If it is too cold or drafty they will be huddling together. If it is too hot they hold their wings out and pant with their mouths open. If ill, they will be depressed, inactive and usually have diarrhea. I will cover some of the common illnesses later.

DUCKS

Ducks are hardy and self-sufficient. They provide good meat and lots of good-quality down for making comforters or other warm articles. Their eggs are good for baking but not frying or boiling.

The Pekin duck is the familiar, large white one with a yellow bill. They average 8 to 9 pounds when mature and lay an average of 160 eggs a year. The Kahki Campbell is a smaller duck. They lay around 200 eggs a year but are poor setters. Indian Runners are white to fawn with patterns. They lay lots of eggs and are also smaller than Pekins. White Muscovies are large white birds with fleshy appendages around their faces, making them rather strange looking. They are not true ducks. They are usually around 9 pounds when mature and they lay 40 to 50 eggs per year.

If you have a nice farm pond, you will probably attract some wild ducks. Many people like to get a few Mallards because of their beautiful markings. You should become familiar with your state game laws in case they pertain to keeping wild waterfowl.

If you raise a lot of ducks, you should provide a large well-drained yard. They are happy with a very modest pond or even a big tub of water but a farm pond is ideal and will enable them to be self-sufficient. Even though they are very hardy, I would advise you to provide a small shed or hut so they can find shelter in bad weather. In their natural environment, they avoid severe weather by their long migrations. Since they will be staying with you year-around, you must take care of their needs. Put nest boxes in the hut up off the floor.

Ducklings raised domestically are very sensitive to cold and wet conditions. You can incubate them artificially or let their mothers do it. You can also let a broody hen incubate and brood them. If you brood them artificially do it just like chicks. Their litter must be kept very clean. Change or add to the litter daily. Surprisingly, ducklings are prone to getting chilled from getting wet. They love to jump in the water but they don't have the natural oils to keep themselves dry. For this reason your waterers must be very small or too narrow for them to get into. If they get wet, they often get pneumonia and die. Keep them away from ponds or deep water until they are over 6 weeks old. They are also sensitive to too much sunshine.

Start the hatchlings on wet chick mash, feeding 5 or 6 times a day with a little grit. Their watering container must be deep enough that they can stick their entire bill into it in order for them to get a drink. Get them started eating and drinking just like with chicks.

If you decide to let a broody hen hatch out some duck eggs, you must sprinkle the eggs with water every day because they require more humidity than chicken eggs. If the hen is small, such as a Bantam, you must turn the eggs for her. It usually takes 28 days to hatch them. After hatching, the ducklings won't be able to keep up with their foster mother very well. You can either confine her to a pen or put her in a wire cage for 4 weeks.

GEESE

Geese are beautiful creatures. They are excellent "watch-dogs" because they honk loudly whenever an intruder enters their yard. They will even attack. Ganders are especially strong and could injure a child, or even an adult, so instruct your children not to pester them. Goose down is the ultimate insulation material for weight and efficiency. If you slaughter a goose or gander, be sure to save the down even if it's for future use. It should never be wasted.

Geese are very self-sufficient. They will subsist entirely on forage but be sure to keep them away from young trees or saplings. They will destroy them by eating the bark. Goose beats turkey in flavor and they are much easier to raise. The Embden is the large, white breed of geese. They average 15 to 20 pounds. They are good mothers and they produce white goose down. The Toulouse is the large grey breed. They average 20 to 25 pounds and produce grey goose down. The Africans are extremely noisy geese, so I don't recommend them. Most of the other breeds are smaller than the Embden or Toulouse.

I would recommend that you give your geese a yard of their own because their manure is so messy and because of their destruction of young shrubs. The simile, "loose as a goose," is certainly a good one. Because of their sanitary habits and appetites, it is very easy to overcrowd geese. You should pasture no more than 10 adults to an acre if raising a large number. They will crop the grass clear to the ground if they are overcrowded.

You can supplement their forage diet with corn, corn meal, oats, wheat, and other grains. Also provide them with oyster shell. In winter, they will eat legume hays along with their grain.

If you wish to fatten a goose for slaughter, you can do so by feeding moist mash of yellow cornmeal and oats for 1 or 2 months. Wet the mash with skim milk or buttermilk. Increase the fattening ration gradually.

DISEASES AND PARASITES

Poultry have several problems that make disease-control difficult. They easily acquire diseases from wild birds either from their droppings or from transfer by biting insects. Some of their diseases are egg-borne and therefore hard to eliminate. They tend to build up disease and parasite organisms in their litter and pastures. These become progressively worse in the flock. Chickens, ducks and geese are fairly easy to raise, but turkeys are very sensitive and delicate.

The general principles of poultry disease-control are the prevention of contamination, a closed system, proper sanitation and good nutrition, just as with your other livestock.

Since some poultry diseases are transmitted by egg passage, you should start your flock with eggs or chicks from a reputable hatchery. Be sure to get a certificate or guarantee that they are "Pullorum-clean" or "Pullorum tested *and passed.*" When adding outside stock to your farm, it would be ideal to isolate the new birds for a 3-week period to be sure you do not introduce a serious disease.

Since many diseases and parasites are transmitted to healthy flocks from wild birds and animals, it will pay you well to screen the poultry houses against birds and insects and to take steps to keep out rodents and wild animals.

Don't use old poultry equipment or housing until you sterilize and disinfect everything.

Many diseases can be prevented or eradicated by merely spreading the organisms too thin for them to reproduce and continue their life cycle. Do this by rotating your pastures and by occasionally de-populating your flocks. Put your birds on a different yard (pasture) every 3 months or so. De-population, the planned re-stocking with clean birds on clean land and complete elimination of the old flock, should be done every 2 or 3 years.

Maintain cleanliness by scrubbing and disinfecting feeders and waterers at least monthly for adult birds. Scrub them daily for brooders. Disinfect the poultry house yearly. Many diseases cause livestock losses only because large concentrations of the organisms are allowed to build up on equipment or in the litter. Only then can the bird get a large enough dose of the organism at one time to cause illness or death. Be sure to burn birds that die in case they had a dangerous disease. However, if several birds are ill, save one for post-mortem examination by a veterinarian or laboratory. Burn or bury unused offal from slaughtering. Don't feed it to the livestock unless it is well-cooked first.

Many of the diseases and problems are caused, or contributed to, by faulty nutrition. The most practical prevention is to calculate your rations for protein, calcium and phosphorus and to provide a wide variety of fresh foods to supplement their dry grains. Sunshine and a clean, grassy range should allow the birds to supplement their diet themselves. Remember if their range becomes dirty and bare of vegetation it is too small or you are not rotating and managing it properly. Sunshine provides Vitamin D and the ultraviolet radiation kills many pathogenic organisms.

Here are a few of the specific problems and diseases of poultry and some suggestions for control and prevention.

Cannibalism
Cause:

This is a psychological problem caused by over-crowding, boredom, excess heat or light in the brooder, hunger or disputes in their social (pecking) order. One or more birds will peck at a victim (or several victims) until they severely injure or kill it.

Action:
Let the birds have more room and let them wander in the yard. Check their housing for temperature, etc. Put pine tar on the victim's wounds so the others will leave them alone.

Aspergillosus or Brooder Pneumonia

Cause:
This is a fungal disease caused by *Aspergillus* species, a group of fungi that grow well in chicken manure and wet feed. This fungus is commonly present in soil and air and causes disease only when the litter or the feeders and waterers aren't properly cleaned.

Signs:
Signs of pneumonia slowly spread through the flock. This is most common in brooders and young birds, causing dullness, labored breathing and loss of weight. Sometimes you can hear the heavy breathing or rattling in the throat.

Postmortem:
On postmortem examination, you may be able to see button-like growths of fungus in the lungs or furry mold growth in the trachea, bronchi, air sacs or sometimes in the mouth.

Action:
Prevent this by using good, clean litter and cleaning the roosting pits frequently. Burn dead carcasses and be careful because the disease can be transmitted to humans.

Botulism

Cause:
Botulism is caused by ingesting the toxins from the organism *Clostridium botulinum,* which grows in spoiled food such as dead animals or decaying vegetation.

Signs:
Botulism causes paralysis of the legs, wings and neck. The birds may be seen with the neck limp and the head lying on the ground or over the shoulder. Or feathers may begin to drop out and diarrhea may occur. Birds may recover in 2 or 3 days if they did not receive a lethal dose of toxin. If they did, they will become comatose and die.

Prevention:
Prevent contact with spoiled animal or vegetable matter. Even the maggots of blowflies, which feed on dead carcasses, may contain the toxin. Don't allow your birds access to swampy areas or ponds that are drying up.

Treatment:

Give a laxative such as molasses to the flock. Put 1 pint of molasses in 5 gallons of water and put it out for 4 hours. If they can't drink it by themselves, feed them with a syringe or put a small rubber tube down their throats. Wash your hands well after handling these birds and don't smoke or touch your mouth. This toxin is one of the world's strongest poisons. You can also use epsom salts as a laxative. Mix 1 pound in enough bran or wet mash for 100 chickens and withhold other feed.

Fowl Cholera

Cause:

Pasturella multocida, a contagious bacterial disease, affects a wide variety of birds and mammals including man. It is especially common in waterfowl.

Signs:

Sudden deaths occur. You will find dead chickens in their nests or on roosts in the *peracute* form of the disease. In the *acute* form, many of the birds become ill with signs of listlessness, loss of appetite and weight loss. Diarrhea is copious and watery. Egg production falls, of course. After a period of illness, survivors develop difficulty breathing. *Chronic* forms of the disease produce swelling of the face and wattles, which become fiery red and hot. They may also get swellings of the foot pads and ear lobes and show lameness.

Postmortem:

Birds dead of the peracute form show almost no lesions. The acute form shows pinpoint hemorrhages in the internal organs, the heart, the liver, proventriculus, gizzard and intestines. These signs are not diagnostic, however. There may also be grey streaks and spots on the liver. The chronic form often has yellow, putrid pus resembling cooked egg yolk around the ovary or in the body cavity. There may be external swellings that are full of pus. Positive diagnosis requires laboratory identification of the causative organism.

Prevention and Treatment:

Prevent the introduction of the organism. Rotate the ranges and eliminate swampy areas. *Pasturella multocida* survives at least 3 months in the soil and in decaying carcasses. Scrub and disinfect or steam the housing and equipment regularly. Dispose of dead birds immediately. Screen out wild birds and keep domestic or wild mammals out of their area. Avoid stress in cold, wet weather. When an outbreak starts, sulfa medications in the drinking water may reduce the flock mortality. If cholera is a problem in your area, the commercial cholera bacterins, given usually at 12 weeks and 9 to 12 months of age, may help reduce losses.

Fowl Pox
Cause:

This is a virus-caused disease affecting poultry and wild birds.

Signs:

The *skin form* of fowl pox starts with white bumps on the comb, face and wattles and sometimes on the legs, feet, and elsewhere. These bumps turn yellow, then brown and turn to scabs in 2 to 4 weeks. In the *wet pox form* of the disease, the birds get yellowish cankers in the mouth, on the tongue and in the esophagus. They may have a discharge from the eyes or nose, facial swelling and develop difficulty breathing. Wet pox produces rapid mortality. You may see one or both forms of pox in the same flock. The virus usually attacks adult birds in the fall and winter. Skin pox losses are not high but production suffers for several weeks.

Prevention:

The virus is spread by mosquitos and wild birds. The virus stays alive in scab tissue for years. Vaccine is available if it starts in your area.

Newcastle Disease
Cause:

This is a virus disease. Foreign varieties are particularly dangerous. It affects most species of fowl, some mammals and even man (as an eye infection).

Signs:

In acute attacks, nearly all the young birds in a flock die in 3 to 4 days. Respiratory signs appear with gasping, coughing, hoarse chirping and rattling sounds. These signs last 2 weeks or more in survivors. They also lose their appetites, huddle near the heat and are very thirsty. Nervous signs may appear after 1 or 2 days with partial or complete paralysis of the wings and legs in about 50% of a group of chicks. Adults rarely get the nervous signs. The chicks may be seen with their heads down between their legs or straight back between their shoulders. They may have head tremors, rotating of the head, walking backwards or in circles and tumbling. In adults, egg laying stops for 4 to 6 weeks. Mortality may be either high or low, starting 3 to 4 days after the first signs. Older birds may have less severe signs. Young birds may have up to 90% mortality. Laboratory testing is required for positive diagnosis.

Postmortem:

Lesions are not diagnostic. There may be mucus or pus in the trachea and bronchi. There may be hemorrhages in the gastrointestinal tract and, in layers, egg follicles may be broken with yolk in the body cavity.

Prevention:

The virus spreads in body discharges. It may be carried by wild birds and recovered birds are often carriers. Eggs may carry the virus either within or on the outside of the shells. If Newcastle is present in your area, vaccinate your chicks as early as 1 day of age and repeat the vaccinations later. Isolate an affected flock and depopulate it. Don't try to treat it. Never visit another poultry operation if it has had Newcastle disease because of the carrier danger.

Infectious Bronchitis

Cause:

Infectious bronchitis is an acute, highly contagious disease affecting chickens caused by a virus.

Signs:

It spreads rapidly through the flock, causing depression, loss of appetite, coughing, sneezing, gasping and respiratory noises. Nasal and occular discharges are common. Chicks huddle around the brooder. Layers decrease production except for some misshapen or soft-shelled, poor quality eggs. Layers seldom return to full production and egg quality is poor for a long period of time. Mortality is usually lower than with Newcastle, but chicks may have up to 60% mortality. Bronchitis never has nervous system symptoms like Newcastle.

Postmortem:

Chicks have inflammation and mucus in the air passages. Dead chicks often have cheesy plugs in the lower trachea and the bronchi. You must submit specimens to a laboratory for a positive diagnosis.

Prevention:

There are no medications that stop the bronchitis virus, but sulfas or antibiotics may help prevent additional losses from secondary infections. The virus is airborne and can be spread by any means. Do not visit other poultry farms and protect your flock from wild birds and mammals. The disease can be controlled by regular vaccinations but I would rather that you keep the disease off your property and prevent it by sanitation and isolation. I would depopulate an affected flock because of the prolonged, sometimes permanent damage to layers.

Laryngotracheitis

Cause:

Larynogtracheitis is a virus respiratory disease of chickens and pheasants.

Signs:

It is most severe in adults, seldom affecting chicks under 4 weeks of age. Egg production of layers drops but egg quality is not affected. It spreads slowly through the flock, usually over a week or two, causing coughing, sneezing and difficulty in breathing. The birds sit depressed, stretch their necks to breathe and often make characteristic cawing sounds. They may cough up bloody mucus. The mortality is usually low, with most of the birds recovering in a couple of weeks.

Postmortem;

Birds that die usually have severe inflammation of the trachea and sometimes of the lungs, with bloody mucus inside. There may be cheesy plugs in the upper trachea. It is necessary to send specimens to the laboratory for a positive diagnosis.

Prevention:

The virus is airborne and can be spread by birds, people and equipment. Recovered birds may be carriers and it tends to recur on the same farm. Although it can be controlled by regular vaccinations, I would recommend de-population and control by strict isolation and sanitary measures if at all possible.

Fowl Typhoid

Cause:

Typhoid is caused by *Salmonella gallinarum,* a bacteria affecting chickens and turkeys.

Signs:

Affected birds are listless and lose their appetites but are very thirsty. They have greenish-yellow diarrhea and rapid breathing. Sudden death often occurs after 2 days of illness. A flock will have heavy losses, but the deaths stop in about 5 days. A flock may have recurring outbreaks. This disease is usually seen in adults, as contrasted with Pullorum disease and Paratyphoid.

Postmortem :

A dead bird usually has a swollen, red spleen and kidneys and greyish spots on the heart, lungs, gizzard and liver. The liver is often discolored, ranging from green to bronze. Chronic cases often show a swollen, bronze-colored liver. The intestines may have ulcers with a slimy, greenish ingesta. There may be malformed, developing eggs in the ovaries and oviduct. Positive diagnosis requires laboratory isolation of the organism.

Prevention:

Recovered adults are carriers, so don't bring adult birds onto your place. The organism can be spread by insects, man and equipment. The organism is also spread in eggs so be sure to get your eggs or hatchlings from a reputable source. Use good sanitation to try to prevent its spread if it occurs. If you do get typhoid, de-populate and start again on clean ground. Antibiotics are not very effective for treating it and they don't eliminate the carriers.

Paratyphoid

Cause:

Salmonella typhimurium and other *Salmonella* species cause disease in young chicks, turkey poults, ducklings and other species. These bacteria can affect man and other mammals but they rarely affect goslings.

Signs:

Paratyphoid is usually mild in adults but often severe in young birds. It usually appears at either 4 to 5 days of age or at 10 to 12 days. Losses may vary anywhere from 10% to 80%. Chicks will usually be seen standing with drooping wings and ruffled feathers. They may have diarrhea and show difficulty breathing.

Postmortem:

The lesions of paratyphoid are usually non-specific. They may show swollen liver and spleen. There may be yellow fluid in the sac surrounding the heart. There may be an exudate-like pus on the liver and lungs. A laboratory examination is necessary to identify the organism.

Prevention:

Paratyphoid is transmitted in the eggs and recovered adults are carriers. It is also carried and spread by rats, mice, wild birds and man. To avoid getting it on your place, get your new birds from a reputable hatchery. If you get it, I would advise you to depopulate and replace your flock on clean ground with sterilized equipment.

Pullorum

Cause:

Pullorum disease is caused by *Salmonella pullorum,* a bacterium which affects young chickens and turkeys. Ducks and geese are usually resistant. This is the most destructive of the Salmonella diseases.

Signs:

Pullorum causes sudden death in newly hatched chicks and poults if it was transmitted in the eggs. If it is introduced to brooder birds, they usually show signs by 5 to 10 days of age. They huddle near the heat with their heads and wings drooping and their feathers ruffled. They may develop labored breathing. They usually have diarrhea with manure pasted over their vents. Mortality in a flock of brooders is often 100%. If there are survivors, they may have another attack later. Adult birds usually do not show any signs but they become carriers.

Postmortem:

Newly hatched chicks that die of Pullorum usually show no lesions. Cases that start in the brooder may show grey spots on the liver and spleen and grey bumps on the heart, gizzard, intestines or lungs. The liver and spleen may be enlarged. There may be raised, white plaques on the inside of the large intestine and rectum. Chronic infection in adults may cause malformed, discolored eggs. The eggs may have oily or cheesy green or brown material in them. Developing eggs may be found imbedded in the abdomen. The body cavity may be filled with a straw-colored fluid. The sac surrounding the heart may be thick and white and filled with fluid. Laboratory testing is necessary to identify the causative organism.

Prevention:

This is one of the most important diseases for you to avoid when you get new birds. It is transmitted in the eggs and it can be spread by adult birds, other animals and man. Breeding chickens can be blood-tested so a reputable hatchery should be able to guarantee their birds Pullorum-free. If you do get it, depopulation and complete sterilization are absolutely necessary. Antibiotics are not very helpful in the treatment of birds affected with Pullorum.

Tuberculosis

Cause:

Tuberculosis in poultry is caused by *Mycobacterium avium,* a bacillus closely related to human tuberculosis. It affects chickens, turkeys and many wild birds. Ducks and geese are relatively resistant.

Signs:

Affected birds have little energy and slowly lose weight. Egg production declines. Their feathers become dull and the comb, wattles and ear lobes become pale. The signs develop slowly. Chronic cases may develop lameness and drooping of the wings.

Postmortem:

Occasionally, sudden death occurs due to avian T.B. and the bird's abdomen is filled with blood. Usually, though, you will find it when dressing a carcass of an older bird. There will be characteristic granular growths or nodules on the internal organs, usually the liver, spleen and intestines, although any tissue can be affected, even the bone marrow. The lesions are irregular, greyish-white to white nodules from pin-head size to an inch or more. The nodules are firm but easily cut. They usually have a soft, yellow center surrounded by a fibrous capsule. Laboratory confirmation is required for a positive diagnosis.

Prevention:

The avian tuberculosis bacillus can infect swine and sheep and it can sensitize cattle to human T.B. Occasionally it infects humans and cattle. Since tuberculosis is a chronic disease, it builds up in older birds. They then can spread great numbers of the infective bacilli and contaminate the ground and the other birds and animals. This disease is the main reason you should kill off the older birds and depopulate your flock every two or three years. Fortunately, avian T.B. is not very common in wild birds but it does exist and this is probably the way you would get it in your flock. It is such a dangerous and destructive disease that it will pay you to take regular steps to prevent it. If T.B. is or was present on your land or your neighbors', don't keep any birds past 2 years of age and don't let them wander over the entire farm. Try to keep them fenced on clean ranges. Rotate the ranges regularly but don't put other species of livestock on land that had infected poultry on it. Sterilize your equipment regularly and keep wild birds out of the hen house. If you happen to open a carcass and see lesions that you think are T.B., don't handle it further. Put it in several plastic bags and take it to a veterinarian or poultry diagnostic laboratory. Burn any other suspected carcasses. Wash and disinfect your hands and clothing after handling them. In the case of T.B., an ounce of prevention is worth a ton of cure.

Perosis

Cause:

This is a nutritional deficiency disease. It is usually due to a deficiency of calcium or phosphorus but may also be a deficiency of manganese, choline, niacin, biotin, or maybe others.

Signs:

Perosis is a deformity of the leg bones with puffy hock joints and lameness. The leg bones become twisted and deformed and the Achilles tendon slips out of place at the hock. The bird then becomes unable to stand.

Prevention:

Perosis usually cannot be treated successfully so it must be prevented by a well-balanced ration of good variety.

Coccidiosis

Cause:

Coccidiosis is caused by various species of protozoal parasites that infect the intestines of all types of fowl. One species infects the kidneys of geese.

Signs:

Signs of coccidiosis vary from unthriftiness and lowered egg production to bloody diarrhea and death. Different species of coccidia have their own characteristic signs and postmortem lesions, such as the following: white patches or a bright red lining to the intestine; swollen, ballooned intestines with a jelly-like mass inside; swollen ceca filled with a solid, bloody mass; bloody, clotted masses filling the intestines and ceca.

Prevention:

This is a chronic, tenacious disease once it is introduced to a poultry operation. Because of their methods, most commercial operations are forced to live with it. They often control it with drugs in the feed or water. Surprisingly, the built-up litter system allows young birds to get a gradual exposure to the coccidial organisms and build up their resistance. A huge dose all at one time, however, would be fatal. The organisms are passed in the feces and can then be mechanically carried by man, birds, insects or other methods. I would recommend that you try to completely avoid the coccidiosis problem by avoiding the introduction of the organisms. If a bird is ill with coccidiosis, a veterinarian or laboratory can identify the organisms in a fecal sample. But in an adult carrier bird, the organisms will be few in number and a fecal test will probably not pick it up. This is just one more reason to avoid bringing adult birds, such as culls from a commercial farm, onto your place. Fortunately, each species of coccidia is host-specific. That is, coccidia of chickens doesn't infect other species of birds and vice-versa.

Poultry Internal Parasites or Worms

Poultry are affected by a large variety of internal worms. Here are the major classes of the most common ones:

Roundworms

Cause:

These are intestinal parasites of the species *Ascaridia galli* which infect chickens and turkeys. Roundworms are 1½ to 3" long, white, and round. They are found in the central portion of the small intestines. The worm eggs are passed in the feces and birds become infested by ingesting the eggs.

Signs:

Roundworms may cause unthriftiness and sometimes diarrhea. They make birds more susceptible to other illnesses. Young birds may die of heavy infestations. You can diagnose the disease by finding the parasites in the intestines on post-mortem examination.

Treatment:

Piperazine and other drugs are available for worming poultry.

Cecal Worms

Cause:

The cecal worm, *Heterakis gallinae,* is a round worm about ½" long that lives in the ceca of chickens, turkeys and other birds. The worms are transmitted by microscopic eggs which are passed in the feces of an infected bird and then ingested by another bird. Cecal worms can carry and trasmit the organisms of the disease, Blackhead, which is especially deadly in young turkeys.

Signs:

Cecal worms can cause unthriftiness, weakness and loss of weight. On post-mortem, the ceca may be thickened. When you open them you will find the fat, often s-shaped worms. The ceca are the 2 long, blind-ended appendages attached to the hind end of the small intestines. Both roundworms and cecal worms may be diagnosed by a microscopic examination of a fecal sample.

Treatment:

Phenothiazine poultry wormer will kill cecal worms and range rotation will help control it on most farms. Don't raise turkey poults on ground that had adult turkeys or chickens within the last 3 years.

Tape Worms

Cause:

There are at least eleven different species of tapeworms infecting poultry in the U.S. These are flat, segmented intestinal parasites. Some are very small and others are up to 6 or 7 inches long. They are found in the small intestines. Segments of the worm, when mature, break off and pass in the feces. The eggs are carried in these segments. These eggs are not directly infective for poultry but must first go through an intermediate host such as certain insects, earthworms, slugs or snails, depending on the species of tapeworms. These intermediate hosts eat the eggs and later become infective to a chicken. The chicken gets the tapeworms by eating the infected intermediate host.

Signs:

Tapeworms can cause poor growth and production. They are usually diagnosed only on post-mortem examination of the intestines. They can be treated with several commercial preparations but it usually isn't necessary since tapeworms are seldom present in sufficient numbers to cause losses.

Capillary Worms or Threadworms

Cause:

There are various species of small, thin roundworms of the *Capillaria* genus. Each species has its own area of the intestine, crop or ceca. They are very fine, some hair-like, some microscopic. Some are transmitted directly from eggs in the feces, others require an intermediate host, the earthworm.

Signs:

Severe capillary worm infestations may cause loss of weight and poor production. Lesions vary from just a little inflammation of the lining of the gut to severe thickening and sloughing.

Treatment:

They can be treated with Hygromycin or thiabendazole, but this should not be necessary with proper range rotation and regular depopulation.

Gizzard Worms

Cause:

Cheilospirura hamulosa, a reddish-brown worm ½ to 1" long, burrows into the lining of the gizzard. The horny lining of the gizzard must be removed from the organ to find them. They require intermediate hosts, insects like grasshoppers, beetles, or weevils, to complete their life cycle.

There is no treatment for gizzard worms.

Gapeworms

Cause:

Syngamus trachea is a species of roundworm that inhabits the trachea of chickens, turkeys, and guinea fowls. They are small red worms. Often a smaller male worm is seen attached to a female worm so that they form the letter 'Y.' The female is ¼" to 3/4" long.

Signs:

Young birds may be seen shaking their heads, gasping and coughing. They may suffocate. On post-mortem, or when dressing a carcass, you may see the worms in the trachea and the inflamed tracheal lining.

Treatment:

Severe infestations can be treated with thiabendozole, a commercial wormer, in the feed for 2 weeks at the rate of 0.1% of the feed. Gapeworms can be carried by "transport" hosts such as insects, earthworms, snails and slugs and live several years in these. Keep your ranges well drained, rotate the ranges, avoid overcrowding, keep the litter clean and dry and exclude wild birds and insects from the henhouse.

Poultry External Parasites

Poultry are affected by a huge variety of external arthropod parasites such as lice, ticks, bedbugs, fleas, mites, mosquitos and flies.

Lice

These are small, flat, usually light-colored critters, several millimeters long, that live on the skin. You will usually see the lice eggs in clusters attached to the feathers. These are called "nits." There are at least 25 species of poultry lice in the U.S., many carried by wild birds.

Avoid the problem of lice as much as possible by disinfecting the housing when depopulating. You can spray or dust with commercial insecticides which are approved for poultry.

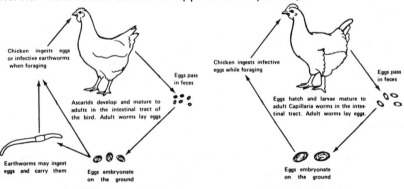

Chicken ingests eggs or infective earthworms when foraging

Eggs pass in feces

Ascarids develop and mature to adults in the intestinal tract of the bird. Adult worms lay eggs

Earthworms may ingest eggs and carry them

Eggs embryonate on the ground

Lifecycle of *Ascaridia galli,* the Poultry Ascarid

Chicken ingests infective eggs while foraging

Eggs pass in feces

Eggs hatch and larvae mature to adult Capillaria worms in the intestinal tract. Adult worms lay eggs.

Eggs embryonate on the ground

Lifecycle of *Capillaria* species Worms of Poultry

Bedbugs

These are small, yellowish, brown or red insects. They move very fast and hide in cracks except at night when they come out to feed. A large population of bedbugs can cause severe anemia and loss of rest by scratching.

This parasite requires that you spray the henhouse thoroughly with insecticide such as malathion according to the directions on the container.

Fleas

These are small, dark brown insects about 2mm long. They are flat from side to side and have long legs which enable them to jump. Heavy infestations cause anemia and irritation to the birds. You can dust the birds and spray the house with insecticide if necessary.

Fowl Ticks

These are 8-legged arthropods with large, hard bodies. They are usually reddish brown and can be up to ½"long. The fowl tick is mainly in the Southwestern U.S. They suck blood at night and retreat to the cracks in the daytime. Large numbers can cause anemia and toxicity in the flock, decreasing production. If you get fowl ticks in your flock, you should spray the house thoroughly with insecticide such as 3% malathion, 1 gallon per 1000 square feet of surface. These are hard bugs to kill.

Fowl tick, *Argus persigus*, adult female. 4 to 10 mm. long. Larval ticks several mm. long. Blue or purple in color.

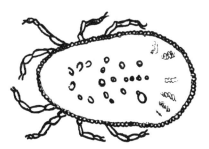

Mites

These are small, 8-legged arthropods no larger than a small pinhole. They can be seen with a magnifying glass. Various species of mites attack different parts of the bird and do different types of damage. They can also carry disease organisms.

Red or Roost Mites: These are the most common external

parasites of poultry. They suck blood and cause anemia and poor production. Birds may refuse to set their nests. The mites live off the bird, in the henhouse, most of the time. You can get rid of them by dusting with a non-residual insecticide such as malathion. Don't use nicotine sulfate (Black-Leaf 40) like most sources recommend because it is too toxic for the birds.

Feather Mites: These mites stay on the birds and damage the skin and feathers. They suck blood and cause a great deal of irritation. You can dust the birds with insecticide or put a pound of 4% malathion dust in a box and let them take dust-baths in it.

Depluming Mites: These live in the feather follicles of the skin. They cause such intense itching that birds pull out their feathers. An insectcide ointment is usually required to get down to the mites in the follicles.

Scaley Leg Mites: These mites burrow into the skin of the feet, legs, comb and wattles, causing scaling, crusting and thickening of the skin. The damage may progress to deformities of the legs and lameness. This mite is so deep in the skin that it is hard to treat. You will find it easier to cull affected birds. You can treat it with preparations of insecticides such as rotenone in oil or with 2 parts raw linseed oil with 1 part kerosene. Paint the insecticide on the roosts and dip the birds' legs in it weekly. It will take weeks to improve. Even if they are culled, the roosts should be changed or treated so other birds don't get it.

Chiggers: Chiggers, red bugs, or harvest mites live in the grass and get on the poultry. They cause severe itching and emaciation in young birds. You should mow the range if the growth gets very tall. You can dust the birds with insecticide if chiggers are a problem.

Flies and Mosquitoes

Some flies are blood-suckers. Flies and mosquitoes can cause severe irritation and anemia if they are numerous. They also carry many disease organisms and parasites. Try to control mosquitoes on your poultry operation by filling in any nearby swampy areas or pouring a small amount of light oil on pooled water, which kills the larvae. Screen the henhouse and avoid garbage or manure piles that attract flies.

13
Sheep Management and Veterinary Care

Sheep are very self-sufficient creatures. Along with beef cattle, they are among the lowest-maintenance animals you can raise. They can do quite well on little more than pasture alone.

SELECTION

If you are striving for self-sufficiency, you have no doubt considered raising your own sheep for wool. Of course, you will need to learn how to shear, clean, spin and weave the product but there are books and classes on this subject. Don't be fooled into thinking you can make comfortable clothing out of just any sheep's wool. The wool from many of our common sheep breeds is more suitable for making carpets than shirts and socks and that is just what it is used for. People automatically think that fine, clothing-grade wool must sell for more and therefore be better to raise commercially. However, the coarse grades of wool often get just as high a price, or higher, because of supply and demand factors. Most commercial farmers raise the more popular medium-wool breeds, which also produce good meat carcasses as lambs.

If you have rather sensitive skin, like I do, I'd advise you to choose one of the fine-wool breeds for home wool production.

Unfortunately, there is a trade-off between the mutton-type, medium-wool sheep and the fine-wool types whose carcasses are not as good. But before we discuss breeds and their wool types, let's discuss choosing individuals.

I would recommend that you choose young healthy individuals. Check the mouth and teeth. Like other ruminants, they have front teeth only in the lower jaw and a dental pad in the upper. You can "age" the individual by it's front teeth. The larger adult teeth come in at the central (middle) pair at 1½ years of age. The next pair of intermediates come in at 2 years of age. The next pair come in at 3 years and the corner or "canine" pair at 4 years. These, of course, replace the smaller baby teeth or milk teeth which drop out. Make sure the teeth are even and sound. Open the mouth in good light and inspect the back teeth, the premolars and molars, too. If these don't meet well, they will get sharp ridges and points which cut the cheeks and tongue, making the animal a "poor-doer." Check the condition of the animal's body by working your fingers straight down into the fleece, carefully parting the wool. Feel along the animal's rump, back, neck, ribs and legs. Skinny, bony sheep are probably wormy or ill. Don't choose them. On mature females, check the udders carefully. They need to be able to milk well to support their suckling lambs. Check the udders for internal lumps, scars or other indications of past or present mastites, just as with dairy goats.

The most important consideration for your satisfaction with raising sheep is your breed selection. Sheep breeds vary tremendously in their attributes. Here are some of the most common breeds and some of their important characteristics.

First, let's discuss the ones called medium-wool breeds. These are considered mutton-type sheep. Their wool is suitable for outer clothing as it is medium-coarse to medium-fine. Their carcasses dress out well for lamb or mutton.

Dorsets:

These are large sheep, usually 150 to 175 lbs. for ewes (females) and 175 to 250 lbs. for rams. Both sexes have horns but there is a polled (hornless) variety. Their eyes, noses and legs are bald of wool; therefore they are easier to take care of. Many people consider Dorsets the best mothers. But they require a little better quality of feed for good health than some other breeds. They usually produce 6 to 8 lbs. of fleece a year. They are often polyestrus and can be bred both spring and fall, producing 2 lamb crops.

Cheviots:

These are smaller sheep, often around 140 lbs. for ewes and 175 lbs. for rams. They have bald white faces and legs so they are also easy to care for. They are also hornless. They are very hardy sheep and do well on rough pasture.they usually produce 5 to 7 lbs. of fleece per year.

Hampshires:

These are exceptionally large sheep, ewes weighing 150 to 200 lbs., rams 225 to 300 lbs. They are hornless. They have dark-colored wool on their heads and sometimes they have black fibers in the fleece, which is undesirable. They produce a small fleece for their size, usually 6 to 8 lbs. per year. But they are popular commercially because they are prolific, good mothers and produce good carcasses for market lamb production or mutton. For a small family operation, Hampshires are too big to handle easily for shearing and other care.

Oxfords:

These are the largest of the medium-wool breeds, weighing 175 to 250 lbs. for ewes, 250 to 350 lbs. for rams. They require heavy feeding and have excessive wool on the head and legs. Their wool is usually more coarse than other medium-wool sheep but they are a strong rugged breed. They produce a large heavy fleece.

Shropshires:

These are of medium size with ewes 135 to 175 lbs., rams 200 to 250 lbs. They are hornless. Their excessive face wool requires trimming but they have a good fleece, 8 to 10 lbs. a year and finer than most medium-wool breeds. Ewes are very prolific and good mothers. They have the highest percentage of twins. They are popular with farmers for their good fleece, good carcasses and early maturing for market lambs.

Suffolks:

These are large sheep with woolless, black-haired heads and legs. They are polled (hornless). Ewes will weigh 160 to 225 lbs., rams 225 to 300. They are good range sheep and are prolific but produce a very light fleece, usually 4 to 5 lbs. They have good mutton conformation and grow fast so they are popular for lamb production. For our purposes, they are probably too large and don't produce enough wool, although they are good range sheep.

Southdowns:

They produce a good-quality fleece, usually 5 to 7 pounds

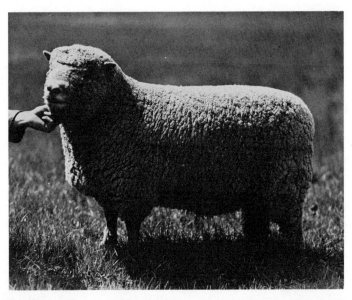

Southdown Ram

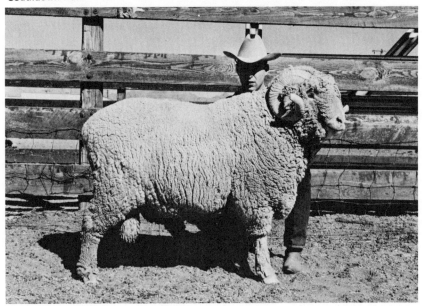

Rambouillet Ram

per year. Lambs mature early with excellent carcasses. These sheep usually don't do well on pasture alone. They need grain supplementation most of the time. They are one of the oldest breeds of sheep, from England as are most breeds.

There are quite a few crossbred breeds of sheep in the U. S. Most of them were started by crossing long-wool sheep with fine-wool sheep. Long-wool sheep produce a very coarse wool that is usually used for things like carpet. These crosses were usually for the objective of producing a good range animal for the western U. S. ranges.

Columbia:

This is a large medium-wool crossbred, originally from Lincoln rams and Rambouillet ewes. They produce a heavy fleece, usually 11 to 13 lbs. They are polled with white open faces. They are vigorous and good range sheep. They are also prolific and produce good carcasses.

Targhee:

This is a medium-sized breed from crosses of three other breeds. They are white-faced and polled. Fleeces average about 11 lbs. and the wool is medium-fine to fine, a very good grade for medium-wool sheep.

There are others, Corriedales, Panamas, Romeldales, Southdales and others. I doubt if any of the other crossbreds or straight old breeds have anything to recommend them for our particular use.

Then there are the long-wool breeds. These are the largest sheep. Their wool is long and very coarse. It is used for carpets and other heavy uses. Some of these breeds are the Cotswolds, Leicesters, Lincolns and Romneys.

Now we come to the fine-wool sheep. These sheep are from the Old Country, originating in Spain. They are strictly wool-type sheep with thin boney carcasses. The lambs, however, still have carcasses that are acceptable for food. As far as American tastes go, most of us can enjoy lamb but very few of us are fond of mutton, the meat of mature sheep, anyway. No matter what breed, mutton has a very distinctive strong flavor and aroma.

The wool from fine-wool sheep is of the smallest diameter, of excellent quality for clothing. It is much finer and softer than that from most medium-wool breeds. Wool from the fine-wool breeds is the standard for grading all wool, according to the old Blood Grade system of grading.

All the fine-wool breeds originally came from the Spanish Merino. The French developed the Rambouillet from it. We have developed the American Merino and the Delaine Merino. There is also an Australian Merino. Besides their fine wool, the Spanish Merino had the characteristics of being very hardy and able to travel great distances. Their shepherds moved them seasonally between mountains and valleys. They have an exceptional flocking tendency which keeps them close together when traveling.

Merinos:

Rams average 150 to 225 lbs., ewes 90 to 150 lbs. They are a relatively small thin breed with large horns on the rams only. Their eyes get covered with wool and must be kept trimmed. Delaine Merinos have fewer body-skin folds and are thereby easier to shear but they have the coarsest wool for Merinos. Delaines are the largest Merinos with the best mutton qualities. Merinos are very hardy and good grazers. They can thrive on poor pastures. They may produce 11 to 18 pounds of wool per year. Merinos are less prolific than medium-wool sheep with fewer twins.

Rambouillets, the French-bred Merinos are large, rugged,hardy sheep. The rams weigh over 250 lbs. with large curled horns. Ewes weigh over 150 lbs. and are hornless. They have good carcasses. Rams may produce up to 25 lbs. of wool a year, ewes up to 18 lbs. They are good grazers, very hardy and adaptable. They are very popular in the Western U. S. as range sheep. They are a little large for easy handling, though, and their wool is more coarse than Merinos.

For our purposes, for raising a few sheep for high-quality wool for our own clothing, for low maintenance and perhaps using some excess lambs for meat, I would recommend one of the fine wool breeds, Merinos or Rambouillets. I would pick one that is popular in your locality. As for the medium-wool breeds, probably the Dorsets, Cheviots or Targhees are the only ones I would want. Their wool is more coarse than the fine-wool breeds but most people are more familiar with medium wool and mutton-type sheep so they tend to choose them.

I'll just mention the Karakul, a Russian fur-type breed of sheep. They are medium-sized with poor carcass quality. Their fleece has a long coarse outer coat and a fine short under-coat. It is used mostly for carpets. Very young lambs produce the typical pelts with the black curly hair, Persian lamb and Karakul.

FEEDING

Sheep generally do well on nothing but pasture except during pregnancy and lactation, when they should be given more grain. They graze the forage very close to the ground so their pasture should be rotated often enough to prevent damage to the pasture. In average areas, you can count on carrying about 15 ewes with their lambs per acre of pasture. They usually do very well on mixtures of legumes and grasses.

During the second half of pregnancy and during lactation, when they are nursing their lambs, I would give each ewe ¼ to ½ pound of grain per day.

During the winter or non-pasture season, I would give them 2 to 4 pounds of hay per day each, depending on their sizes. If the weather is cold and they are on hay, you may need to give them up to a pound of grain per day so that they can maintain their health and body condition.

"Flushing" is the process of feeding extra food for several weeks before breeding time. For typical sheep that are on hay or pasture and are in mediocre condition, flushing will raise the lamb crop to around 150%, an average of 1½ lambs per ewe, which means that half of the ewes give birth to twins. But if the ewes are in top condition, flushing won't help. If your ewes are fat, over-conditioned, you must decrease their food for 6 weeks before breeding or you will get a poor lamb crop. Flushing generally consists of feeding ½ to ¾ pound of grain per ewe per day or putting them on lush pasture or top quality legume hay free-choice. Some farmers feed as high as 2 pounds of grain per day for flushing, especially if the pasture was poor. Grain rations for sheep consist of a mixture of local grains such as oats, corn, wheat, milo or others.

Farmers that have trouble with ketosis in their ewes at lambing time add a half-pint or more of molasses per ewe per day to their grain ration.

BREEDING

In most climates, sheep have a breeding season of about August to January. Their estrous cycle takes from 13 to 19 days.

They may be in heat for from 3 hours to 3 days during each cycle.

If you have been feeding your sheep well, you can safely breed the ewes their first year if they are over 9 months old. Before breeding, trim all the sheep around their eyes and under their tails. This is called tagging. While you're at it, check all their feet to see if they need trimming.

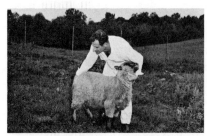

Catch sheep by loose skin of flank. Hold it with left hand under jaw, right hand over its dock.

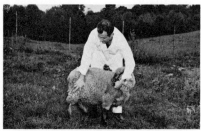

Slip left thumb into sheep's mouth behind incisor teeth. Move right hand to sheep's right hip. Turn its head around .

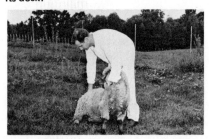

Holding its lower jaw tightly, bend its head back over its right shoulder and press its rear end down and toward you.

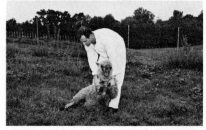

Lower sheep to the ground, then grab its front legs and lift its front end up between your knees

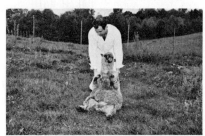

Position for examination and trimming of feet.

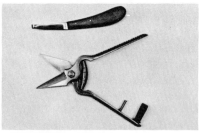

Hoof knife and hoof shears

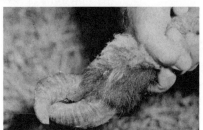

Excessively overgrown hoof, causing lameness

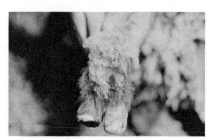

Same hoof after proper trimming

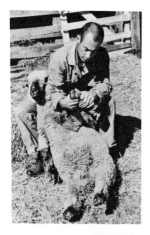

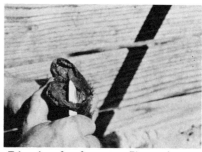

Trimming for foot rot. First, trim overgrown hoof wall with sharp knife. Remove ragged and separated parts of hoof from diseased foot.

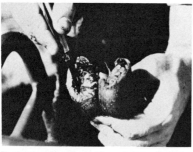

Probe hoof with knife point to find deep pockets of infection. Tap on sole to locate hidden pockets under the sole.

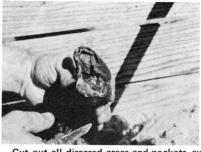

Cut out all diseased areas and pockets, even if it requires cutting through healthy tissue and drawing blood.

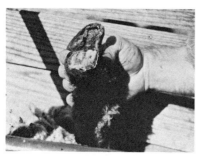

Appearance with all diseased tissue removed from the one claw.

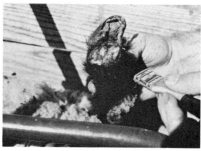

Paint trimmed area with fresh disinfectant

You can use a young ram, over 10 months old, for up to 10 or 12 ewes. Older, mature rams can efficiently service up to 30 ewes. Their fertility decreases after about 5 years of age.

The ewes' gestation periods vary with the breeds. Fine-wool breeds have gestation periods of 150 to 155 days. Southdowns usually have 144 days. Shropshires are usually 145 days and Hampshires 146.

You must try to be on hand at lambing time to assist the ewes and care for the lambs. Neither ewes nor lambs seem to have very much sense at this time.

In cold climates, set up a lamb brooder. This is often just a piece of plywood covering a corner of a stall with a light or heat lamp hung through a hole. Just be sure you don't burn down the barn. The important thing is that you must prevent chilling of the lambs. Assist the ewe if she has difficulty with birth. Be sure to scrub her rear end and your hands and arms before helping. Dry each lamb as soon as it is born and put it in the brooder. Give it warm milk or water, 103°F (39.4°C), and give each one an enema with warm water with a little mild soap in it. *Don't* use detergent in the enema! Use a bulb syringe with a soft tip on it.

You should dock the tails and castrate the ram lambs at 7 to 10 days of age. Follow the suggestions for goat kids for castrating. You must dock their tails because they naturally have long wooly tails that collect loads of manure and are then attacked by fly maggots. Dock the tails with a scissors or other cutting instrument and cauterize them with a hot iron. In fly season, paint them with a fly repellent smear after docking and castration. An early-castrated sheep is called a wether.

DISEASES AND PARASITES

The cardinal rule to avoid problems is to purchase young healthy stock and prevent exposure to outside sources. Sheep have several parasite and disease problems that you can't prevent but you can minimize these with preventive action. Check your sheep carefully on a regular basis. Since they are self-sufficient and need only pasture, people often neglect them. Clip off any wool that is matted with manure. Clip around any wounds and treat them immediately. Use fly repellent on wounds if needed. Trim their feet as needed. Rotate their pastures at least every 60 days to break the life cycles of the internal parasites. Pasture your sheep where someone can keep a close watch on them. Sheep are defenseless against dogs and, for some reason, even pet dogs will often attack them for no apparant reason. Put your sheep in a barn at night if you have any problems at all with roaming carnivores.

Sheep are susceptible to some of the same diseases as goats. Especially common are foot rot, pinkeye, sore mouth and ketosis. These are discussed under goat diseases. The courses and treatments are about the same as for goats. Let's discuss a few of the more common sheep diseases.

Enzootic Ataxia:
Cause:

This is a nutritional copper deficiency, seen mostly in Colorado, Montana, California, Ohio and Florida.

Signs:

The first signs are frequent stillborn lambs and lambs that are so weak they can't nurse. If it affects one-to-four-month old lambs, they get posterior paresis (partial paralysis in the hind quarters), staggering, incoordination, then progression to complete paralysis and death. Older lambs get diarrhea, loss of color to the wool, loss of crimp to the wool (steely wool), then progressive weakness, anemia and weight loss. Adults get the same steely wool, loss of color to the wool, anemia and weakness.

Prevention:

If this nutritional deficiency is present in your locality, give 1 gram of copper sulfate mixed in 1 ounce of water to each ewe 60 days before lambing. Give it by mouth with a dose syringe. Injectable copper is available to treat the disease.

White Muscle Disease:
Cause:

This is a nutritional deficiency of vitamin E and/or the mineral selenium. The deficiency occurs in calves and lambs in the springtime in certain areas of the U.S. West Coast states and in a few other states. There seem to be sporadic outbreaks of this problem for some unknown reason.

Signs:

The animals develop a stiff, straddling gait. It becomes difficult for the lambs to get up and keep up with the ewes. They may develop rapid pulse and rapid breathing. Some may die.

Post-mortem Examination:

When you open the animal and incise the muscles, you will see areas of pale color or white streaks in the muscle tissue. There may be whole groups of muscles with the light color. These lesions will be the same on both sides (bilaterally symmetrical).

Prevention:

Veterinarians can provide injections of vitamin E and selenium if the problem is common in your area. There are presently no legal feed supplements for selenium, so you would have to ship in feed from an area of the U.S. with high soil selenium. You can give supplemental vitamin E. In most outbreaks the animals are being fed very poor-quality feed. It is seldom seen in animals getting a good quality green leafy hay or pasture with some cereal concentrate.

Enterotoxemia (Overeating Disease):

Cause:

This is a disease caused by toxins from intestinal bacteria of the species *Clostridium perfringens* type C or D. Production of the toxins is usually stimulated by overfeeding, especially with lush feed or pasture such as young grass, grain or milk.

Signs:

Sudden acute illness occurs with signs of colic (stomach pains), frequent getting up and down and kicking at the belly. These signs progress to tetanic (stiff) spasms, convulsions, then prostration and death. Those few that live over 24 hours will show diarrhea but most of the affected lambs will die within 2 to 24 hours.

Post-mortem Examination:

The walls of the stomach and intestines are hemorrhagic. There are hemorrhages resembling paint-brush marks on the intestines, diaphragm or lining of the abdominal cavity. There are hemorrhages on the outside and inside of the heart. Most of the lymph nodes are swollen and reddened.

Prevention:

Unfortunately, treatment is usually not successful even with specific antitoxin unless it is given immediately at the first hint of an outbreak. There are enterotoxemia toxoids types C & D available with which you can immunize feedlot lambs prior to putting them on rich feed. If you suspect you are getting it in your suckling lambs, cut down the feed for the ewes to reduce their milk production. You should be able to easily avoid this disease because you will not be trying to fatten your lambs as a commercial operator would do in a feedlot.

Caseous Lymphadenitis (Pseudotuberculosis):

Cause:

This is a chronic infectious disease caused by the bacteria *Corynebacterium pseudotuberculosis* (or *C. ovis*). Goats and deer can also get it. Cattle can get skin nodules from it that resemble tuberculosis. It is a worldwide disease. Nearly 20% of all sheep condemned at slaughter are condemned because of this disease.

Signs:

It develops slowly so it is seen more in older sheep and it is more common on permanent feedlots than in range flocks. The sheep can develop no resistance or immunity to this organism. The bacteria pass into the feces and usually infect another sheep through a skin wound such as during shearing. Affected sheep may develop a chronic cough with pneumonia. They gradually become weak and thin. Their lymph nodes on the shoulders and under the legs may be enlarged enough to easily feel them as hard lumps. The lumps or abcesses may be opened. They contain a greenish-yellow pastey material. Old lesions contain a sandy calcified pus with concentric layers. These lesions are diagnostic. On post-mortem you may find the abcesses in any lymph nodes or in any other tissue, even the brain or eye. The abcesses can reach 12 inches in diameter but are usually only 1½ inches. Affected sheep are easily killed by other stresses.

Control:

There is no treatment because the lesions are walled off by a thick capsule that won't admit drugs or antibiotics. Vaccines and bacterins don't do much to prevent it. The best control once you get it in your flocks is scrupulous sanitation and marketing or destroying any animals that show lesions. The bacteria are killed by sunlight and disinfectants so disinfect all the indoor pens. When shearing, do the lambs first. After each sheep, dip the clipper blades in barbers' disinfectant. During the shearing, check each adult sheep for swollen lymph nodes in front of the shoulder blades and in the flanks. Get rid of any with "lumps." Shear these last! Control biting insects as these might transmit the disease mechanically.

Ulcerative Dermatosis, Lip and Leg Ulceration or Venereal Disease of Sheep:

Cause:

This is a virus disease that is transmitted during the breeding and by body contact. It is seen mostly in yearlings and adults. It occurs worldwide and is common in the western U.S.

Signs:

Affected sheep may get lesions on the legs between the hoof and the knee or hock joint. Females may get lesions around the vulva and males may get inflammation and swelling of the prepuce or the penis or both. They may also get lesions on the upper lip, usually between the lip and nostril, and on the chin below the lower lip. The lesions start as ulcers and become covered with scabs. Under the scab is a creamy, odorless pus. These ulcerations can go quite deep, even clear through the lip.

Control:

There are no vaccines or antiserums for this virus. Treatment consists of caring for the wounds and keeping insects off them until they heal. Topical antiseptics may help a little but the most important thing is to prevent fly maggot infestation. Prevent the disease by examining all new rams and ewes and quarantining them to prevent introducing this problem to your flock.

Nose Bots:

Cause:

A certain fly of the species *Oestrus ovis* lays its live larvae on the noses of the sheep. The larvae enter the nose and mature there. They then drop out and pupate in the ground. They live in the nose for 2 weeks to 9 months!

Signs:

Infested sheep show a profuse clear mucous, then muco-purrulent, nasal discharge. There may be streaks of blood in the

Oestrus ovis **adult fe-male. Sheep nasal fly.**

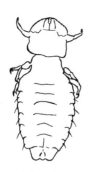

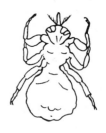

Biting louse of sheep, *Damalinia ovis.* **About 1.5 mm. long.**

Oestrus ovis **larvae, about 3 mm. long.**

Sheep ked, *Melophag-us ovinus,* **4 to 6 mm. long.**

discharge. They sneeze a lot and lose weight. Severe infestations can lead to fatal infections or to blockage of the nasal passage with convulsions and death. When the flies are trying to lay their larvae on the sheeps' noses, you will see the sheep running wildly and stamping their feet with their noses down. They may be vigorously shaking their heads. You may see a group of sheep standing with their heads down in the middle of a circle. All these activities are to avoid the flies.

Treatment:
There are several commercial insecticides available to instill in their noses or to give orally. Unfortunately, if nose bots are common in your area, you will have continual problems.

Sheep Ked or Sheep Tick:

Cause:
This is actually a wingless fly (insect) of the species *Melophagus ovinus* that attacks only sheep. It is dark brown, 4 to 6 mm long and it sucks blood.

Signs:
The sheep will be restless, biting and scratching. They will damage their fleeces, become anemic and show poor growth. If you examine the animals you can find the keds in the fleece around the neck, shoulders, belly and thighs. Keds are more abundant in the winter.

Prevention and Treatment:
The keds are passed directly by contact. They are passed from ewes to lambs. Shearing removes most of them so if the weather is warm, you may shear the ewes before lambing. You can also use commercial powder or spray insecticides *after* shearing to eradicate them from your flock. Again, inspect new livestock and don't bring sheep ked onto your place.

Lice:

Sheep commonly are infested with lice. There are 4 species of biting and sucking lice that infest sheep. Use nontoxic insecticide powder after shearing if your sheep have them.

Screwworms and Myiasis, also called Strike, Wool Maggots, Fleeceworms or Blowflies:

Cause:
Various species of flies lay their eggs on wounds or on filthy wool. The eggs hatch into maggots which may simply irritate the animal or may actually burrow into the flesh. Some species attack just dead flesh of wounds. Others, screwworms, attack living flesh,

burrowing into the tissue, causing severe damage and even death. Fly strike is common after castration and tail docking and on wounds from insect bites (keds, etc.) or other injuries. Any type of maggots will attack a glob of wool that is matted to the skin with wet manure. The activities of the maggots then cause great local irritation and can lead to a severe infection. The maggots then enter the infected tissues.

Signs:

Affected sheep lose their appeties and become depressed and toxic. You may see a large or small open pink wound or round hole with serum or pus draining from it. Close inspection may reveal small round holes in the flesh where maggots have burrowed in. You may see maggots in the holes. This is screwworm. The U.S. & Mexican governments are presently carrying out distribution of sterilized male screwworm flies to re-eradicate this pest from the United States. You may also see strike as a large number of maggots on a tag or spot of wet or dirty wool or on a wound, without them burrowing into the flesh.

Prevention:

If screwworms are presently in your locality, you must constantly check all your livestock for wounds. Every wound must be treated with an insecticide smear or a pine tar repellant. These are available at rural stores. In cold climates you should do all your tail docking and castrating in cold weather before fly season. Shear any dirty or matted wool, especially around the tails. When an animal is affected, trim all around the area to find any more lesions. Pick out all the maggots and apply an insecticide. Be sure to crush the maggots so they don't pupate.

Scabies or Sheep Scab:

Cause:

Sheep can be affected by various species of parasitic skin mites. These are extremely small 8-legged arthropods. You need a magnifying glass just to see them. The species of mite can only be identified under the microscope. Psoroptic scab is so contagious and destructive to fleeces that it is under U.S. eradication control.

Signs:

The mites bite and burrow and cause extreme itching. The Sheep destroy their fleeces with their vigorous scratching and biting. Affected sheep are restless with the continuous biting and scratching. You will see bald areas where the wool is almost gone. There are usually tags or clumps of wool hanging from the bare spots. The bald areas spread and the affected skin becomes irritated with red or yellow sores and crusts. You can find the mites at the edges of the bare spots if you use a strong magnifying glass.

Treatment and Prevention:

Scabies is so contagious that it requires isolation or quarantine of the whole flock and dipping in insecticides to clear it up. Dip the flock at least two times, 10 to 14 days apart, in a commercial sheep dip, available at rural stores.

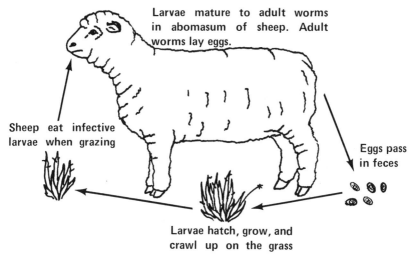

Lifecycle of *Haemonchus contortus,* the Stomach worm or Wire worm of Sheep, Cattle and Goats

Internal Parasites (Worms)

Cause:

Sheep can be infested with many different types of worms. There are 10 different genus groups and many more species of stomach and intestinal roundworms of sheep. All are more or less damaging. They also get tapeworms, flukes and lungworms but these should not be very common on most small farms. Keep dogs out of the sheep pasture except when using them to herd sheep. Dogs can carry several species of tapeworms that are harmful to sheep.

Signs:

Worms can cause all levels of slow growth, weight loss and even death. Severely infested sheep may be thin and depressed.

They may have dry, poor wool and even edema or swelling of lower parts of the body or under the jaw. Young stock can easily die of severe worm infestation. One species of worm is so debilitating that it has long been called the "bankrupt worm."

Treatment:

Phenothiazine and thiabendazole are the least toxic effective drugs. Phenothiazine should be used only as the "microfine" type. This smaller particle size is more effective. Phenothiazine is green and stains the wool green. It comes through the urine red which then stains the wool. It can easily be toxic to sick or weak individuals. You can give an adult sheep 25 grams and a lamb over 2 months old 12½ grams. Most commercial preparations are mixed to contain 12½ grams per ounce so it comes out to two ounces for adults and 1 ounce for lambs. Don't withhold the feed before worming. Give it by mouth with a dose syringe.

Thiabendazole suspension is very safe and doesn't stain the wool. It is given at the rate of 3 grams for large adults, 2 grams for smaller adults, such as the smaller breeds, and 1 gram for lambs under 50 pounds.

Prevention:

Try to build a flock that is free of worms if possible although this is hard to do. Quarantine new stock and worm them several times before putting them on your regular pastures. Don't mix sheep and goats as they can cross-infest each other. New sheep should be wormed probably every 3 months for a year and you should practice good pasture rotation to try to get them free of worms. If you don't get rid of them, you will have to worm regularly, usually every spring and fall.

14
Notes on Beef and Dairy Cattle

BEEF CATTLE

If your place is large enough, with some unused range or pasture, beef cattle might be a good addition. You certainly don't want to raise them the way commercial operators do, crowding them into feedlots, carrying them hay and grain. Beef cattle are very self-sufficient if there is decent forage available. They need a grassy or legume type of forage, not just brush and scrub trees. In dry desert areas it may take several hundred acres of natural unirrigated land to support a single beef but since they are ruminants they can utilize natural low-quality forage that might otherwise be wasted. If you have the land, use it. Consider range beef cattle as a semi-wildlife species. You simply put them out on the range and let them fend for themselves. Then when you want a beef you have to go round one up. At this point it will be rather wild and you will have to play cowboy. The drawback to this range-cattle approach is that you need some natural or manmade barriers to keep them on or near your property or else you will never see them again. If you use fencing, you must ride the fenceline regularly to find and repair damage that might let them escape. If you have a box canyon, fence off the opening. Either way you must check regularly to be sure they have adequate water and forage. In dry or cold weather you may have to haul water or hay to them to be sure you don't lose them.

Rounding up range cattle is tougher than you might imagine. For one thing, they learn to hide and blend into the bushes just like the wildlife. They breed, reproduce and raise their young in a wild state. You probably will need a horse or stock dogs to harvest your occassional beef. If you are in an open range area with other beef owners then you must round up your cattle yearly to brand your calves unless you want them to become a part of someone else's herd. You may need to vaccinate them at this time depending on the disease prevelance in your area.

Working cattle for branding and vaccinating on open range with no corrals is exceptionally hard work which calls for experienced cowhands. I would highly recommend that you build a corral with a chute and maybe a loading dock. A loading dock is a narrow chute built onto a pen or corral with a treaded incline or some other type of dock so you can back a truck up to it and drive the cattle onto the truck. The loading chute should be long enough to move a number of animals into it and close a gate behind them. They will move up into the truck more easily this way than if you

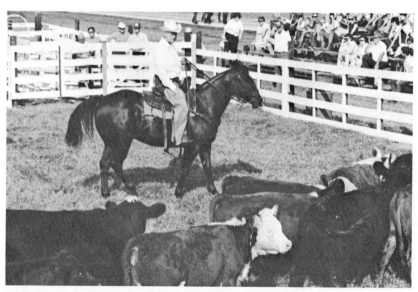

Tom Lockwood demonstrating cutting at the 1970 Ohio Farm Science Review

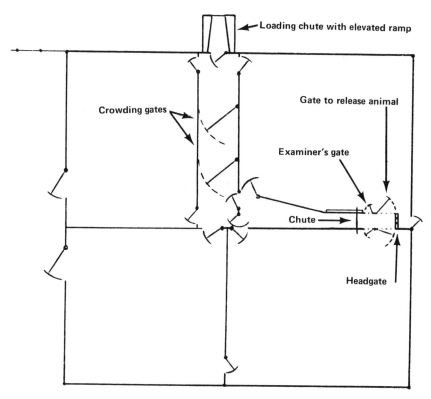

Design of cattle corral for sorting, vaccinating, pregnancy examining, treating, and loading.

try to drive them in one-at-a-time. The ones in the rear can be prodded and they push the ones in front into the truck. A loading dock is a necessity if you plan to sell any beef or send yours somewhere to be slaughtered. If you are near a cold-storage plant, you may just send your beef there to be slaughtered, butchered and stored.

Although the commercial beef raisers have been taking a financial beating for a number of years, the time may come when those people controlling food production have the upper hand. At that time, you may find that commercial beef production is a real gold mine. I certainly hope it works out this way because I feel

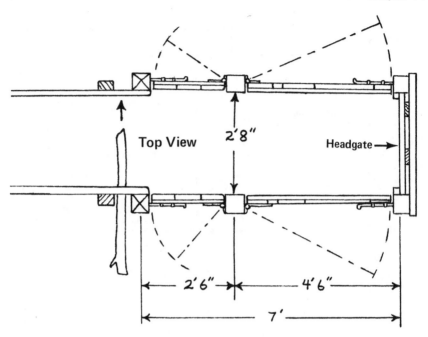

Top View

2'8"

Headgate →

2'6"   4'6"

7'

Cattle chute for treatment and examination

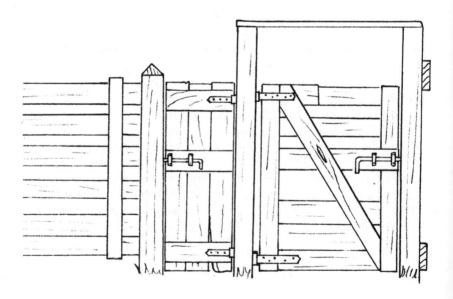

that this is the natural scheme of things.

The squeeze chute is a narrow aisle inside of, or attached to, the corral. This chute has a number of gates or removable parts so that you can run a cow into it, restrain her and work on her. Ideally it should have a head gate which is like a very strong stancheon. She is driven into the chute and her head is locked into the head gate. Then there are other gates or slats on both sides and the rear of the chute that can be opened to give you access to the cow. There are lots of variations and refinements of these corrals and chutes to make the work of handling cattle easier. Often there is

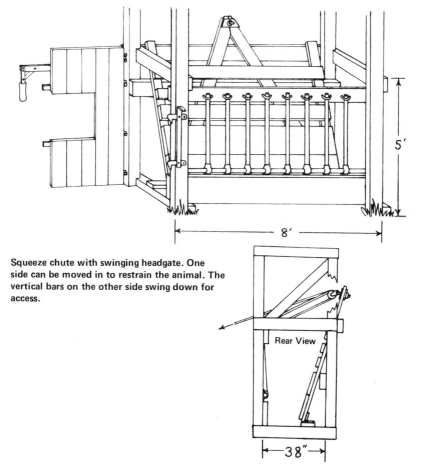

Squeeze chute with swinging headgate. One side can be moved in to restrain the animal. The vertical bars on the other side swing down for access.

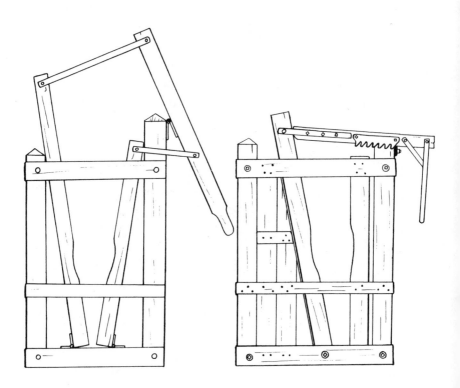

Various designs for cattle headgates

a wide lane leading up to the chute and the sides of the lane swing in to move the cattle forward. These are called crowding gates. Squeeze chutes of tubular steel are available commercially. You can design your corral around the types of loading and squeezing chutes that you can buy or build. You must design it so that you can sort them from the chute. That is, after you have examined the cattle you can let them out of the chute into one of at least two different areas for sorting purposes. this may be to cull or just to separate them. Commercial breeders often have a veterinarian rectally palpate all the cows in the fall. Those that are not pregnant may be culled, in order to avoid feeding them all winter. This is commonly done in northern areas with severe winters that require a lot of supplemental feed.

If you don't have the size of ranch to run range cattle, perhaps you can keep a few head of breeding stock on a pasture. The acreage they will require is quite variable, according to the productivity of your land. For a rough estimate you can figure that most mature beef cattle will wiegh 1,000 to 1,500 pounds. In most climates they will need about 2% of their body weight in dry roughage per day. This may vary from 1½% in warm climates to 3½% in severe climates. They won't need grain or supplements except salt and mineral until you wish to fatten them for slaughter.

An average requirement then would be 25 pounds of dry roughage per day or 9,125 pounds per year per head. This may require anywhere from a little under an acre on extremely productive land to several acres on poorer land, for one adult beef. Most areas require over an acre per head. Reproduction will require a little more, of course. Growing calves, from weanlings to yearlings, will consume about 3 pounds of dry roughage per 100 pounds of body weight. If you have extra grain, give each calf about 2 lbs. of grain per day the first year. Do this with a creep feeder. A creep feeder is a small corral or shed with narrow openings. The calves can walk through the openings to get to the grain but the adult cattle cannot. Start feeding soft grains at 2 to 4 weeks of age.

For a small farm I would recommend at least one beef bull and several cows to assure a continuing breeding stock. Fortunately, beef bulls are fairly manageable, especially if they are handled regularly when they are young. You can put a halter on a young beef bull and teach him to lead quite well. If you have your cattle in a pasture where they see you and you work with them regularly to check for wounds and injuries, they will be quite manageable. Of course, a beef cow or bull, especially a cow with a calf, can hurt you because of its size and strength. Don't let young children play in the beef pasture in case a cow might get upset and charge or accidentally run over someone.

Range beef cattle are more wild and unpredictable. A range cow with a calf is definitely dangerous. Don't try to approach her on foot. Round her up and drive her into a corral on horseback or with stock dogs.

Be sure your beef have plenty of water available at all times. Don't rely on a small spring or stream unless you check it regularly.

Provide a regular supply of salt, preferably trace-mineralized, iodized salt. Cattle can get by with block salt but I would recommend that you use loose salt in a waterproof feeder. This is a salt box with a waterproof protective roof, overhanging the opening. These can be built like a weathervane so rain doesn't blow in on the salt. Check the salt box regularly. With loose salt they can get as much as they need. In hot weather they may not get enough salt from licking a salt block. You can anticipate needing anywhere from 1 to 2½ pounds of salt per month per cow on pasture. This means you should stock probably 25 pounds of salt per head of beef per year.

When you decide to slaughter a beef you should put it in a separate lot or corral so you can feed it grain for fattening.

For fattening a beef for slaughter you usually give them about 2% of their body weight in grain per day, 1% in hay, and one or two pounds of protein supplement per day. Protein supplements include soybean oil meal, cottonseed and linseed meals, surplus milk and meat products, and surplus eggs. Steers on full feed such as this will usually gain two pounds per day. Usually three to four weeks of grain feeding will put a nice firm "finish" on them and they will be ready for slaughter.

Horned breeds should be de-horned before 4 weeks of age.

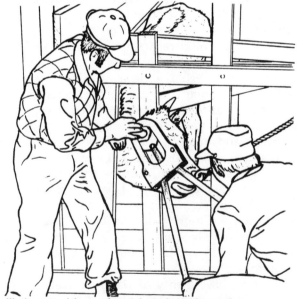

Use of guillotine-type dehorner for adult cattle and large calves

I would recommend that you use an electric dehorning iron. Done properly this is safer and simpler than either caustic paste or stick or dehorning gouges. Don't leave their horns on them or you will get a lot of injuries.

You should castrate your male beef calves at 3 to 8 weeks of age. A male beef castrated at a young age is called a steer. Castration causes a change in growth and development. Steer beef is higher in quality and more tender than bull meat. Steers are easier to handle, too.

For a family-sized self-sufficient farm I definitely recommend that you stick to the *Bos taurus* or European breeds of beef cattle, mainly the Aberdeen Angus, Hereford, and Shorthorn breeds. Galloways are black like Angus. They are hardy and good grazers but are rare in the U.S. Scotch Highlands are very rugged cattle with long, shaggy hair and long horns. Few have been imported. Some are being raised on the Aleutian Islands. I recommend that you not try to raise any of the Brahman or Zebu breeds or their crosses unless you have the experience and facilities. These are a different species of cattle, *Bos indicus*, mostly from India. These are the breeds that have a large fatty hump on their shoulders, drooping ears, and excessive folds of skin under the neck and underline. They are resistant to ticks and well-adapted to tropical climates, but they are very large, nervous, and unpredictable. Brahman bulls are too mean to be handled except by an experienced person with the proper equipment. Some of the crossbred Brahman breeds are the Brangus, Beefmaster, Braford, Charbray, and Santa Gertrudis.

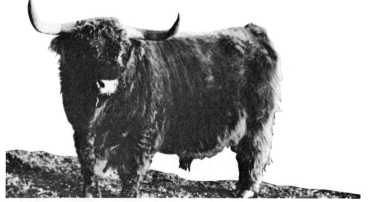

Scotch Highland Bull. A very hardy breed

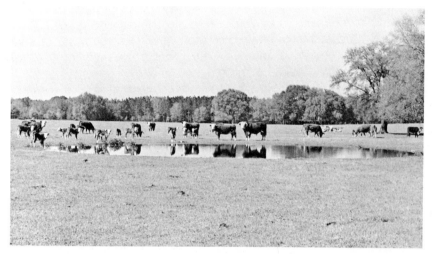

Photos courtesy, American Hereford Association

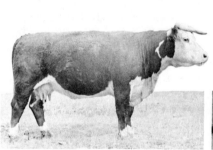

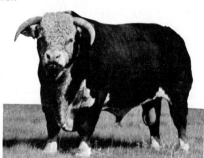

Hereford Cow   Hereford Bull

DAIRY CATTLE

If your place is large and you prefer, you may want to keep dairy cattle instead of goats for milk production. Dairy cattle have several drawbacks for a small operation. You have a very large animal to maintain and she won't give any milk unless she is successfully bred and "freshens" or gives birth. So you have a larger maintenance unit and a larger gamble. If you have been around dairy cattle and you are attached to them and their docile manners, you may wish to keep a few dairy cattle on your place. The only drawback to keeping dairy cattle is the bull. Under no circumstances could I advise anyone to keep a dairy bull. These creatures are without a doubt the meanest, most dangerous animals in the country. They aren't simply dangerous like a wildcat, which will fight if cornered. They are agressive killers. I can't tell you how many farmers and veterinarians have been attacked, injured or killed by dairy bulls! Many a veterinarian has been "retired" from large-animal practice by a dairy bull. Most dairy farms today don't keep a bull. They use artificial insemination (A.I.) for all their breeding. The A.I. companies keep a selection of exceptionally well-bred and good-producing bulls of different breeds. They collect the semen, treat it and freeze it in ampules for artificial insemination by veterinarians and trained A.I. technicians.

The A.I. companies don't take any chances with the handling of their dairy bulls. The bulls are kept in pens made of welded heavy steel pipe and concrete. The pen gates open into aisles of steel-pipe fencing. The bulls are handled with long-handled bull-clamps which grasp the nose or the ring in the nose in conjunction with a chain from the nose-ring or a chain around the horns. The bull handler never gets on the same side of the steel fence as the bull. The aisles are made with gates that can be arranged to take the bull wherever they want him for semen collection, treatment or exercise. Treatment is done in heavily-built stocks where the bull can be completely restrained. Dairy bulls are so mean that they may become agitated and charge the fence just because someone walks by. In the old days dairy bulls kept on farms were forever breaking down the wooden fences and getting out. Contrary to popular opinion the bull does not usually injure you by attacking with his horns. That is, he is not trying to gore his victim. Rather he tries to get you down on the ground and crush you with his head or chest. Cows, that is females, are the ones more likely to gore a person or another animal with their horns.

There are several ways to get around this dairy bull problem. If you are in a farming community you can just use A.I. like every-one else. But if you really want to become self-sufficient or if you are quite isolated then you are going to want some type of breeding stock of both sexes. One solution is to use a beef bull to breed your dairy cows since beef bulls are relatively docile and easy to manage. Of course, you cannot use a small bull like an Angus on a huge cow like a Holstein. Many self-sufficient farmers like to keep Jersey cows because of their high butterfat production. These cows are small enough for a beef bull to breed. The only drawback to using a beef bull on a dairy cow is that the female calves won't grow up to be good dairy cows like their mothers. You will get good steers for beef but you won't get good replacement milk cows. The best solution to the dangerous dairy bull problem is to raise a dual-purpose breed of cattle which will provide manageable bulls and cows, an adequate milk supply and good beef.

Originally Milking Shorthorns, Red Polls and Devons were the breeds of cattle raised and promoted as dual-purpose with the ability both to give lots of milk and to produce good beef. These breeds were popular on small family farms. Unfortunately all these breed associations have officially abandoned the dual-purpose type in favor of changing their breeds either to a dairy type or a beef type. This is because the family farms have been largely replaced by large commercial operations and the commercial producers need animals that are extremely efficient either at milk production or beef production. You can't get top efficiency for both types of production out of the same animal.

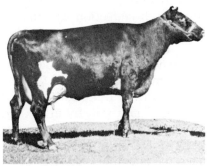
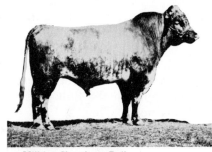

Milking Shorthorn Cow   **Milking Shorthorn Bull**

The American Milking Shorthorn Society is now promoting their breed mainly as dairy but they still point out their dual-purpose background. They also promote them for crossbreeding with beef breeds to improve the milk production of beef cow mothers in order to get greater gains from the calves. In England they are called Dairy Shorthorns; in Canada, Dual-Purpose Shorthorns; in the U.S. and New Zealand, Milking Shorthorns. The Society also recognizes the Australian Illawarra Shorthorns although these are a separate dairy breed not closely related to the other Milking Shorthorns. In Colonial days the forerunners of Milking Shorthorns were called Durhams.

The Red Poll Cattle Club of America declared their breed

a beef breed in 1970 but some breeders are still milking them and are carefully maintaining the traditional milking qualities. While Red Polls were still being raised as a dual-purpose breed their recorded milking average was 7,627 pounds of milk per year at 4.19% butterfat. This is about three gallons of milk a day.

Devons used to be a dual-purpose breed but now the Devon Cattle Association is promoting them as a beef breed. Most individuals still retain some of their dual-purpose dairyness, however, and they could very well be milked.

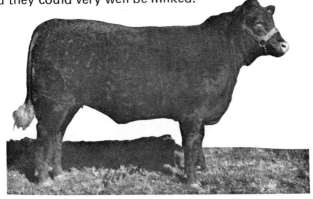

Devon Heifer, courtesy Devon Cattle Association, Inc.

Another breed you might consider is the Irish Dexter. This is the smallest breed of cattle in America. Cows average 650 pounds

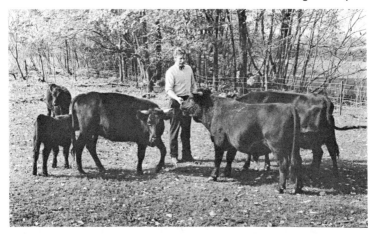

Irish Dexter adults and calves. Courtesy *Organic Gardening and Farming,* Emmaus, PA 18049

and bulls, 800 pounds. They are usually around 40" tall at the withers. The American Dexter Cattle Association promotes them as a dual-purpose breed. They were originally a hardy mountain breed, excellent grazers and able to thrive on rough forage. The Association claims that they require only three-fifths the feed of a 1,200-pound dairy cow and that Dexter cows will produce 400 to 600 gallons of milk per year, which is about one-and-one-third to two gallons per day. Because of their efficiency at digesting forage the Association claims that they need less grain per gallon of milk than the larger breeds of dairy cows. Unfortunately some Dexters carry genes for bulldog calves. This is a lethal recessive trait so that an occassional calf will die and be aborted during the fifth to ninth month of pregnancy. The cow may still give some milk on this aborted pregnancy, however, and future production is not harmed. Both cows and bulls are exceptionally gentle and easy to handle.

A family farm, or a small self-sufficient farm or ranch doesn't need and can't even utilize the huge quantities of milk produced by a good dairy cow. An acceptable commercial dairy cow will produce over 60 pounds (7 gallons) of milk per day! And you should always breed at least two cows per season in case one fails to freshen. That's an awful lot of milk to find a usage for.

Since the dual-purpose types of cattle breed true to their type they can be selectively bred by a discerning breeder to improve their desirable characteristics. This is something you can hardly do if you are crossing beef on dairy cattle. A dual-purpose type will cut down the breeding stock you must keep for beef and milk production so they are especially recommended for a small place. The bulls are usually docile and manageable which is another factor to recommend them. Moreover they are very hardy and require less attention and less concentrate feed than dairy breeds. You should expect to get around 4% butterfat and 20 pounds (2½ gallons) of milk per day on pasture or roughage alone from a dual-purpose cow. If fed grain they should produce more. Many cows of dual-purpose breeds that lean heavily toward the dairy type have achieved record-breaking milk production. But this is not your goal. In fact, you should stay away from record-breaking producers and their attendant problems.

Dual-purpose or dairy cows should be fed 2% of their body weight per day in dry roughage if they are not on pasture. If you have the facilities to put up silage you can replace half the hay with three times that much silage. Silage is very high in moisture so a heavier amount must be fed to get the same amount of nutrients. If a cow is lactating give her extra hay and about a pound of concentrate (grain) for every 5 pounds of milk she is producing.

When choosing your breeding stock, choose healthy cows with good, well-attached udders and a record for regular and easy calving in her line. Choose a bull with a docile, manageable disposition, good conformation and from a line with good producing cows.

15
Notes on Pets and Animals that Help With the Work

PETS IN GENERAL

Do you live in an urban environment? Take a look at your pet dog. Is he a contented, healthy, well-adjusted and obedient animal? If so he is lucky. Probably you spend a lot of time with him and give him regular attention and outlets. Or is he a nervous, yappy animal that goes berserk when someone comes to the door? Or how about the lethargic dog that looks like a watermelon on legs and sleeps or eats most of the time? These two extremes are poorly-adjusted house pets who probably have no jobs or "responsibilities" of their own. They have no outlets for their inherited tendencies to be helpers and part of the family life. Dogs were traditionally bred selectively for given jobs. The man who raised a working breed only bred the best performers. The others were neutered or disposed of. In the old days when dogs had jobs and had to earn their keep, selective breeding was an economic or even a survival necessity. Now our economic sucesses allow us to salve our soft hearts. We all tend to nurse the runt of the litter and save the physically defective individuals for pets. This is fine if you have the means to support the defectives as well as the superior performers. But just consider two points. First, during your busy days on a self-sufficient farm or ranch, will you have plenty of time to spend developing the talents of your superior animals as well as to take care of the poor doers? This applies to all your working animals, dogs, horses or any other species that require training. As long as you have the time and food for them, then go ahead and collect all the pets you want. But don't let your place be turned into a one-family welfare society because of feelings of guilt or a soft heart. Remember that stray and sick animals can bring diseases onto your place. Taking in a sick stray could wipe out all your other animals of that species or even of unrelated species. Also remember to plan ahead. You may be able to support lots of pets this year but what about a future year when you have drought, wind damage or other disasters that force you to cut back and live on your stores. Then you will wish you were supporting only your best working animals, the ones that carry their own weight, plus maybe a few favorite pets. The second point, as I suggested at first, is that the animal without a job or a purpose is probably very frustrated and perhaps even neurotic. This seems to account for many of the bad habits of housepets such as unreasonable barking, chewing, housebreaking accidents, digging in the yard and others. Just the simple procedure of obedience training a dog and working with him a few minutes every day gives him some purpose and satisfaction because he finds that he can do things that get attention and please his owner. Even cats frequently bring their masters "gifts" of birds or rodents they have caught.

Consider the plight of the bird in the little cage. Many people keep birds in tiny cages like prison cubicles. If you keep a trainable bird such as a parakeet, budgie or even a wild bird of prey, for Pete's sake take the fellow out every day for training and exercise. Let him have something to do. Remember that most of the small psitticine birds (birds with parrot-like beaks) are fruit tree pests so don't let them loose to establish themselves in your orchard! If you have birds that aren't usually trained such as canaries then have several of them and build a big, easily-cleaned flight cage. This is a large or long cage with natural shrubs or branches and room to fly back and forth.

I want to exhort you not to adopt or try to tame any wild creatures, that is, species of wildlife other than the domestic animals. So many people think it would be glamorous to have wildlife pets. They sometimes even try to keep them in an urban area. I can't tell you how many times people tell me about their unhappy experiences with their "pet" wild animal or exotic cat. Exotic cats, by the way, are all the wild species of cats. They have become the "in" pets especially since some well-known personalities raise or harbor them. The difference, which the average person doesn't realize, is that the "personalities" have the resources to provide housing and equipment for a satisfactory habitat for their wild species. Then there are the people who want to achieve status or ego trips with exotic species but they don't take the time and effort to research the subject to find out the animal's needs and habits. These people, as well as the misinformed ones, often try to make a house pet out of, for instance, a male racoon and then someone, usually a child, ends up severely bitten and scratched after the nasty fellow reaches sexual maturity, or maybe even before.

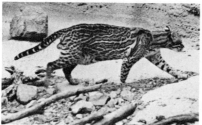

Ocelot, *Felis pardalis*. People often try to make a "pet" of this wild species.

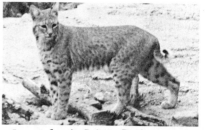

Lynx rufus, the Bobcat. Don't try to make a baby bobcat into a pet!

And then there was the fellow who called his veterinarian and wanted to know at what age and for what price he could get his prospective "pet" racoon de-clawed, de-fanged and castrated! All he wanted to do was take a naturally independent creature and cut out his teeth, his claws and his testicles so it could "vegetate" around the house. Let me say about both wildlife and exotic species that you should not consider keeping them unless you thoroughly research the subject and build a completely comfortable and natural housing situation so that the animals can have a relatively natural life. Only *after* you provide this can you morally proceed to try to tame the wild animal such as you might a domestic animal. Never trust a wild-species creature around children or unfamiliar people no matter how much you may personally trust the animal. There is one more tremendous, overriding reason why you should not adopt wild animals, even orphans, and that is the danger to you and your family of rabies. Pet skunks have been known to have been taken from the nest as babies (sucklings), raised, bitten friends or family and then tested positive for rabies. There are several documented cases of this type. Those people who were exposed were no doubt frightened for their lives because rabies is a horrible and deadly disease.

CATS

Now let's talk about a few pets that can work and help around the farm and ranch. One of the more underrated helpers is the cat. Farm cats generally take on two varieties, that is, house cats and barn cats. House cats are like any other pet cats but barn cats often become rather wild. In a large barn they can find their own food and shelter and reproduce with little or no contact with people so some of them are just not tame. Of course if you have the time to work with them you can tame the young ones with a little feeding, handling and affection. But tame or wild, your cats will do an admirable job of controlling the rat and mouse population.

Cats are susceptable to a viral disease called feline panleucopenia or feline distemper. This virus is distributed world-wide in domestic and wild cats. No matter where you live it is likely that your cats will be exposed to the distemper virus. On many farms, the barn cats are plagued by distemper and frequently all the young ones become ill, with many of them dying. Because of this I would recommend that you vaccinate your pet cats and, hopefully, your barn cats annually. If you live in an area that is endemic for rabies in the wildlife, I would also vaccinate the cats yearly for rabies. This is to protect both your animals and you and your family.

STOCK AND WORKING DOGS

Dogs are no doubt one of our oldest domestic species. For thousands of years dogs have been selectively bred and trained to help with the work. Probably at first this was the work of hunting. Then no doubt as men learned to herd livestock they taught their dogs to help. I'm sure you have seen a demonstration or at least a movie of herding dogs at work. They follow the cues of their master to move almost any type of animal from a ground squirrel to a herd of cattle.Their speed and intelligence enable them to herd more animals more efficiently than men on horseback. But training a dog to herd is no casual job. First, the master must know more than his charge. As with most skills, the best way to learn is to go to someone who does it. Even where I am from, Ohio, which still has one of the highest concentrations of sheep, few farmers train working stock dogs. But you can certainly find people who are still doing it. Contact the National Stock Dog Registry listed in the last chapter or contact the Animal Science Department and the

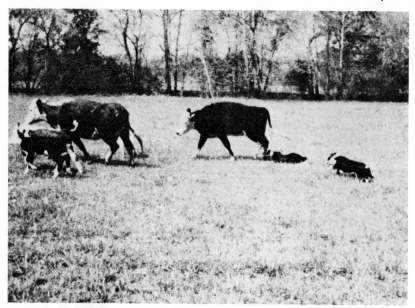

Team of Border Collies herding cattle. Courtesy Ben Means, Walnut Grove, Missouri

sheep herdsman at the nearest agricultural college.

In Ohio one of the most popular stock dog breeds is the Border Collie but many other breeds, such as Australian Shepherds, English Shepherds, and Queensland Blue Heelers and others, are suitable and have been selectively bred for sheep herding ability for years. Dogs that are bred for herding have natural tendencies for the job. Some individuals take to it so naturally that they need minimal training. A good stock dog can be taught to round up and move any of your livestock, sheep, cattle, goats, hogs or what-have-you.

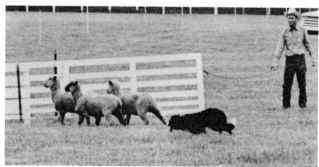

Border Collie herding sheep on command. Courtesy H.J. Cannon, Fairfield, Texas

The shepherds or stock dogs are not the only dogs that can be useful for a farm or retreat. A self-sufficient farm may be able to support other working dogs such as hunting dogs and guard dogs. Hunting dogs come in all varieties and sizes. The hunt takes full advantage of the dog's instinctive food-hunting traits so this is a natural job for him. Still, it takes a lot of skill, time and patience to train a dog to his specific job as a hunter's helper. Good dog-training books are helpful but I would recommend you go to an experienced trainer to get a good hunting dog or to have a good dog trained.

The true guard dog is supposed to be the most thoroughly-trained dog of all, contrary to popular conception. The idea of using vicious dogs, that even the trainer fears, to guard a store or yard is repugnant to any serious dog lover. This is widely done in this country but it is a dangerous short-cut. In the Old Country, the guard dog is a family protector and bodyguard and is respected as a perfectly trained obedience dog. In German kennel clubs a dog may not proceed to guard or attack training until it is so well obedience trained that it *never* fails to follow a known command. Then the dog is trained to protect its master from an agressor without command. However, even in the middle of the dog's attack, a command from his master will stop him. During training, on the master's command, the dog will submit to handling or examination by a person who was previously "assaulting" his master. This dog is also taught to enter and search an area or building with the command to either attack any intruder or just find him. This is then the "complete dog" as they call him. What a far cry from the "guard dogs" we see in the movies which must be lured into the "trainer's" truck with food or a chain. There are a few good books and a few clubs in the U.S. that do a good job with this type of training. They usually use the German title, schutzhund, for "the complete dog." This type of training, by the way, can only be done on a group basis. An owner must never "agitate" his own dog to attack him or a member of his family. This training requires experienced supervision in order to catch any bad habits before they become serious or dangerous. Consult the last chapter for organizations and books on this subject.

If there is no way that you can participate in a group to train a guard dog, simply do your best to train your dog for good obedience. Dogs naturally have an instinct for property and they will learn to guard or defend their property naturally. Just be watchful that they do not become too vicious about it. You don't want them attacking members of your family or the neighbor children. You can't afford to have a mean dog that is controlled only by a perimeter fence. Some day it may get over or through the fence and injure innocent people or livestock. Any breed of dog can be made vicious by an ignorant owner and this is how some of our good breeds get their bad reputations. So many insecure, inadequate people want a mean dog so that they can intimidate other people. They seem to get a morbid pleasure from having control of an animal that scares people. So what do they do? They choose a breed that has a reputation as a guard or attack dog such as a German Shepherd or a Doberman Pinscher since these dogs have been used by the military and police. Then they proceed to take a normal puppy and make him into a mean, vicious dog as they could well do to most any breed. What a crime!

The most satisfying way to handle any dog, for both the dog and its master, is to give it lots of time and attention and a job to do. Obedience training is the starting point for all types of canine occupations.

Dogs are susceptable to a number of serious diseases and parasites. Their habits of roaming and hunting are responsible for their contracting many of the canine diseases.

Canine distemper and infectious canine hepatitis are diseases caused by specific viruses. Both these viruses are world-wide in distribution. Distemper virus can be passed by aerosol, that is, can be airborne from an animal that is carrying it. It can occur naturally in wolves, foxes, coyotes and other canine species. Infectious canine hepatitis virus is usually spread in the urine from a sick or recovered dog.

Leptospirosis is a bacterial disease that is also passed in the urine from sick or recovered animals. Many species of animals, both wild and domestic, may catch it and spread it, including humans, dogs, hogs, cattle, sheep, goats and horses. Dogs commonly pick it up from the urine of rodents or from drinking water that was contaminated by infected urine.

Fortunately a combination vaccine is widely available for all three of these dangerous illnesses. Because these diseases can be picked up even in an isolated area and because they are so destructive I would recommend that you take the precaution of vaccinating your dogs annually. Start your new puppies on their vaccination program at six to eight weeks of age. Don't let them get half-grown and catch one of these diseases by failing to vaccinate them.

Because dogs like to roam and hunt they are more likely to catch rabies than are your livestock. Rabies is transmitted by the bite of a rabid animal. When a wild animal is coming down with the symptoms of rabies and is shedding the virus, it is more likely to be caught by a dog or even to attack one. Cattle and other domestic animals occasionally get rabies by being attacked by a rabid wild animal. Wildlife such as foxes, coyotes, wolves, skunks, racoons, bats and many others can acquire and transmit rabies. Be sure to vaccinate your dogs regularly for rabies. In most areas you can vaccinate every three years with a modified live virus vaccine but in areas that have a high incidence of rabies in the wildlife you should vaccinate annually. This is one disease you cannot take any chances with because it is so dangerous to you and your family.

Because of their hunting habits dogs often contract tapeworm infestations. The intermediate stages of many species of dog tapeworms are carried in the flesh and internal organs of various wild animals, from rabbits to caribou. The tapeworms normally carry out half their life cycles between these animals and wild carnivores such as wolves and coyotes. But dogs can certainly become heavily infested. This is one reason you shouldn't feed your dogs raw meat or entrails after you clean your wild game.

Other internal parasites are common in dogs besides tapeworms. I would recommend that you have your dogs checked for parasites before you take them to a new farm or retreat and before you breed them. You can have them checked by taking a fecal sample to your veterinarian.

GEESE

Geese are probably more pets than poultry on most farms. Geese by nature mate for life. People who are familiar with them and their habits often just keep them around rather than use them for food. The fine insulation feathers, goose down, make the world's best insulation for clothing, quilts and sleeping bags.

Geese make excellent "watchdogs." They start honking loudly whenever a stranger or a wild animal enters their area. Some people have a fenced area around the farmhouse or the chicken house and they let the geese roam free. Their alarm is loud enough to wake the dead! Some geese or, especially, ganders will attack an intruder. Unfortunately they will often attack a young child as well. A goose or gander is quite heavy and its bite is very strong. It can injure a child especially around the face or eyes so be careful about roaming geese if you have small children.

HORSES

Another type of work for animals is, of course, draft or pulling. Horses, mules and oxen have traditionally been used for draft work. This includes pulling all types of implements and wagons and powering various types of static machinery. Training and using draft animals probably requires more patience and skill than any other job on a farm or ranch. Although I hate to repeat it, you must go to someone who is doing it in order to learn it right. You simply cannot learn to harness, train, handle and keep horses by reading it in a book. But of course you can add to your knowledge and skills by studying the subject if you are careful to critically analyze everything you read. There is probably as much written about horses as any other single subject. There are many clubs and organizations promoting breeds of horses including draft breeds. Contact these associations to find someone who will help you learn. See the last chapter for their addresses.

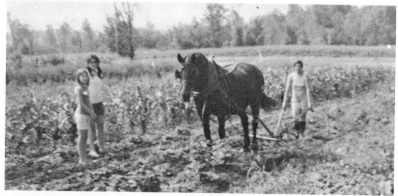

One-horse cultivator in family garden. Courtesy John Donaghy, Philadelphia, New York

I won't discuss oxen because I feel they are too limited for a self-sufficient farm. I would recommend a light draft horse or a strong light horse breed for several reasons. For self-sufficiency, you need efficient, multi-purpose animals. Your horses should be able to pull your wagons and farm implements and provide transportation as well. You may wish to use them to pull a family-sized surrey or you may at some time need them to provide you with fast, maneuverable mounts. This may be for flight, combat or hunting. The horse was the original and perhaps still unmatched combat transportation save the helicopter. Men charging on horseback present a psychologically terrifying sight and sound. Horses are considered one of the best police tools in crowd control because the physical stature of a man on a horse demands respect.

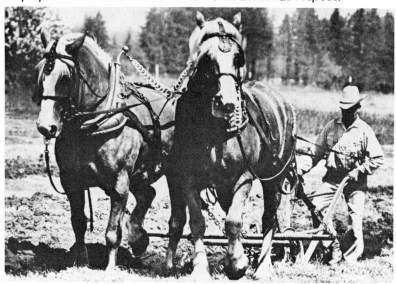

Two Belgians pulling a walking-plow. Photo by Fred Bay, courtesy David Horner, Forest Grove, Oregon

Mules were very popular for agricultural and commercial usage for a number of reasons. American mule breeding became quite an art from Colonial days. Mules are especially well suited to hard work in hot climates. They are more resistant to hot weather and they can eat a lower-quality ration than horses. They are usually less nervous than horses and they can take more abuse from an unskilled handler. Their feet and legs are often stronger and tougher than horses'. If a mule gets loose in the corn field or the grain bin he won't over-eat and get sick like a horse. However, mules are phlegmatic and difficult to train and handle. They do not have the spirit of a horse. They will not pull as hard and so they cannot pull as heavy a load as a horse of comparable size. Mules have small, narrow feet like light horses while light draft horses have large wide feet. The draft horses can therefore work much better in soft, wet fields. Mules were most popular for plantation and farm work in the South and for mountainous and mining jobs.

The biggest drawback to mules is that they are sterile. Females are always sterile and males don't usually get a chance to find out as they are castrated young. There are only a few fertile mules on record. This fact of sterility means that you would have to keep a good large jack (male ass, *Equus asinus*) and one or more mares (female horse, *Equus caballus*) of the appropriate type for the type of mule you wish to raise. Technically, any hybrid cross is called a mule but in practice in America the draft mules were always a cross between a jack and a mare. The cross between a stallion (male horse) and a jennet (female ass) is called a "hinny." This tradition no doubt originated in the old days when mules were very popular. Many mares could be procured and bred to a single good jack to produce the desired type of mule. The good mule-producing jack, called the American Jack, was an unusually large specimen, the result of careful importations and selective breeding by stockmen mostly in the Southeastern U.S. Mules were divided into many market classes for many types of draft work according to their size and type. My wife's grandfather was an officer in the U.S. Cavalry. He has said that a good saddle mule was unsurpassed for comfort on a long, hard ride. Nevertheless, I would recommend that you seek the right type of horses for your place, according to your specific needs. Unless you have a large place with room for lots of people and animals, horses are more efficient because of the mule's reproductive problem. I would recommend a general-purpose type of horse for self-sufficiency. It should be large enough to pull your implements in the type of soil you have and yet no larger than necessary. Draft and light draft breeds come in all sizes. The type you want will depend on the work they must do. Read the old, beloved children's book, *Justin Morgan Had a Horse* by Marguerite Henry. This is what you want but it may not necessarily be of the Morgan breed.

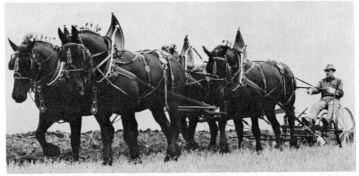

Four Percherons pulling a riding gang-plow. Courtesy Big Ed's Photos, Davenport, Iowa

The purebred draft breeds in the U.S. include the Belgian, Percheron, Shire, Clydesdale and Suffolk.

The Shires are the largest breed, weighing in at well over a ton! They came from England where they were originally bred for pulling large carts. Shires have dark colors, brown, black and bay. Bay is a reddish chestnut colored body and legs with black mane, tail and black above the hooves. Shires have very long hair on the legs from below the knees and hocks down to the feet. This long hair is called "feather." It protects the legs from sharp grasses and weeds.

Belgians are the next largest breed. They originated in Belgium from Flemish horses. They are usually of a light color such as sorrel, chestnut or red roan but there are some that are brown, black or grey.

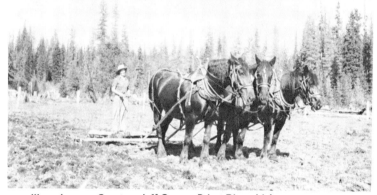

Horses pulling a harrow. Courtesy Jeff Gevrez, Priest River, Idaho

Percherons are a French breed. They originated from Flemish, Arab and Barb horses. They were originally bred as smaller coach horses but were then bred up to a heavy draft type in the late 1800's as large draft horses became more popular. Now they are usually more of a general-purpose type. Percherons are usually black or grey, often with a beautiful dappled pattern. They are one of the most stylish of draft breeds in their appearance and action.

Clydesdales are from Scotland. They originated from Flemish and Shire horses. They are smaller than Shires and they are often very striking in appearance with long, fluffy white feather on their legs above the feet. Anheuser-Bush, Inc. has for years used teams of perfectly-matched chestnut Clydesdales with white legs and blazes on their faces. Their eight-horse hitches are the trade mark of their advertising. Clydesdales are very stylish in action and appearance.

Suffolks are the oldest pure breed of draft horses. They come from Suffolk County, England, where they have been bred as a pure breed for centuries. They are always chestnut in color with perhaps a little white on the face or feet. Suffolks, often called the Suffolk Punch, are short legged with muscular bodies. They are the smallest of the draft breeds and are just about the perfect draft animal for farming. One reason that there were never many Suffolks in this country is that the English farmers would seldom part with one. They are well known for longevity, fertility, strength in drawing (pulling) and the ability to work continuously from dawn to dusk with only two meals daily, one before and one after work.

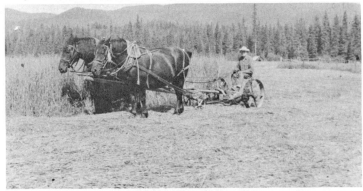

Team pulling a mower. Courtesy Jeff Gevrez, Priest River, Idaho

If your farm work will be light with light-weight implements you may not even need a draft breed. You may be able to find a large, heavy-boned light horse. You will see many chunky grade (not pure-bred) horses on farms and ranches. Often you can tell by the shape of their feet, heads and necks that they have some cold (draft) blood in their lineage. The draft breed horses are traditionally called "cold blooded" while the light horse breeds, mostly descending with some amount of Arab, Turk or Barb blood, are called "hot blooded." This traditional nomenclature originated with their relative temperaments.

Harness for draft horses must all be hand-made. The type of harness you need depends on the type and size of implements you use. Harness for a team of horses will cost more than a tractor! For best results the collars should be fitted individually for each horse. The collars provide a cushion for the wood-and-steel hames which bear all the force of pulling. Properly fitted collars and hames spread the contact evenly over the muscles of the shoulders. Improperly fitted collars and hames cause sores and nerve and muscle damage. Damage to a certain nerve in the shoulder causes wasting of the muscles on the front of the shoulder blade, called "sweeny," which ruins the horse for life.

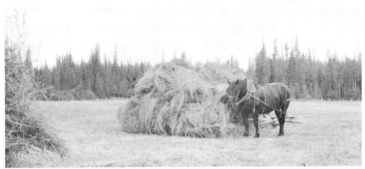

Heavy team pulling a sweep. Note second horse's head behind stack. Courtesy Jeff Gevrez

Let me emphasize that you must find someone who is using horses for draft and get them to teach you the fine points of the proper harnessing, hitching and use of horses.

If you have a large place with room for both draft and saddle horses, I would recommend keeping some light, agile saddle horses. There are many breeds suitable for riding for livestock, for transportation and for pleasure riding. There are Quarter Horses, Arabs, Appaloosas, Morgans, Pintos, Tennessee Walkers, and many others. Choosing a riding horse is invariably done by personal taste but you should still remember to look for any unsoundnesses, lamenesses or weaknesses that would make the horse break down early.

Horses are susceptable to some special problems due to their anatomy, physiology and type of work. These problems mainly fall into the catagories of nutrition and unsoundness but they really originate from either hereditary weaknesses or poor management.

The old-timers, the farmers, ranchers and cowboys didn't know what we know today about the anatomy, physiology and heredity of the horse yet they got a lot of work and a lot of years out of each of their horses. First, they learned how to select a horse for its form, its ancestors and its way-of-going. Then they took constant great care of each animal. The stockman who failed to care for his horses was an early failure!

If you can, visit the stables of a racetrack some day and

look closely at the horses' legs. Chances are that on many of the horses you will see a lot of scars and bumps where there should be smooth, unblemished lines. For reasons of economics, mostly misguided, as well as tradition on the track, most racehorses are pushed too hard too soon, before their bones, joints, tendons and ligaments are fully formed and strong enough to take the stresses of racing.

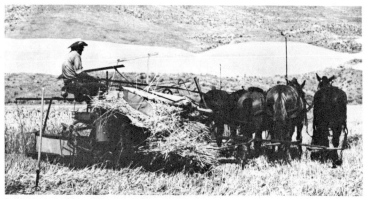

Four Percherons pulling a binder. Photo by Durland, Courtesy David Horner

Then go to an average riding stable and look at the condition of the horses, especially their feet. At many riding stables you will see thin, poorly groomed horses. Their feet are often cracked and in need of attention. Again, these problems are blamed on misguided economics because good horse feed is expensive and farriers (blacksmiths) must be paid for their services.

If you talk to an old-timer he will tell you that any horseman worth a nickel spent most of his time caring for his horses. He made sure their needs were met before his own. Every morning he would feed and groom his horses before working them. He would carefully clean their feet to be sure there were no pieces of sharp gravel in them. After work he would groom them again, sponging and drying them if they had worked up any lather. Then he would clean their feet again with a hoofpick. A true horseman paid a great deal more attention to his animals than we pay to the machinery that has replaced them in modern agriculture and transportation.

According to some engineers upon calculating the efficiency of energy consumption by petroleum-fueled agricultural implements, the horse is a much more efficient animal for our environment. Horses pulling farm implements produce more energy in terms of crops than they consume. But petroleum-burning implements

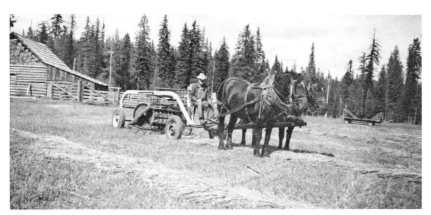

Home made hitch cart used to pull a standard hay rake.   Courtesy Jeff Gevrez

consume more stored energy from the earth than the resulting crops replace!

If you are seriously considering using horses for farm work there is only one main problem and that is the difficulty of finding or adapting implements for them to work the land. You will have very little difficulty finding draft horses as there are many breeders and fanciers all over the country. There are many harness shops making draft horse harnesses and there are even some shops making buggies and wagons. Check the last chapter for horse associations and magazines. Breeders and craftsmen advertise in their publications. But no one is making horse-drawn farm implements to speak of. You may be able to pick up something now and then from farm auctions or by contacting draft horse users. One of the best solutions is to make a "hitch cart" or "fore cart." This is, in essence, a draw-bar on wheels with a seat on it that you hitch to the horses and use to pull standard farm implements that were made for a tractor. You can even pull something like a hay baler, which requires a power take-off from the tractor, by mounting a small gas engine on it. The best design for a fore cart would have adjustable tread, that is, the width between the wheels would be adjustable for various uses. Be sure to mount the seat high enough for good control and visibility and to keep you out of the dust. The only drawback to the fore cart is that you are in front of the implement and thus in a dangerous position in case of a fall or accident.

I highly recommend making use of some type of draft animals on any farm. They are efficient and a lot of fun. They can pull many implements just as fast as a tractor and you don't have to worry

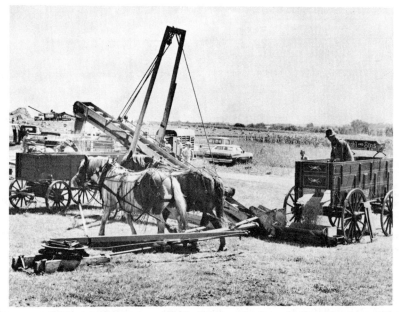

"Horsepower" being used to power a grain elevator. Photo by Waltner, Freeman, South Dakota

about a shortage of spare parts or petroleum. In today's energy shortage they are ideal for anyone who wants to approach self-sufficiency. Just ask any Amishman — the times they are a-changing — after years of being laughed at for sticking to the old-fashioned, self-sufficient methods, the energy crunch is finally giving the Amish and other self-sufficient farmers the last laugh.

16
References
And Sources

If you are serious about achieving self-sufficiency then you must be serious about learning. If you are serious about learning then you will want a good selection of references and textbooks. This won't come cheap. Many of the technical references and textbooks you may want are quite expensive. But of course there are numerous publications available free or at minimum cost from universities, county and state agricultural extension services, agricultural experiment stations, the U.S. Department of Agriculture and the U.S. Printing Office.

There is so much valuable information available that your biggest problem will be to select the publications you want from the vast assortment. My list of references is just a cross-sectional sample of what is available. I would recommend that you write to all the agencies and publishers and ask for their lists of publications in the specific area in which you are interested. You will probably have to write more than once to each of the governmental agencies. They have so many publications available that unless you know the specific titles, you will have trouble finding what you need. Some governmental offices will send only a limited number of free publications for each request.

If you are really serious, start collecting your library of references now. Here is a partial list of references that might be of assistance. Some of them are very technical for background information and basic understanding while others are completely practical. I have not included a review or description of their contents because of the space this would require. I have not included their current prices because prices change so often and I don't want to misquote them. For descriptions of the contents and for current prices, write to the publishers. Most of them will send a complete catalog. These catalogs are full of tantalizing titles on every imaginable subject. You can spend hours just leafing through the catalogs!

Following the list of references is a list of groups, clubs, associations and their journals that may help you locate information, equipment and people that can help you. The last, of course is always the most important.

I would make only one suggestion about your references. When you are considering methods of management recommended in a reference on livestock, keep in mind whether that recommendation is for commercial production. You must carefully sift through these recommendations to choose those that are relevant to your self-sufficient, closed-system farm or ranch.

General Animal Science

Animal Agriculture, The Biology of Domestic Animals and Their Use by Man
H. H. Cole and M. Ronning, 1974
W. H Freeman and Co., San Francisco, CA 94104

Animal Breeding, 5th Ed.
L. M. Winters, 1954
John Wiley & Sons, Inc., N.Y., NY 10016

Animal Science
M. E. Ensminger   1969
The Interstate Printers & Publishers, Inc., Danville, IL 61832

Breeding and Improvement of Farm Animals, 6th Ed.
V. A. Rice *et. al.,* 1967
McGraw-Hill Book Co. N.Y., NY 10020

Improvement of Livestock Production in Warm Climates
R. E. McDowell, 1972
W. H. Freeman and Co., San Francisco, CA 94104

Introduction to Livestock Production Including Dairy and Poultry
H. H. Cole, Editor, 1966
W. H. Freeman and Co., San Francisco, CA 94104

Introductory Animal Science, 4th Ed.
A. L. Anderson & J. J. Kiser, 1963
MacMillan Publishing Co., Inc., 866 Third Ave.,N.Y.,
NY 10022

Modern Breeds of Livestock
H. M. Briggs, 1969
MacMillan Publishing Co.,Inc., 866 Third Ave., N.Y.
NY 10022

Raising Livestock on Small Farms, Farmers' Bulletin No. 2224
U.S.D.A.
Supt. of Documents, U.S. Gov. Printing Office, Wash., D.C.
20402

The Science of Animals that Serve Mankind
J. R. Campbell and J. F. Lasley, 1975
McGraw-Hill Book Co., N.Y., NY 10020

The Stockman's Handbook
M. E. Ensminger   1970
The Interstate Printers and Publishers, Inc., Danville, IL 61832

Livestock Housing, Equipment, Fencing and Farmsteads

Agricultural Engineers' Handbook
C. B. Richey, P. Jacobson & C. W. Hall, 1961
McGraw-Hill Book Co., N.Y., NY 10020

Farm Service Buildings
H. E. Gray, 1955
McGraw-Hill Book Co., N.Y., NY 10020

Fences for the Farm and Rural Home, Farmers' Bulletin No. 2247
U.S.D.A.
Supt. of Documents, U.S. Gov. Printing Office, Wash., D.C.
20402

Handbook of Livestock Equipment
E. M. Juergenson, Ph.D., 1971
The Interstate Printers and Publishers, Inc.,Danville, IL 61832

Mechanics in Agriculture
Lloyd J. Phipps 1967
The Interstate Printers and Publishers, Inc., Danville, IL 61832

Practical Farm Buildings
J. S. Boyd 1973
The Interstate Printers and Publishers, Inc., Danville, IL 61832

Nutrition

Animal Growth and Nutrition
E. S. E. Hafez, Ph.D. & I. A. Dyer, Ph.D.
Lea & Febiger, Phila., PA 19106

Animal Nutrition, 6th Ed.
L. A. Maynard and J. K. Loosli, 1969
McGraw-Hill Book Co. N.Y., NY 10020

Applied Animal Nutrition, 2nd Ed.
E. W. Crampton and L. E. Harris, 1969
W. H. Freeman & Co., SanFrancisco, CA 94104

Atlas of Nutritional Data on United States and Canadian Feeds
National Academy of Sciences, 1972
Printing and Publishing Office, 2101 Constitution Ave.
Wash., D.C. 20418

Effect of Processing on the Nutritional Value of Feeds
National Academy of Sciences, 1973
Printing and Publishing Office, 2101 Constitution Ave.,
Wash., D.C. 20418

Feed Formulations
T. W. Perry 1975
The Interstate Printers and Publishers, Inc., Danville, IL

Feeds and Feeding, Abridged, 9th Ed.
Professor Frank B. Morrison, 1958
The Morrison Publishing Company, Box 130, Orangeville, Ontario, Canada L9W 2Z5

Nutrients and Toxic Substances in Water for Livestock and Poultry
National Academy of Sciences, 1974
Printing and Publishing Office, 2101 Constitution Ave., Wash., D.C. 20418

The Handbook of Foodstuffs
R. Seiden, 1957
Springer Publishing Co., Inc., N.Y., NY 10003

The Scientific Feeding of Chickens
H. W. Titus & J. C. Fritz 1971
The Interstate Printers and Publishers, Inc., Danville, IL 61832

United States - Canadian Tables of Feed Composition
National Academy of Sciences, 1969
Printing and Publishing Offices, 2101 Constitution Ave., Washington, D.C., 20418

Veterinary Sciences and Disease and Parasite Control

Adaptation of Domestic Animals
E.S.E. Hafez, PhD, 1968
Lea and Febiger, Philadelphia, PA 19106

An Introduction to General and Comparative Animal Physiology
E. Florey, PhD, 1966
W.B. Saunders, Co., Philadelphia, PA 19105

Anatomy and Physiology of Farm Animals, 2nd ed.
R.D. Frandson. D.V.M., 1974
Lea and Febiger, Philadelphia, PA 19106

Animal Agents and Vectors of Human Disease, 4th Ed.
Faust, Beaver and Jung, 1975
Lea and Febiger, Philadelphia, PA 19106

Diseases Transmitted from Animals to Man, 6th Ed.
W.T. Hubbert *et al.,* 1975
Charles C. Thomas, Publisher, Springfield, IL 62717

Dorland's Illustrated Medical Dictionary, 25th Ed., 1974
W.B. Saunders, Co., Philadelphia, PA 19105

Farm Animal Health and Disease Control
J.H. Galloway, B.V.Sc., 1972
Lea and Febiger, Philadelphia, PA 19106

Livestock Health Encyclopedia, 3rd Ed.
R. Seiden, D.Sc., 1968
Springer Publishing Co., Inc., NY, NY 10003

Merck Veterinary Manual, 4th Ed., 1974
Merck and Company, Inc., Rahway, N.J. 07065

Pets and Human Development
Boris M. Levinson, 1972
Charles C. Thomas, Publisher, Springfield, IL 62717

Reproduction in Farm Animals, 3rd Ed.
E.S.E. Hafez, Ph.D., 1974
Lea and Febiger, Philadelphia, PA 19106

Sisson and Grossman's Anatomy of the Domestic Animals, 5th Ed.
R. Getty, D.V.M., M.D., Ph.D., 1975
W.B. Saunders Co., Philadelphia, PA 19105

The House Fly-How To Control It, Leaflet 390
U.S.D.A.
Supt. of Documents, U.S. Gov. Printing Office, Wash. D.C.
20402

Meat Production

A Complete Guide to Home Meat Curing
Morton Salt Company, 1975
Morton-Norwich Products, Inc., 110 N. Wacker Dr.
Chicago, IL 60606

Meat for the Table
Sleeter Bull, 1951
McGraw—Hill Book Co., NY, NY 10020

Meat Hygiene, 4th Ed.
J.A. Libby, D.V.M., 1975
Lea and Febiger, Philadelphia, PA. 19106

Principles of Meat Science
J.C. Forest *et al.,* 1975
W.H. Freeman and Co., SanFrancisco, CA 94104

The Meat We Eat
Professor P. T. Zeigler and J. R. Romans, 1974
The Interstate Printers and Publishers, Inc., Danville, IL 61832

The Science of Meat and Meat Products, 2nd Ed.
J.F. Price and B.S. Schweigert, 1971
W.H. Freeman and Co., SanFrancisco, CA 94104

Poultry

A Guide to Better Hatching
Janet Stromberg, 1975
50 Lakes Route , Pine River, Minn. 56474

Farm Poultry Management, Farmers Bulletin No. 2197
U.S.D.A.
Supt. of Documents, U.S. Gov. Printing Office, Wash. D.C. 20402

Nutrient Requirements of Poultry
National Academy of Sciences, 1971
Printing and Publishing Office , 2101 Constitution Ave., Wash.
D.C. 20418

Poultry Production, 11th Ed.
>L.E. Card, Ph.D., 1972
>Lea and Febiger, Philadelphia, PA 19106

Poultry Science
>M.E. Ensminger 1971
>The Interstate Printers and Publishers, Inc. Danville, IL 61832

Poultryman's Manual
>J.W. Bailey, 1957
>Springer Publishing Co., Inc., NY, NY 10003

Poultry Health Book, 2nd Ed.
>L. Dwight Schwartz, D.V.M.
>John H. Thiele
>P. O. Box 1545, Hobe Sound, Fla. 33455

The Fowl Tick—How To Control It, Leaflet No. 382
>U.S.D.A.
>Supt. of Documents, U.S. Gov. Printing Office, Wash. D.C. 20402

Rabbits

A Practical Beginning to Successful Rabbit Raising
>The American Rabbit Breeders Association, Inc.
>2401 East Oakland Ave., Bloomington, IL 61701

Commercial Rabbit Raising, Agricultural Handbook No. 309
>Agricultural Research Service, U.S.D.A.
>Supt. of Documents, U.S. Gov. Printing Office, Wash. D.C. 20402

Domestic Rabbit Production
>George S. Templeton 1968
>The Interstate Printers and Publishers, Inc., Danville, IL 61832

Nutrient Requirements of Rabbits
>National Academy of Sciences, 1966
>Printing and Publishing Office, 2101 Constitution Ave., Wash., D.C. 20418

Official Guide to Raising Better Rabbits,
 The American Rabbit Breeders Assoc,. Inc., 1973
 2401 East Oakland Ave., Bloomington, IL 61701

Raising Small Meat Animals
 Victor M. Giammattei, 1976
 The Interstate Printers & Publishers, Inc., Danville, IL 61832

Standard of Perfection
 The American Rabbit Breeders Association, Inc., 1971
 2401 East Oakland Ave., Bloomington, IL 61701

Hogs

Breeds of Swine, Farmers Bulletin No. 1263
 U.S.D.A.
 Supt. of Documents, U.S. Gov. Printing Office, Wash. D.C.
 20402

Nutrient Requirements of Swine, 7th Ed.
 NationalAcademy of Sciences, 1973
 Printing and Publishing Office, 2101 Constitution Ave., Wash.,
 D.C. 20418

Raising a Few Hogs, Leaflet No. 537
 U.S.D.A.
 Supt. of Documents, U.S. Gov. Printing Office, Wash. D.C.
 20402

Slaughtering, Cutting and Processing Pork on the Farm, Farmers
 Bulletin No. 2138, U.S.D.A.
 Supt. of Documents, U.S. Gov. Printing Office, Wash., D.C.
 20402

Swine Production, 4th Ed.
 J.L. Krider and W.E. Carroll, 1971
 McGraw-Hill Book Co., NY, NY 10020

Swine Production in Temperate and Tropical Environments
 W.G. Pond and J.H. Maner, 1974
 W.H. Freeman and Co., SanFrancisco, CA 94104

Swine Science
    M.E. Ensminger 1970
    The Interstate Printers and Publishers, Inc., Danville, IL 61832

Milk Production, Dairy Cattle and Dairy Goats

A Dairy Goat for Home Milk Production, Leaflet No. 538
    U.S.D.A.
    Supt. of Documents, U.S. Gov. Printing Office, Wash., D.C.
    20402

Aids to Goatkeeping
    Corl A. Leach
    American Supply House, Box 1114, Columbia, MO 65201

Biology of Lactation
    G.H. Schmidt, 1971
    W.H. Freeman and Co., SanFrancisco, CA 94104

Dairy Cattle Feeding and Management, 5th Ed.
    Paul M. Reaves and H.O. Henderson, 1963
    John Wiley and Sons, Inc., NY, NY 10016

Dairy Cattle: Principles, Practices, Problems, Profits
    R.C. Foley, Ph.D., *et al.*, 1972
    Lea and Febiger, Philadelphia, PA 19106

Dairy Cattle Science
    M.E. Ensminger 1971
    The Interstate Printers and Publishers, Inc., Danville, IL 61832

Dairy Goat Management, Extension Bulletin No. 334
    G.W. Vander Noot and D.M. Kniffen
    College of Agriculture, Rutgers Univ., New Brunswick, N.J.

Guide Book of Rules and Services
    American Dairy Goat Association
    Spindale, North Carolina 28160

Handbook for Dairymen
    A. Colletti, 1966
    Iowa State University Press, Ames, Iowa 50010

Milk and Milk Products, 4th Ed.
C. H. Eckles *et. al.,* 1951
MgGraw-Hill Book Co., N.Y., NY 10020

Nutrient Requirements of Dairy Cattle
National Academy of Sciences, 1971
Printing and Publishing Office, 2101 Constitution Ave., Washington, D.C. 20418

Principles of Dairy Science
G. H. Schmidt and L. D. Van Vleck, 1974
W. H. Freeman & Co., San Francisco, CA 94104

The Illustrated Standard of the Dairy Goat
Nancy Lee Owen
American Supply House, Box 1114, Columbia, MO 65201

Veterinary Handbook for Cattlemen
J. W. Bailey, D.V.M., 1972
Springer Publishing Co. Inc., N.Y., NY 10003

What You Can Do About Bovine Mastitis,
Farmers Bulletin No. 2253
U.S.D.A.
Supt. of Documents, U.S. Gov. Printing Office, Washington, D.C. 20402

Sheep

Nutrient Requirements of Sheep, 5th Ed.
National Academy of Sciences, 1975
Printing and Publishing Office, 2101 Constitution Ave., Washington, D.C. 20418

Sheep and Wool Science
M. E. Ensminger 1970
The Interstate Printers & Publishers, Inc., Danville, IL 61832

Beef Cattle

Beef Cattle, 6th Ed.
 A. L. Neuman & R. R. Snapp, 1969
 John Wiley & Sons, Inc., N.Y., NY 10016

Beef Cattle Breeds
 Farmers Bulletin No. 2228
 U.S.D.A.
 Supt. of Documents, U.S. Gov. Printing Office,
 Washington, D.C. 20402

Nutrient Requirements of Beef Cattle, 5th Ed.
 National Academy of Sciences, 1975
 Printing and Publishing Office, 2101 Constitution Ave.,
 Washington, D.C. 20418

Beef Cattle Science
 M. E. Ensminger 1976
 The Interstate Printers and Publishers, Inc., Danville, IL 61832

Commercial Beef Cattle Production
 C. C. O'Mary, Ph.D. & I. A. Dyer, Ph.D., 1972
 Lea & Febiger, Philadelphia, PA 19106

Dehorning, Castrating, Branding and Marking
 Farmers Bulletin No. 2141
 U.S.D.A.
 Supt. of Documents, U.S. Gov. Printing Office,
 Washington, D.C. 20402

Feedlot and Ranch Equipment for Beef Cattle
 Farmers Bulletin No. 1584
 U.S.D.A.
 Supt. of Documents, U.S. Gov. Printing Office,
 Washington, D.C. 20402

The Farm Beef Herd
 Farmers Bulletin No. 2126
 U.S.D.A.
 Supt. of Documents, U.S. Gov. Printing Office,
 Washington, D.C. 20402

Dogs

Behavior Problems in Dogs
William E. Campbell, 1975
American Veterinary Publications, Inc., Drawer KK, Santa
Barbara, CA 93102

Genetics of the Dog, the Basis of Successful Breeding, 2nd Ed.
M. Burns and M.N. Fraser, 1966
J.B. Lippincott Co., Philadelphia, PA 19101

Happy Herding Handbook
Maryland E. Little
P.O. Box 2404, Riverside CA 92506

How to Breed and Whelp Dogs
J.S. Hansen, 1973
Charles C. Thomas, Publisher, Springfield, IL 62717

Nutrient Requirements of Dogs
National Academy of Sciences, 1974
Printing and Publishing Office, 2101 Constitution Ave., Wash.,
D.C. 20418

The Farmer's Dog
John Holmes
Animal Research Foundation, Quinlan, Texas 75474

The Koehler Method of Guard Dog Training
William R. Koehler
Howell Book House, Inc., 730 Fifth Ave., NY, NY 10019

The Natural Method of Dog Training
Leon F. Whitney, D.V.M., 1963
J.B. Lippincott Co., Philadelphia, PA 19101

The Perfect Stock Dog
Ben Means, 1970
Rt. 1, Walnut Grove, MO 65770

Training and Racing Sled Dogs
World Champion George Attla, 1975
Arner Publications, 8140 Coronado Lane, Rome, NY 13440

Training Dogs: A Manual
Colonel Konrad Most, 1974
Popular Dogs Publishing Co., Ltd., 3 Fitzroy Square,
London, W1, United Kingdom

Horses

Breeding and Raising Horses, Agriculture Handbook No. 394
M.E. Ensminger
U.S.D.A.
Supt. of Documents, U.S. Gov. Printing Office, Wash., D.C.
20402

Horse Handling Science
Monte Foreman
P.O. Box 105, Little Rock, AK 72203

Horses and Horsemanship
M.E. Ensminger 1969
The Interstate Printers and Publishers, Inc., Danville, IL 61832

Horsemanship and Horse Care, Agriculture Information Bulletin
No. 353, U.S.D.A.
Supt. of Documents, U.S. Gov. Printing Office, Wash., D.C.
20402

Lameness In Horses, 3rd Ed.
O.R. Adams, D.V.M., 1974
Lea and Febiger, Philadelphia, PA 19106

Nutrient Requirements of Horses
National Academy of Sciences, 1973
Printing and Publishing Office, 2101 Constitution Ave.,
Wash., D.C., 20418

The Anatomy of the Horse, A Pictorial Approach
R.F. Way, V.M.D., M.S., and D.G. Lee, V.M.D., 1965
J.B. Lippincott Co., Philadelphia, PA 19105

The Art and Science of Horseshoeing
R.G. Greeley, B.S., M.S., D.V.M., 1970
J.B. Lippincott Co., Philadelphia, PA 19105

The Complete Book of the Quarterhorse
Nelson C. Nye
A.S. Barnes and Co., Inc., NY, NY

The Harness Maker's Illustrated Manual
W.N. Fitz-Gerald
Caballus Publishers, P.O. Box 2307, Ft. Collins, CO 80522

The Master Farrier
Bud Beaston, 1975
The Master Farrier, P.O. Box 7098, Tulsa, OK 74105

Understanding and Training Horses
A. James Ricci, 1964
J.B. Lippincott Co., Philadelphia, PA 19101

Using the American Quarter Horse
L.N. Sikes with Bob Gray
The Saddlerock Corporation, 602 N. Main, Dayton, TX 77535

Miscellaneous Publications

Crop Production, Principles and Practices
S.R. Chapman and L.P. Carter, 1976
W.H. Freeman and Co., SanFrancisco, Ca 94104

Diseases of Field Crops, 2nd Ed.
J.G. Dickson, 1956
McGraw-Hill Book Co., NY, NY 10020

Forage Crops, 2nd Ed.
G.H. Ahlgren, 1956
McGraw-Hill Book Co., NY, NY 10020

Grain Crops, 2nd Ed.
H.K. Wilson, 1955
McGraw-Hill Book Co., NY, NY 10020

Grow It!
    Richard W. Langer, 1972
    Saturday Review Press, 230 Park Ave., NY, NY 10017

Horticultural Science
    Jules Janick, 1972
    W.H. Freeman and Co., SanFrancisco, CA 94104

Law and the Farmer, 4th Ed.,
    Jacob H. Beuscher and Harold W. Hannah, 1975
    Springer Publishing Co., Inc., NY, NY 10003

Nature and Prevention of Plant Diseases, 2nd Ed.
    K. Starr Chester, 1947
    McGraw-Hill Book Co., NY, NY 10020

Principles of Farm Management
    J.N. Efferson, 1953
    McGraw-Hill Book Co., NY, NY 10020

Restraint & Handling of Wild and Domestic Animals
    Murray E. Fowler, 1978
    Iowa State Univ. Press, Ames, IO 50010

The Homesteader's Handbook to Raising Small Livestock
    Jerome D. Belanger, 1974
    Rodale Press, Inc., Book Division, Emmaus, PA 18049

Wild Orphan Babies, 2nd Ed.
    William J. Weber, D.V.M.
    Holt, Rinehart and Winston, New York, N.Y. 10017

Clubs, Associations and Journals

Affiliated Schutzhund Club of America
P.O. Box 216, Northbrook, IL 60062

American Dairy Goat Association
Spindale, N.C. 28160

American Working Dog Federation
Rochester Bank and Trust
16th Ave. and 4th St., Rochester, Minn.

Animal Research Foundation
Quinlan, TX 75474

Blair and Ketchum's Country Journal
Richard M. Ketchum, Dorset, VT

Countryside and Small Stock Journal
Rt. 1, Box 239, Waterloo, WI 53594

Dairy Goat Journal
Box 1908, Scottsdale, AZ 85252

Domestic Rabbit, The Official Publication of the A.R.B.A.
American Rabbit Breeders Assoc., Inc.
2401 E. Oakland Ave., Bloomington, IL 61701

Northern Dog News Magazine
Box 310-L, Snohomish, WA 98290

OFF-LEAD, The National Dog Training Monthly
Arner Publications, 8140 Coronado Lane, Rome, NY 13440

Organic Gardening and Farming
Rodale Press, Inc., 33 E. Minor St., Emmaus, PA 18049

Team and Trail, The Musher's Monthly News
Center Harbor, NH 03226

The American Rabbit Breeders Association, Inc.
2401 E. Oakland Ave., Bloomington, IL 61701

The Draft Horse Journal
Rt. 3, Waverly, IO 50677

The Mother Earth News
P.O. Box 70, Hendersonville, NC 28739

The National Stock Dog Magazine
    Rural Rt. 1, Butler, IN 46721

The National Stock Dog Registry
    Division of International English Shepherd Registry, Inc.
    Rural Rt. 1, Butler, IN 46721

The Schutzhunder Magazine
    P.O. Box 216
    Northbrook, IL 60062